Biomarkers: Diagnostic Applications

Biomarkers: Diagnostic Applications

Editor: Ralph Bowen

AMERICAN
MEDICAL PUBLISHERS
www.americanmedicalpublishers.com

AMERICAN
MEDICAL PUBLISHERS
www.americanmedicalpublishers.com

Cataloging-in-Publication Data

Biomarkers : diagnostic applications / edited by Ralph Bowen.
p. cm.
Includes bibliographical references and index.
ISBN 978-1-63927-539-7
1. Biochemical markers. 2. Biochemical markers--Diagnostic use. 3. Biochemistry.
4. Indicators (Biology). I. Bowen, Ralph.
R853.B54 B56 2021
610.28--dc23

American Medical Publishers,
41 Flatbush Avenue,
1st Floor, New York,
NY 11217, USA

ISBN 978-1-63927-539-7 (Hardback)

Contents

Preface

The measurable indicators of a biological condition or state are termed as biomarkers. They can be evaluated and measured through the soft tissues, urine and the blood. Biomarkers can be used to study pathogenic processes, normal biological processes and pharmacological reaction to a therapeutic intervention. Biomarkers are broadly categorized into diagnostic biomarkers, predictive biomarkers and prognostic biomarkers. A diagnostic biomarker is a traceable substance which is introduced into an organism to evaluate organ function as well as other aspects of health. It can also be used to detect a particular disease state. General characteristic changes or complex organ functions in biological structures may also serve as biomarkers. This book traces the progress of the research in the field of biomarkers and highlights some of its key concepts and applications. It will also provide interesting topics for research which interested readers can take up. This book is a resource guide for experts as well as students.

The researches compiled throughout the book are authentic and of high quality, combining several disciplines and from very diverse regions from around the world. Drawing on the contributions of many researchers from diverse countries, the book's objective is to provide the readers with the latest achievements in the area of research. This book will surely be a source of knowledge to all interested and researching the field.

In the end, I would like to express my deep sense of gratitude to all the authors for meeting the set deadlines in completing and submitting their research chapters. I would also like to thank the publisher for the support offered to us throughout the course of the book. Finally, I extend my sincere thanks to my family for being a constant source of inspiration and encouragement.

Editor

1

Biomarkers of Common Childhood Renal Diseases

Samuel N. Uwaezuoke

Abstract

Novel biomarkers are now used in the diagnostic and prognostic evaluation of common kidney diseases in children. The increased scientific interest in these biomarkers is partly due to the remarkable progress in their discovery techniques, and their validation in clinical subjects. However, the wide variation in their sensitivity and specificity is still a major concern. In the identification of biomarkers of kidney injury, an ideal biomarker should be produced after organ injury in concentrations which directly correlates with the degree of injury; should be easily measured in body fluids; and should serve as a potential tool to monitor therapeutic response which is predicated upon a post-injury decrease in its concentration. This book chapter aims to highlight and discuss the novel biomarkers used in the diagnostic and prognostic evaluation of common acute diseases of the kidney in children, such as urinary tract infection (UTI) and acute kidney injury (AKI), as well as chronic kidney disease (CKD) secondary to idiopathic nephrotic syndrome (INS) and diabetic nephropathy (DN).

Keywords: acute diseases, chronic diseases, kidney, children, biomarkers

1. Introduction

Novel biomarkers are now utilized in the diagnostic and prognostic evaluation of common kidney diseases in children [1–3]. Unlike in developing countries where they are scarcely used in medical diagnostics, they are currently used as site-of-care and laboratory tools for disease evaluation in developed settings although some of them have not been fully validated for routine clinical use. The increased scientific interest in novel biomarkers is nevertheless due to the remarkable progress in their discovery techniques, their validation in clinical populations and their utility as diagnostic tests. Despite the reliability of the conventional diagnostic methods for some of these diseases, their limitations as diagnostic tools have underscored the need for a paradigm shift to biomarkers. The attraction of these novel biomarkers lies in the non-invasive nature of their use in disease evaluation. However, the wide variation in their sensitivity and specificity is still a major challenge.

According to the definition by the *National Institute of Health Biomarkers Definitions Working Group*, a biomarker refers to 'a characteristic that is objectively measured and evaluated as an indicator of normal biological processes, pathogenic processes, or pharmacologic responses to a therapeutic intervention' [4, 5]. In other words, it is a measurable indicator of a biological state or condition. Although there are diverse perspectives to the definition of a biomarker, for the purpose of the current topic, a biomarker can be defined as a substance whose detection indicates a particular disease-state, or a change in expression/state of a protein which correlates with the risk/progression of a disease, or with disease susceptibility to a given therapy. In fact, the most actively studied biomarkers presently are the biological macromolecules. For instance, proteins are most easily measured by immunoassays or by mass spectrometry combined with high-resolution separation techniques, while nucleic acids can be amplified by the polymerase chain reaction (PCR) and related techniques.

In the identification of biomarkers of kidney injury, an ideal biomarker should be produced after organ injury in concentrations which directly correlate with the degree of injury; should be easily measured in body fluids; and should serve as a potential tool to monitor therapeutic response, predicated upon a post-injury decrease in its concentration [6].

In this book chapter, novel biomarkers which essentially meet these requirements with respect to evaluating common kidney diseases in children are highlighted and discussed.

2. Acute diseases of the kidney and biomarkers

Biomarkers have been identified for the following acute diseases of the kidney: acute pyelonephritis or upper urinary tract infection (UTI) and acute cystitis/urethritis or lower UTI, as well as acute kidney injury (AKI). UTI ranks third in the hierarchy of common childhood infections in developing countries [7], and remains one of the commonest causes of febrile illness in the pediatric age group [8, 9].

2.1. Biomarkers of UTI

Serum procalcitonin (PCT), urine/serum interleukin 6 (IL-6) and 8 (IL-8), and urine neutrophil gelatinase-associated lipocalin (NGAL) are currently the major biomarkers identified in the evaluation of the disease. Other novel biomarkers include urine interleukin 1-beta (IL-1β), urine 8-hydroxy-2-deoxyguanosine (8-oxodG), and urine total anti-oxidant capacity (TAC) (**Figure 1**).

PCT is one of the inflammatory markers recognized as a biomarker of severe bacterial infection [10]. It is essentially a peptide precursor of the hormone- calcitonin - produced by the thyroid parafollicular cells, as well as the neuroendocrine cells of the lungs and intestines. Its serum level in healthy subjects is below the limit of detection (0.01 μg/L) of laboratory assays [11]. Notably, serum PCT level is not elevated significantly with viral or non-infectious inflammatory process, but may rise up to 100 μg/L in systemic inflammatory response from severe bacterial infection. In fact, estimation of PCT can be used as a marker of severe bacterial

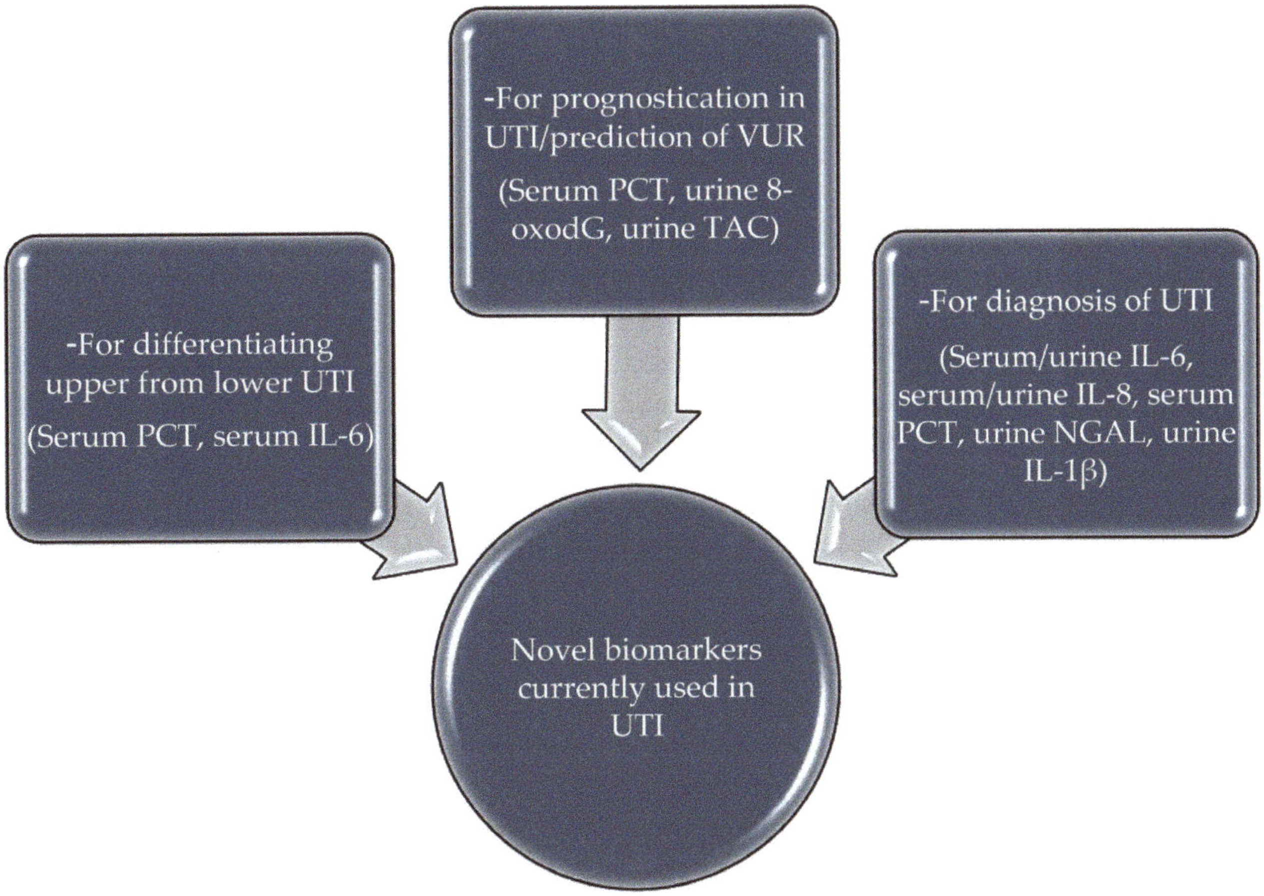

Figure 1. Schematic representation of the list of biomarkers used in the three-fold evaluation of urinary tract infection (UTI).

sepsis, as its levels correlate with the severity of sepsis [12]. In comparison with other acute phase reactants such as IL-2, IL-6, IL-8, C-reactive protein (CRP) and tumor necrosis factor-α (TNF-α), PCT has a high sensitivity (85%) and specificity (91%) for discriminating between patients with systemic inflammatory response syndrome (SIRS) and those with sepsis [13]. It is now well established that serum PCT has a good diagnostic accuracy for the diagnosis of acute pyelonephritis than for lower UTI, with reported high sensitivity and specificity values [14–16]. For instance, sensitivity and specificity values of 94.1 and 89.7% respectively, and sensitivity and specificity values of 83.3 and 93.7% respectively, have been documented [15, 16]. PCT also has a good predictive ability for vesico-ureteric reflux (VUR), as high levels of this biomarker are significantly related to high-grade VUR [17–19]. Again, children with VUR reportedly presented with significantly higher median PCT levels than those without VUR; sensitivity and negative predictive values of 94.3 and 95.4% respectively for predicting high-grade VUR (using the biomarker alone), as well as 97.1 and 97.8% respectively (using a combination of the biomarker and ultrasound studies) have been recorded [18]. Finally, PCT can also serve as an early predictor of renal parenchymal damage in children with UTI [20]. The implication is that the prognostic utility of PCT may in future preclude the need for dimercaptosuccinic acid (DMSA) scan, or better still, may serve as an adjunct to this imaging study.

Similarly, other biomarkers such as urine 8-hydroxy-2′-deoxyguanosine (8-oxodG) and total antioxidant capacity (TAC) are useful in the prediction of renal parenchymal injury in children with UTI [21]. Interestingly, those patients with positive DMSA scan had higher levels of urine 8-oxodG and higher urine TAC than the patients with normal DMSA scan: showing that urine levels of 8-oxodG may directly correlate with renal parenchymal injury.

Urine NGAL is another biomarker for the diagnostic evaluation of UTI. NGAL (also called lipocalin-2) is a protein involved in innate immunity as it is involved in the sequestration of iron which ultimately blocks bacterial growth [22]. It is expressed mainly in neutrophils and in low concentrations in the kidney, prostrate, as well as respiratory and gastrointestinal epithelia [23]. NGAL is currently employed as a biomarker of renal injury [24], given that it is secreted in high concentrations into the blood and urine within 2 hours of AKI [25]. In addition, the biomarker is easily excreted and detected in the urine because it is protease-resistant. Thus, urine NGAL appears to be a specific and sensitive biomarker for the diagnosis of UTI and for the prediction of renal parenchymal injury in the disease [26, 27].

Finally, some interleukins also play a role in disease diagnosis and in differentiating upper from lower UTI. Generally, the infection stimulates both local and systemic cytokine responses [28, 29]. For instance, *Escherichia coli* is known to activate a cytokine response in the uroepithelial cell lines to produce IL-6 and IL-8, and in peripheral blood monocytes to produce interleukin 1-alpha (IL-1α), IL-1β, IL-8, IL-6, and TNF-α [28]. Adherence of this bacterium on the mucosal sites of the urinary tract triggers inflammation, including a mucosal cytokine-response which results in the secretion of IL-6 and IL-8 by activated uroepithelial cells [29, 30]. Thus, since IL-6 and IL-8 are expressed early after a UTI episode and are secreted by uroepithelial cells, these cytokines have clearly fulfilled some of the five characteristics of an ideal biomarker outlined in the introductory section. Reports indeed suggest that urine IL-6 and IL-8 are proven biomarkers for UTI in children [31]. The serum and urine levels of IL-6 were more sensitive and specific for upper UTI than levels of IL-8 [32]. Sensitivity and specificity values for serum IL-6 were noted to be 88 and 83% respectively, while for urine IL-6, sensitivity and specificity values were 86 and 81%, respectively [32]. Furthermore, serum IL-6 was able to differentiate upper from lower UTI with a sensitivity of 88% and specificity of 74%, while serum IL-1β was known to have a sensitivity of 97% and a specificity of 59% for detecting upper UTI [14].

2.2. Biomarkers of AKI

Serum creatinine represents a poor traditional biomarker for AKI due to some limitations. First, its levels are only altered when renal function diminishes by 50% [33]. Second, there are well-known confounders to serum creatinine levels such as muscle size, chronologic age, gender, drugs and state of hydration [34]. Third, a sudden reduction in renal function may not be shown by a rise in serum creatinine until after 24–48 hours. Finally, it provides little information about the underlying cause and nature of kidney injury, and is less accurate for patients with small muscle mass and unusual diets [1]. These draw-backs have resulted in a paradigm shift to novel biomarkers.

Generally, there are two main types of AKI biomarkers: *biomarkers of kidney function* and *biomarkers of kidney injury*. Irrespective of the type of kidney injury and the clinical scenario, an inflammatory response appears to play a significant role in the pathogenesis of AKI [34]. The major triggers of AKI (ischemia, nephrotoxins, and bacterial endotoxins) stimulate the release of inflammatory mediators from renal endothelial and tubular cells. As AKI progresses, a number of causative factors result in the accumulation of biomarkers in plasma and urine, and possibly indicate different pathophysiologic events during the process of kidney injury and repair [1]. For example, biomarkers like NGAL, interleukin-18 (IL-18), N-acetyl-β-D-glucosaminidase (NAG), kidney injury molecule-1 (KIM-1), accumulate in urine due to an induced tubular epithelial synthesis in different parts of the nephron, or as a consequence of reduced reabsorption of the filtered load in the proximal tubule (NGAL, cystatin C) [34]. Furthermore, production of biomarkers from transmigrated, activated immune cells into the tubular lumen may be contributory (NGAL, IL-18), while increased production of some biomarkers in other tissues (NGAL, IL-18) also occurs, thus raising concerns about their diagnostic value in the disease [35]. Biomarkers of AKI have been classified as follows: *functional markers* (serum cystatin C, urine albumin and NGAL), *up-regulated proteins* (KIM-1, liver-type fatty-acid binding protein [L-FABP], IL-18, β-trace protein and asymmetric dimethyl arginine), *low-molecular weight proteins* (urine cystatin C, NAG, glutathione S-transferase, γ-glutamyl-trans peptidase [γGT]) and *enzymes* (alanine amino-peptidase and lactate dehydrogenase) [36]. Other markers which have shown diagnostic ability include hepatocyte growth factor (HGF), vasoactive endothelial growth factor (VEGF), interferon gamma-induced protein 10 (IP-10) and total protein [37]. Some of the novel biomarkers are highlighted as below.

First, KIM-1 is a transmembrane tubular glycoprotein which is upregulated approximately 50- to 100-fold in the kidney, and is secreted into the urine after proximal tubular injury. KIM-1 is highly expressed in renal tubules, and is typically seen in areas of fibrosis and inflammation. The results of a meta-analysis indicate that urine KIM-1 represents a promising biomarker for early detection of AKI, with a good predictive value, especially in cardiac surgery patients [38]. Furthermore, in comparison to other biomarkers used as indicators of drug toxicity, KIM-1 significantly performed better than serum creatinine and blood urea nitrogen at detecting renal tubular injury in murine models; this makes it a useful marker for determining drug toxicity [39].

Second, NAG (another biomarker of kidney injury) is a large (>130 kDa) lysosomal enzyme which is located in several human cells including the renal tubule [34]. Its size hinders glomerular filtration, and elevated urine levels are thus presumed to emanate from the tubules, indicating tubular injury. In fact, during active renal disease, urine NAG activity is increased [40]. This feature makes it a potential and sensitive biomarker of AKI.

Third, cystatin C is a low-molecular-weight protein produced by all nucleated cells in the body at a constant rate, freely filtered by the glomeruli but completely reabsorbed and catabolized by the renal tubule [41]. Thus, its elevated urine levels are also seen in a tubulopathy because of the reduced re-absorptive capacity of the proximal tubules: making it a non-specific biomarker of AKI [42]. However, urine cystatin C could correctly predict the need for dialysis in intensive care unit (ICU) patients with established AKI [43]; could be an early predictor of AKI in children and in pediatric RIFLE classification, as well as a predictor of reduced estimated GFR (eGFR) after cardiac surgery [44]; while serum cystatin C could be used alone or in combination with serum creatinine and eGFR for early and accurate diagnosis of AKI in patients at emergency settings [45].

Finally, NGAL (which plays a role in the evaluation of UTI as previously mentioned) is a universal iron-transporter protein expressed in the tubular epithelium of the distal nephron and released into the blood and urine following tubular injury. This biomarker was first identified as a 25 kDa protein in the secondary granules of human neutrophils which is released into the bloodstream in response to bacterial infection. Interestingly, its elevated level in the urine may be diagnostic of AKI using the Acute Kidney Injury Network (AKIN) criteria: although with a moderate predictive value [46, 47]. In addition, its combination with another urine biomarker such as L-FABP resulted in early detection of AKI after cardiac surgery in a sample of adult patients before a rise in serum creatinine was noted [48]. Similarly, in murine models of ischemic and toxic AKI, NGAL was identified as one of the most speedily-induced proteins; its level was elevated by several folds in both serum and urine within hours of the insult [49].

3. Chronic kidney disease (CKD) and biomarkers

Several novel biomarkers have also been identified in the evaluation of childhood CKD: especially CKD secondary to idiopathic nephrotic syndrome and diabetic nephropathy (DN) [2, 50]. Remarkably, an overlap exists between some of the biomarkers of CKD and those of AKI and acute pyelonephritis. For instance, urine NAG, NGAL, cystatin C and L-FABP all play a role in the evaluation of both CKD and these acute kidney diseases. Similar to the grouping of biomarkers of AKI, biomarkers of CKD can be broadly classified into *biomarkers of kidney function* and *biomarkers of kidney damage*.

GFR is the most important marker of kidney function in CKD, although it is poorly estimated in most clinical and research settings. Thus, equations for its estimation are predicated upon filtration biomarkers such as serum creatinine and serum cystatin C [51]. However, equations for eGFR based on cystatin C appear more reliable because this biomarker is not affected by muscle mass and gives a better representation of GFR, in addition to having a more stable rate of production compared to creatinine [52].

Although albuminuria represents the traditional biomarker of kidney damage, it may only be present after significant damage has occurred, or may be absent in other types of kidney damage such as tubulointerstitial disease and hypertensive kidney disease. Therefore, there is now a paradigm shift to novel biomarkers which could identify patients with CKD early enough so that prompt interventions could slow down the progression of the disease.

3.1. Biomarkers of diabetic nephropathy (DN) and other causes of CKD

The major pathogenic components of DN consist of renal fibrosis, mesangial expansion, glomerular hypertrophy, oxidative stress and tubular inflammation [53]. Myriad novel biomarkers of DN have now been identified. An attempt to categorize them has also been made [50]. *Glomerular biomarkers* include transferrin, immunoglobulin G (IgG), ceruloplasmin, type IV collagen, laminin, glycosaminoglycans (GAGs), lipocalin-type prostaglandin D synthase (L-PGDS), fibronectin, podocytes-podocalyxin, and VEGF. *Tubular biomarkers* include NGAL, α-1-microglobulin, KIM-1, NAG, cystatin C, and L-FABP. *Biomarkers of inflammation* comprise TNF-α, IL-1β, IL-18, IP-10, monocyte chemoattractant protein 1 (MCP-1), granulocyte colony-stimulating factor (G-CSF), eotaxins, RANTES (regulated on activation, normal T cell expressed and secreted) or CCL-5, and orosomucoid. A typical example of *biomarkers of oxidative stress* is 8oHdG, while *miscellaneous biomarkers* include some tubular markers such as urine heart fatty acid-binding protein and urine retinol-binding protein 4 (RBP4), and podocyte biomarkers such as podocalyxin, nephrin, and VEGF, and urine advanced glycation end products (AGEs). Notably, these podocyte biomarkers are also regarded as glomerular markers. Some of the biomarkers of DN are shown in **Table 1**, and will be briefly discussed below.

Biomarkers	Clinical significance	Comments
• Kidney injury molecule-1	• Diabetic nephropathy‡	• Predicts CKD progression to ESKD
• Neutrophil gelatinase-associated lipocalin	• Ig A nephropathy • Polycystic kidney disease	• Predicts CKD progression from early stages to ESKD
• N-acetyl-β-D-glucosaminidase	• Diabetic nephropathy‡,† • Idiopathic glomerulonephritis (MN, FSGS, and MCN)	• Predicts early and late stages of CKD in type 1 diabetics, and early CKD in type 2 diabetics • Predicts proteinuria-induced tubular damage in early stage of disease
• Liver fatty acid-binding protein	• Diabetic nephropathy†,‡	• Predicts early CKD and progression to ESKD in type 1 diabetics and early CKD in type 2 diabetics
• Cystatin C	• Diabetic nephropathy†	• Predicts early CKD in type 2 diabetics
• α-1-microglobulin	• Diabetic nephropathy†	• Predicts early CKD in type 2 diabetics
• Monocyte chemoattractant protein-1 (MCP-1)	• Diabetic nephropathy†	• Predicts CKD and cardiovascular disease risk in type 2 diabetics
• Interleukin-18	• Lupus nephritis • Diabetic nephropathy†	• Elevated urine levels • Same as in MCP-1
• Retinol-binding protein 4	• Tubulointerstitial diseases	• Elevated urine levels

MN, membranous nephropathy; FSGS, focal segmental glomerulosclerosis; MCN, minimal change nephropathy.
‡Among type 1 diabetics.
†Among type 2 diabetics.

Table 1. Novel biomarkers of chronic kidney diseases.

NAG has the ability to predict the onset and progression of CKD in diabetes mellitus. For instance, baseline urine levels of this tubular biomarker can independently predict microalbuminuria and macroalbuminuria in type 1 diabetes mellitus [54]. Furthermore, it is a sensitive biomarker for the detection of early renal damage in type 2 diabetes mellitus [55], while elevated urine levels can precede microalbuminuria in type 1 diabetes mellitus [56].

Furthermore, high levels of KIM-1 have been observed in DN: a disease characterized by renal fibrosis and tubular inflammation, among other components that have been previously mentioned. For instance, majority of type 1 diabetic subjects with DN (stage 1 to 3 CKD) who had higher plasma KIM-1 levels reportedly ended up with end-stage kidney disease (ESKD); only a few of their counterparts who had lower plasma KIM-1 levels developed ESKD [57]. Baseline plasma KIM-1 levels also correlated with the rate of eGFR decline after adjusting for baseline urine albumin-to-creatinine ratio, eGFR, and glycated hemoglobin (Hb1Ac).

Another biomarker of DN is L-FABP, whose baseline urine levels in newly-diagnosed type 1 diabetics not only predicted the development of microalbuminuria but also the progression of microalbuminuria to macroalbuminuria [58]. In type 2 diabetes mellitus, elevated urine level of this biomarker also plays a role in predicting early CKD [59], and also serves as an independent predictor of CKD progression in type 1 diabetics [60]. Thus, L-FABP has the advantage of predicting kidney injury before albuminuria, especially in type 1 diabetics. Serum and urine cystatin C levels are useful biomarkers for early prediction of nephropathy in type 2 diabetes mellitus [61], and for progression of diabetic kidney disease [62]. Furthermore, α-1-microglobulin has been identified as an inexpensive biomarker for the early prediction of DN [63]. Elevated urine levels occur in patients with normoalbuminuric type 2 diabetes mellitus: preceding the onset of microalbuminuria and confirming this tubular biomarker as a more sensitive urine biomarker of CKD [64].

Expression of MCP-1 is upregulated in kidney diseases which present with a continued inflammatory response, such as in DN and lupus nephritis. Some reports indeed indicate that elevated levels of urine MCP-1 were observed in DN [65], as well as in active lupus nephritis [66]. Serum and urine levels of IL-18 were positively correlated with albumin excretion rate, whereas its serum levels were positively correlated with the development of carotid intima-media thickness in type 2 diabetics, and may therefore be a predictor of DN progression and cardiovascular diseases [67].

Finally, urine RBP4 is elevated in patients with tubulointerstitial disease, and may constitute a risk factor for long-term allograft loss, independent of the histology of renal biopsy, as well as for albuminuria [68].

3.2. Biomarkers of idiopathic nephrotic syndrome

The use of biomarkers in childhood idiopathic nephrotic syndrome has been well documented [2]. It represents a non-invasive approach in diagnostic nephrology, as these markers can be used in the prediction and prognostic evaluation of the disease, as well as in differentiating steroid-resistant nephrotic syndrome (SRNS) from steroid-sensitive nephrotic syndrome (SSNS). **Table 2** summarizes the list of identified biomarkers reported for childhood idiopathic nephrotic syndrome. Adiponectin (ADPN) – one of the adipokines, neopterin, β2-microglobulin, and NAG were reported to be diagnostic markers [69–71]. In addition to neopterin and NAG, urine vitamin D-binding protein (u VDBP) and α1β-glycoprotein were able to differentiate SRNS from SSNS [72, 73] while NAG and β2-microglobulin could also predict steroid responsiveness and renal outcome in SRNS [74]. Some of these biomarkers are further discussed as follows. First, elevated serum ADPN levels were documented in SRNS patients in relapse compared to those in remission [69]. Specifically, strong positive correlations were observed between serum ADPN levels and lipid parameters/proteinuria, whereas negative correlations were noted between ADPN levels and serum protein/albumin levels. Second, serum neopterin levels were found to be significantly elevated among SSNS and

Novel biomarkers (body fluids)	Reported role of biomarkers (references)
• Adiponectin (serum)	• Diagnostic[*] (Bakkalŏglu et al. [69])
• Neopterin (serum)	• Diagnostic[**] (Bakr et al. [70]) • Discriminatory[†] (Bakr et al. [70])
• Vitamin D binding protein (urine)	• Discriminatory[†] (Bennett et al. [72])
• N-acetyl-beta-D glucosaminidase (urine)	• Discriminatory[†] (Calişkan et al. [71]) • Prognostic[‡] (Fede et al. [74])
• α 1-β glycoprotein (13.8 kDa fragment) (urine)	• Discriminatory[†] (Piyaphanee et al. [73])
• beta2-microglobulin (urine) • N-acetyl-beta-D glucosaminidase (urine)	• Prognostic[***] (Fede et al. [74])
• beta2-microglobulin (urine) • N-acetyl-beta-D glucosaminidase (urine)	• Diagnostic[¥] (Calişkan et al. [71])

[*]Raised serum levels in steroid-resistant nephrotic syndrome (SRNS) relapse.
[**]Raised serum levels in primary active nephrotic syndrome.
[†]Differentiates SRNS from steroid-sensitive nephrotic syndrome (SSNS).
[‡]Predicts steroid-responsiveness.
[***]Predicts tubular injury and dysfunction in SRNS.
[¥]Elevated levels in SRNS and SSNS.

Table 2. Role of some novel biomarkers in childhood idiopathic nephrotic syndrome.

SRNS patients with the active disease when compared to those in remission and the controls [70]. The diagnostic utility of neopterin for active idiopathic nephrotic syndrome was thus highlighted, but its poor discriminatory ability for SSNS and SRNS were also noted in the report. Third, uVDBP was reported to have a high discriminatory ability in distinguishing SRNS from SSNS [72]. For instance, levels of uVDBP were significantly higher in patients with SRNS than in patients with SSNS and in the controls. Despite the direct correlation between microalbuminuria and uVDBP, the latter exhibited a higher discriminatory ability for differentiating SRNS from SSNS than the former.

4. Conclusion

Many biomarkers have now been identified for the diagnostic and prognostic evaluation of acute and chronic diseases of the kidney in children. However, more evidence-based studies are still required to validate some of the novel biomarkers. Remarkably, a biomarker-panel comprising several of the markers potentially improves their sensitivity and specificity in disease evaluation. Inequities in the availability and accessibility of the laboratory tools between the developed and developing world still remain a challenge. Biotechnology firms should urgently prioritize the mass production of tools for identifying these biomarkers in order to bridge this gap.

Acknowledgements

The author acknowledges the invaluable information obtained from his previous published works in Refs. [1–3], during the preparation of this book chapter.

Conflict of interest

The author declares no conflict of interest in this work.

Author details

Samuel N. Uwaezuoke

Address all correspondence to: samuel.uwaezuoke@unn.edu.ng

College of Medicine, University of Nigeria/University of Nigeria Teaching Hospital, Enugu, Nigeria

References

[1] Uwaezuoke SN. Acute kidney injury in children: Enhancing diagnosis with novel biomarkers. Journal of Acute Disease. 2016;**5**:267-270

[2] Uwaezuoke SN. The role of novel biomarkers in childhood idiopathic nephrotic syndrome: A narrative review of published evidence. International Journal of Nephrology and Renovascular Disease. 2017;**10**:123-128

[3] Uwaezuoke SN. Urinary tract infection in children: Diagnostic and prognostic utility of biomarkers. Journal of Comprehensive Pediatrics. 2017;**8**:e59248. DOI: 10.5812/compreped.59248

[4] Strimbu K, Jorge T. What are biomarkers? Current Opinion in HIV and AIDS. 2010;**5**:463-466. DOI: 10.1097/COH.0b013e32833ed177

[5] Atkinson AJ Jr, Colburn WA, DeGruttola VG, et al. Biomarkers and surrogate endpoints: Preferred definitions and conceptual framework. Clinical Pharmacology and Therapeutics. 2001;**69**:89-95. DOI: 10.1067/mcp.2001.113989

[6] Cruz DN, Goh CY, Haase-Fielitz A, Ronco C, Haase M. Early biomarkers of renal injury. Congestive Heart Failure. 2010;**16**:S25-S31. DOI: 10.1111/j.1751-7133.2010.00163.x

[7] Srivastava RN, Bagga A. Urinary tract infection. In: Srivastava RN, Bagga A, editors. Pediatric Nephrology. 4th ed. New Delhi: Jaypee Brothers Medical Publishers Ltd; 2005. pp. 235-264. DOI: 10.5005/jp/books/11308

[8] Shaikh N, Morone NE, Bost JE, Farrell MH. Prevalence of urinary tract infection in childhood: A meta-analysis. The Pediatric Infectious Disease Journal. 2008;**27**(4):302-308. DOI: 10.1097/INF.0b013e31815e4122

[9] Chang SL, Shortliffe LD. Pediatric urinary tract infections. Pediatric Clinics of North America. 2006;**53**:379-400. DOI: 10.1016/j.pcl.2006.02.011

[10] Assicot M, Gendrel D, Carsin H, Raymond J, Guilbaud J, Bohuon C. High serum procalcitonin concentrations in patients with sepsis and infection. Lancet. 1993;**341**:515-518. DOI: 10.1016/0140-6736(93)90277-N

[11] Dandona P, Nix D, Wilson MF, et al. Procalcitonin increase after endotoxin injection in normal subjects. Journal of Clinical Endocrinology and Metabolism. 1994;**79**:1065-1608. DOI: 10.1210/jcem.79.6.7989463

[12] Meisner M, Tsachaikowsky K, Palmaers T, Schmidt J. Comparison of procalcitonin (PCT) and C-reactive protein (CRP) plasma concentrations at different SOFA scores during the course of sepsis and MODS. Critical Care. 1999;**3**:45-50. DOI: 10.1186/cc306

[13] Balci C, Sungurtekin H, Gürses E, Sungurtekin U, Kaptanoğlu B. Usefulness of procalcitonin for diagnosis of sepsis in the intensive care unit. Critical Care. 2003;**7**:85-90. DOI: 10.1186/cc1843

[14] Gürgöze MK, Akarsu S, Yilmaz E, Gödekmerdan A, Akça Z, Çiftçi I, et al. Proinflammatory cytokines and procalcitonin in children with acute pyelonephritis. Pediatric Nephrology. 2005;**20**:1445-1448. DOI: 10.1007/s00467-005-1941-6

[15] Smolkin V, Koren A, Raz R, Colodner R, Sakran W, Halevy R. Procalcitonin as a marker of acute pyelonephritis in infants and children. Pediatric Nephrology. 2002;**17**:409-412. PMID: 12107804

[16] Pecile P, Miorin E, Romanello C, Falleti E, Valent F, Giacomuzzi F, et al. Procalcitonin: A marker of severity of acute pyelonephritis among children. Pediatrics. 2004;**114**:e249-e254. DOI: 10.1542/peds.114.2.e249

[17] Leroy S, Adamsbaum C, Marc E, Moulin F, Raymond J, Gendrel D, et al. Procalcitonin as a predictor of vesicoureteral reflux in children with a first febrile urinary tract infection. Pediatrics. 2005;**115**:e706-e709. DOI: 10.1542/peds.2004-1631

[18] Sun HL, Wu KH, Chen SM, Chao YH, Ku MS, Hung TW, et al. Role of procalcitonin in predicting dilating vesicoureteral reflux in young children hospitalized with a first febrile urinary tract infection. The Pediatric Infectious Disease Journal. 2013;**32**:e348-e354. DOI: 10.1097/INF.0b013e3182905d83

[19] Rahimzadeh N, Otukesh H, Hoseini R, Shadani S, Hooman N. Serum procalcitonin level for prediction of high-grade vesicoureteral reflux in urinary tract infection. Iranian Journal of Kidney Diseases. 2014;**8**:105-108

[20] Barati L, Safaeian B, Mehrjerdian M, Vakili MA. Early prediction of renal parenchymal injury with serum procalcitonin. Journal of Renal Injury Prevention. 2016;**5**:108-111. DOI: 10.15171/jrip.2016.23

[21] Chien JW, Wang LY, Cheng YS, Tsai YG, Liu CS. Urinary 8-hydroxy2′-deoxyguanosine (8-oxodG) level can predict acute renal damage in young children with urinary tract infection. Biomarkers. 2014;**19**:326-331. DOI: 10.3109/1354750X.2014.910552

[22] Yang J, Goetz D, Li JY, Wang W, Mori K, Setlik D, et al. An iron delivery pathway mediated by a lipocalin. Molecular Cell. 2002;**10**:1045-1056. DOI: 10.1016/s1097-2765(02)00710-4

[23] Cowland JB, Borregaard N. Molecular characterization and pattern of tissue expression of the gene for neutrophil gelatinase-associated lipocalin from humans. Genomics. 1997;**45**:17-23. DOI: 10.1006/geno.1997.4896

[24] Devarajan P. Neutrophil gelatinase-associated lipocalin: A troponin-like biomarker for human acute kidney injury. Nephrology (Carlton). 2010;**15**:419-428. DOI: 10.1111/j.1440-1797.2010.01317.x

[25] Bennett M, Dent CL, Ma Q, Dastrala S, Grenier F, Workman R, et al. Urine NGAL predicts severity of acute kidney injury after cardiac surgery: A prospective study. Clinical Journal of the American Society of Nephrology. 2008;**3**:665-673. DOI: 10.2215/CJN.04010907

[26] Ghasemi K, Esteghamati M, Borzoo S, Parvaneh E. Predictive accuracy of urinary neutrophil gelatinase associated lipocalin (NGAL) for renal parenchymal involvement in children with acute pyelonephritis. Electronic Physician. 2016;**8**:1911-1917. DOI: 10.19082/1911

[27] Yilmaz A, Sevketoglu E, Gedikbasi A, Karyagar S, Kiyak A, Mulazimoglu M, et al. Early prediction of urinary tract infection with urinary neutrophil gelatinase associated lipocalin. Pediatric Nephrology. 2009;**24**:2387-2392. DOI: 10.1007/s00467-009-1279-6

[28] Agace W, Hedges S, Andersson U, Andersson J, Ceska M, Svanborg C. Selective cytokine production by epithelial cells following exposure to *Escherichia coli*. Infection and Immunity. 1993;**61**:602-609. PMCID: PMC302770

[29] Agace W, Hedges S, Ceska M, Svanborg C. Interleukin-8 and the neutrophil response to mucosal gram-negative infection. The Journal of Clinical Investigation. 1993;**92**:780-785. DOI: 10.1172/JCI116650

[30] Svanborg C, Agace W, Hedges S, Lindstedt R, Svensson ML. Bacterial adherence and mucosal cytokine production. Annals of the New York Academy of Sciences. 1994;**730**:162-181. DOI: 10.1111/j.1749-6632.1994.tb44247.x

[31] Jantausch BA, O'Donnell R, Wiedermann BL. Urinary interleukin-6 and interleukin-8 in children with urinary tract infection. Pediatric Nephrology. 2000;**15**:236-240. DOI: 10.1007/s004670000456

[32] Sheu JN, Chen MC, Lue KH, Cheng SL, Lee IC, Chen SM, et al. Serum and urine levels of interleukin-6 and interleukin-8 in children with acute pyelonephritis. Cytokine. 2006;**36**:276-282. DOI: 10.1016/j.cyto.2007.02.006

[33] Coca SG, Yalavarthy R, Concato J, Parikh CR. Biomarkers for the diagnosis and risk stratification of acute kidney injury: A systematic review. Kidney International. 2008;**73**:1008-1016. DOI: 10.1038/sj.ki.5002729

[34] Mårtensson J, Martling CR, Bell M. Novel biomarkers of acute kidney injury and failure: Clinical applicability. British Journal of Anaesthesia. 2012;**109**:843-850. DOI: 10.1093/bja/aes357

[35] Mårtensson J, Bellomo R. The rise and fall of NGAL in acute kidney injury. Blood Purification. 2014;**37**:304-310. DOI: 10.1159/000364937

[36] de Geus HR, Betjes MG, Bakker J. Biomarkers for the prediction of acute kidney injury: A narrative review on current status and future challenges. Clinical Kidney Journal. 2012;**5**:102-108. DOI: 10.1093/ckj/sfs008

[37] Vanmassenhove J, Vanholder R, Nagler E, Van Biesen W. Urinary and serum biomarkers for the diagnosis of acute kidney injury: In-depth review of the literature. Nephrology, Dialysis, Transplantation. 2013;**28**:254-273. DOI: 10.1093/ndt/gfs380

[38] Shao X, Tian L, Xu W, Zhang Z, Wang C, Qi C, et al. Diagnostic value of urinary kidney injury molecule 1 for acute kidney injury: A meta-analysis. PLoS One. 2014;**9**:e84131. DOI: 10.1371/journal.pone.0084131

[39] Bonventre JV, Vaidya VS, Schmouder R, Feig P, Dieterle F. Next generation biomarkers for detecting kidney toxicity. Nature Biotechnology. 2010;**28**:436-440. DOI: 10.1038/nbt0510-436

[40] Endre ZH, Pickering JW, Walker RJ, Devarajan P, Edelstein CL, Bonventre JV, et al. Improved performance of urinary biomarkers of acute kidney injury in the critically ill by stratification for injury duration and baseline renal function. Kidney International. 2011;**79**:1119-1130. DOI: 10.1038/ki.2010.555

[41] Srivastava RN, Bagga A. Evaluation of renal function. In: Srivastava RN, Bagga A, editors. Pediatric Nephrology. 4th ed. New Delhi: Jaypee Brothers Medical Publishers Ltd; 2005. pp. 20-29. DOI: 10.5005/jp/books/11308

[42] Ghys L, Paepe D, Smets P, Lefebvre H, Delanghe J, Daminet S. Cystatin C: A new renal marker and its potential use in small animal medicine. Journal of Veterinary Internal Medicine. 2014;**28**(4):1152-1164. DOI: 10.1111/jvim.12366

[43] Nejat M, Pickering JW, Walker RJ, Westhuyzen J, Shaw GM, Frampton CM, et al. Urinary cystatin C is diagnostic of acute kidney injury and sepsis, and predicts mortality in the intensive care unit. Critical Care. 2010;**14**:R85. DOI: 10.1186/cc9014

[44] Hassinger AB, Backer CL, Lane JC, Haymond S, Wang D, Wald EL, et al. Predictive power of serum cystatin C to detect acute kidney injury and pediatric-modified RIFLE class in children undergoing cardiac surgery. Pediatric Critical Care Medicine. 2012;**13**:435-440. DOI: 10.1097/PCC.0b013e318238b43c

[45] Bongiovanni C, Magrini L, Salerno G, Gori CS, Cardelli P, Hur M, et al. Serum cystatin C for the diagnosis of acute kidney injury in patients admitted in the emergency department. Disease Markers. 2015;**2015**:416059. DOI: 10.1155/2015/416059

[46] Schinstock CA, Semret MH, Wagner SJ, Borland TM, Bryant SC, Kashani KB, et al. Urinalysis is more specific and urinary neutrophil gelatinase-associated lipocalin

is more sensitive for early detection of acute kidney injury. Nephrology, Dialysis, Transplantation. 2013;**28**(5):1175-1185. DOI: 10.1093/ndt/gfs127

[47] Xu SY, Carlson M, Engström A, Garcia R, Peterson CG, Venge P. Purification and characterization of a human neutrophil lipocalin (HNL) from the secondary granules of human neutrophils. Scandinavian Journal of Clinical and Laboratory Investigation. 1994;**54**:365-376. PMID: 7997842

[48] Liu S, Che M, Xue S, Xie B, Zhu M, Lu R, et al. Urinary L-FABP and its combination with urinary NGAL in early diagnosis of acute kidney injury after cardiac surgery in adult patients. Biomarkers. 2013;**18**:95-101. DOI: 10.3109/1354750X.2012.740687

[49] Obermüller N, Geiger H, Weipert C, Urbschat A. Current developments in early diagnosis of acute kidney injury. International Urology and Nephrology. 2014;**46**:1-7. DOI: 10.1007/s11255-013-0448-5

[50] Uwaezuoke SN. The role of novel biomarkers in predicting diabetic nephropathy: A review. International Journal of Nephrology and Renovascular Disease. 2017;**10**:221-231. DOI: 10.2147/IJNRD.S143186

[51] Lopez-Giacoman S, Madero M. Biomarkers in chronic kidney disease, from kidney function to kidney damage. World Journal of Nephrology. 2015;**4**:57-73. DOI: 10.5527/wjn.v4.i1.57

[52] Shlipak MG, Matsushita K, Ärnlöv J, et al. Cystatin C versus creatinine in determining risk based on kidney function. The New England Journal of Medicine. 2013;**369**:932-943. DOI: 10.1056/NEJMoa1214234

[53] Arora MK, Singh UK. Molecular mechanisms in the pathogenesis of diabetic nephropathy: An update. Vascular Pharmacology. 2013;**58**:259-271. DOI: 10.1016/j.vph.2013.01.001

[54] Kern EF, Erhard P, Sun W, Genuth S, Weiss MF. Early urinary markers of diabetic kidney disease: A nested case-control study from the Diabetes Control and Complications Trial (DCCT). American Journal of Kidney Diseases. 2010;**55**:824-834. DOI: 10.1053/j.ajkd.2009.11.009

[55] Patel DN, Kalia K. Efficacy of urinary N-acetyl-β-D glucosaminidase to evaluate early renal tubular damage as a consequence of type 2 diabetes mellitus: A cross-sectional study. International Journal of Diabetes in Developing Countries. 2015;**35**:449-457. DOI: 10.1007/s13410-015-0404-2

[56] Jones AP, Lock S, Griffiths KD. Urinary N-acetyl-β-glucosaminidase activity in type 1 diabetes mellitus. Annals of Clinical Biochemistry. 2006;**21**:142-148. DOI: 10.1177/000456329503200104

[57] Krolewski AS, Niewczas MA, Skupien J, et al. Early progressive renal decline precedes the onset of microalbuminuria and its progression to macroalbuminuria. Diabetes Care. 2014;**37**:226-234. DOI: 10.2337/dc13-0985

[58] Nielsen SE, Sugaya T, Hovind P, Baba T, Parving HH, Rossing P. Urinary liver-type fatty acid-binding protein predicts progression to nephropathy in type 1 diabetic patients. Diabetes Care. 2010;**33**:1320-1324. DOI: 10.2337/dc09-2242

[59] Kamijo-Ikemori A, Sugaya T, Yasuda T, et al. Clinical significance of urinary liver-type fatty acid-binding protein in diabetic nephropathy of type 2 diabetic patients. Diabetes Care. 2011;**34**:691-696. DOI: 10.2337/dc10-1392

[60] Panduru NM, Forsblom C, Saraheimo M, et al.; Finn Diane Study Group. Urinary liver-type fatty acid-binding protein and progression of diabetic nephropathy in type 1 diabetics. Diabetes Care. 2013;**36**:2077-2083. DOI: 10.2337/dc12-1868

[61] Jeon YK, Kim MR, Huh JE, et al. Cystatin C as an early biomarker of nephropathy in patients with type 2 diabetes. Journal of Korean Medical Science. 2011;**26**:258-263. DOI: 10.3346/jkms.2011.26.2.258

[62] Kim SS, Song SH, Kim IJ, et al. Urinary cystatin C and tubular proteinuria predict progression of diabetic nephropathy. Diabetes Care. 2013;**36**:656-661. DOI: 10.2337/dc12-0849

[63] Shore N, Khurshid R, Saleem M. Alpha-1 microglobulin: A marker for early detection of tubular disorders in diabetic nephropathy. Journal of Ayub Medical College, Abbottabad. 2010;**22**:53-55. http://www.ayubmed.edu.pk/JAMC/PAST/22-4/Najla.pdf

[64] Hong CY, Hughes K, Chia KS, Ng V, Ling SL. Urinary alpha-1-microglobulin as a marker of nephropathy in type 2 diabetic Asian subjects in Singapore. Diabetes Care. 2003;**26**:338-342. DOI: 10.2337/diacare.26.2.338

[65] Takebayashi K, Matsumoto S, Aso Y, Inukai T. Aldosterone blockade attenuates urinary monocyte chemoattractant protein-1 and oxidative stress in patients with type 2 diabetes complicated by diabetic nephropathy. The Journal of Clinical Endocrinology and Metabolism. 2006;**91**:2214-2217. DOI: 10.1097/MNH.0b013e32833ce6d5

[66] Noris M, Bernasconi S, Casiraghi F, Sozzani S, Gotti E, Remuzzi G, Mantovani A. Monocyte chemoattractant protein-1 is excreted in excessive amounts in the urine of patients with lupus nephritis. Laboratory Investigation. 1995;**73**:804-809. PMID: 8558841

[67] Nakamura A, Shikata K, Hiramatsu M, et al. Serum interleukin-18 levels are associated with nephropathy and atherosclerosis in Japanese patients with type 2 diabetes. Diabetes Care. 2005;**28**:2890-2895. DOI: 10.2337/diacare.28.12.2890

[68] Amer H, Lieske JC, Rule AD, et al. Urine high and low molecular weight proteins one-year post-kidney transplant: Relationship to histology and graft survival. American Journal of Transplantation. 2013;**13**:676-684. DOI: 10.1111/ajt.12044

[69] Bakkalŏglu SA, Soylemezoglu O, Buyan N, et al. High serum adiponectin levels during steroid-responsive nephrotic syndrome relapse. Pediatric Nephrology. 2005;**20**:474-477. DOI: 10.1007/s00467-004-1770-z

[70] Bakr A, Rageh I, El-Azouny M, Deyab S, Lotfy H. Serum neopterin levels in children with primary nephrotic syndrome. Acta Paediatrica. 2006;**95**:854-856

[71] Calişkan S, Hacibekiroğlu M, Sever L, Ozbay G, Arisoy N. Urinary N-acetyl-beta-D-glucosaminidase and beta 2-microglobulin excretion in primary nephrotic children. Nephron. 1996;**74**:401-404. DOI: 10.1159/000189442

[72] Bennett MR, Pordal A, Haffner C, Pleasant L, Ma Q, Devarajan P. Urinary vitamin D-binding protein as a biomarker of steroid-resistant nephrotic syndrome. Biomarker Insights. 2016;**11**:1-6. DOI: 10.4137/BMI.S31633

[73] Piyaphanee N, Ma Q, Kremen O, et al. Discovery and initial validation of α 1-B glycoprotein fragmentation as a differential urinary biomarker in pediatric steroid-resistant nephrotic syndrome. Proteomics. Clinical Applications. 2011;**5**:334-342. DOI: 10.1002/prca.201000110

[74] Fede C, Conti G, Chimenz R, Ricca M. N-acetyl-beta-D-glucosaminidase and beta2-microglobulin: Prognostic markers in idiopathic nephrotic syndrome. Journal of Nephrology. 1999;**12**:51-55. PMID: 10203005

2

Biomarkers and Heart Failure

Hakan Altay

Abstract

Heart failure (HF) represents fatal endpoint of all cardiovascular diseases. Acute and chronic HF is a complex, heterogeneous syndrome consisting of many overlapping syndromes making its diagnosis and treatment more challenging. There is no single test for diagnosis of HF, and diagnosis is based on clinical judgment driven by a combination of history, physical examination, and appropriate tests. Despite improvements in clinical management within the last 50 years, it has still been a disease of poor prognosis. Attempts to further improve its prognosis can only be achieved by understanding pathophysiology of HF clearly and finding, developing, and using appropriate and new clinical biochemical markers for diagnosis of each different clinical subtype and hence unique intervention of that specific subtype of HF. This review is an overview of biomarkers, which are either currently used in the clinical practice or hold promise for future use in patients with both chronic and acute HF.

Keywords: heart failure, diagnosis, prognosis, biochemical markers

1. Introduction

Heart failure (HF) is the end stage of all the cardiovascular diseases. It is an important mortality and morbidity cause. It is a syndrome that can be defined clinically by a collection of symptoms (dyspnea, fatigue, and exertional intolerance) and signs (edema, rales, and gallop) that are caused by a cardiac disorder [1]. In half of the patients with HF, inadequate pumping action of the heart is the main cardiac disorder forming the HF with reduced ejection fraction (HFrEF). In the other half, abnormality in the relaxation properties of the heart is the main cardiac disorder forming the HF with preserved ejection fraction (HFpEF). HFrEF and HFpEF share the same clinical phenotype. First of all, HF is a clinical diagnosis. Unfortunately, diagnosis of HF is not an easy task and cannot be made only by clinics because symptoms and signs of HF are nonspecific.

Rather, the diagnosis is based on clinical judgment using history, physical examination, and combination of appropriate tests. Biomarkers form complementary information in addition to the clinics and the other tests used, help for the diagnosis, prognosis, and follow-up of the HF patients, and sometimes form the basis for implementing specific treatment.

2. Biomarkers

The definition of biomarker is as follows: biomarkers are parameters which can be measured objectively and assessed as an indicator of normal biologic or pathogenic process or response to treatment. An ideal biomarker should have the capability of reflecting the pathway centrally important to the disease under investigation, thereby providing therapeutic insights. An ideal biomarker should have three important characteristics: (1) It should be measured in a short time with low cost. (2) It should add complementary information to clinical evaluation. (3) It should aid to the treatment of HF. Biomarkers with these characteristics can be used for confirming the presence or absence of HF syndrome, for finding the specific underlying cause of HF, assessing the severity and prognosis of HF, and identifying patients likely to respond to specific treatments. HF does not occur as a result of a single pathophysiologic disease, but a multiple of pathophysiologic mechanisms resulting in volume and/or pressure overload. This makes the use of these biomarkers complex and difficult. Despite significant overlaps,

Biomarkers	
(1) Myocardial stress/injury	
• Myocardial stress	NT-proBNP, BNP, MR-proBNP
• Myocardial injury	Troponin, heart-type fatty-acid protein
• Oxidative stress	Myeloperoxidase, uric acid
(2) Neurohormonal activation	
• Renin angiotensin system	Renin, Angiotensin II, Aldosterone
• Sympathetic nervous system	Norepinephrine, chromogranin A, adrenomedulin
• Arginine vasopressin system	Arginine vasopressin, copeptin
• Endothelins	ET-1
• Parathyroid	Parathyroid hormone
(3) Remodeling	
• Inflammation	C-reactive protein, osteoprotegerin, TNF-alfa, IL-6, adiponectin
• Hypertrophy/fibrosis	ST-2, galectin-3
• Apoptosis	GDF-15
• Miscallenous	microRNA
(4) Comorbidities	
• Renal biomarkers	Kreatinin, BUN, eGFR, cystatin C, beta-trace protein
• Hematologic biomarkers	Hb, Htc, iron deficiency (ferritin, transferrin saturation), RDW
• Liver function tests	AST, ALT, LDH, Albumin

ALT, Alanine aminotransferase; AST, aspartate aminotransferase; BNP, brain natriuretic peptide; BUN, blood urea nitrogen; ET-1, endothelin 1; Hb, hemoglobin: Htc, hematocrit; IL-6, interleukin-6; LDH, lactate dehydrogenase; MR-proADM, mid-regional proadrenomedullin; MR-proBNP, mid-regional proBNP; NT-proBNP, N-terminal proBNP; RDW, red blood cell distribution width.

Table 1. Biomarkers in heart failure.

biomarkers used in HF can be roughly arranged into four categories: (1) myocardial stress/ injury, (2) neurohormonal activation, (3) remodeling, and (4) comorbidities (**Table 1**).

3. Biomarkers for heart failure

3.1. Myocardial stress/injury

3.1.1. Natriuretic peptides (NPs)

In this group, there is robust evidence for both brain natriuretic peptide (BNP) and NT-proBNP regarding HF. The most potent inducer of release of BNP from the left ventricle is left ventricular (LV) wall stretch from increased pressure or volume. A prohormone (proBNP) is degraded to BNP and NT-proBNP, forming three distinct subtypes in the circulation as BNP, NT-proBNP, and proBNP. BNP acts on natriuretic peptide receptor system resulting in natriuresis, diuresis, vasodilation, inhibition of renin and aldosterone, and inhibition of fibrosis [2]. BNP is cleared from circulation by a receptor-mediated mechanism as well as degradation by neutral endopeptidases such as neprilysin. The half-life of BNP is significantly shorter than that of NT-proBNP (approximately 20 vs. 60–120 minutes). Conventional assays for BNP detect proBNP and BNP, as well as various degraded fragments of BNP, while NT-proBNP assays detect NT-proBNP and proBNP [3].

Analytical studies have shown that ratio of BNP to proBNP may have superior prognostic value compared to single BNP assay [4]. In a normal healthy individual, BNP and NT-proBNP serum levels are low, but in a HF patient, serum levels rise proportionately to excess volume overload. The Breathing Not Properly Multinational Study demonstrated that the optimal cutoff value of BNP to diagnose HF was 100 pg/mL, with high accuracy at 85% [5]. Similar findings were seen for NT-proBNP in the ProBNP Investigation of Dyspnea in the Emergency Department (PRIDE) Study in which elevated NT- proBNP concentrations were the strongest predictor of HF compared with traditional assessment [6].

Based on accumulating evidence, BNP and NT-proBNP have been generally used for the differential diagnosis of acute dyspnea [7]. These two peptides have especially high negative predictive value; therefore, they have been generally used for exclusion of HF. The exclusion thresholds of these peptides are different in acute HF in the emergency department than chronic HF in the outpatient setting. For patients presenting with acute onset HF, the optimal exclusion cutoff point is 300 pg/ml for NT-proBNP and 100 pg/ml for BNP, whereas the exclusion cutoff values are 125 and 35 pg/ml, respectively, in the outpatient setting. The sensitivity and specificity of BNP and NT-proBNP for the diagnosis of chronic HF are lower in the outpatient setting [8]. Natriuretic peptide levels increase with age. Therefore, age-stratified cutoff points for NT-proBNP (≥450 for ages <50 years, ≥900 for 50–75 years, and ≥1800 pg/ml for >75 years) performed the best diagnostic accuracy (**Table 2**) [7]. The negative predictive values are high in both acute and non-acute outpatient settings, but the positive predictive values are lower in both situations. Therefore, the use of NPs is recommended more to rule out HF, but not to establish the diagnosis.

Acute HF		Sens.	Spec.	PPV	NPV
BNP	<100 pg/ml	90%	76%	79%	89%
NT-proBNP, overall	<300 pg/ml	99%	68%	62%	99%
NT-proBNP, age-stratified approach		90%	84%	88%	66%
	<450 pg/ml for <50y				
	<900 pg/ml for 50–75y				
	<1800 pg/ml for >85y				
Outpatient screening for symptomatic HF					
BNP	<35 pg/ml	–	–	–	96%
NT-proBNP	<125 pg/ml	–	–	–	98%

BNP, brain natriuretic peptide; HF, heart failure; NPV, negative predictive value; PPV, positive predictive value; Sens., sensitivity; Spec., specificity.

Table 2. Natriuretic peptide exclusion threshold cutoff points (modified from reference 7).

There are some shortcomings of natriuretic peptide biomarkers. HF is not the only disease that increases these peptides. Other diseases that can cause a rise in natriuretic peptides are as follows: acute coronary syndrome, myocarditis, valvular heart disease, hypertrophic cardiomyopathy, cardiotoxic drugs, atrial fibrillation, or flutter and pulmonary embolism. Other conditions that are associated with higher BNP or NT-proBNP levels may be related to comorbidities such as advanced age, renal dysfunction, stroke, and high-output states. HFpEF is associated with lower than expected natriuretic peptide levels compared with HFrEF. The other condition which is associated with lower than the expected NP level is obesity. The explanation for this is suppression of natriuretic peptide synthesis or release in obese people. Therefore, the diagnostic sensitivity of NPs in obese patients is modestly lower. With respect to HFpEF, the same cutoff points for BNP or NT-proBNP can be utilized to diagnose HF with the understanding that the sensitivity is somewhat decreased and HFpEF is associated with lower NP levels compared to HFrEF [9]. Apart from BNP and NT-proBNP, another natriuretic peptide called mid-regional proANP (MR-proANP) has been tested in a large prospective trial [10]. In this large trial, MR-proANP was reported to be a better biomarker in conditions like obesity and chronic renal failure where BNP and NT-proBNP could be less reliable. It has also a diagnostic utility in acute HF same as BNP and NT-proBNP.

Natriuretic peptides are, to date, the best predictors of prognosis in HF. HF therapies, both disease-modifying agents like angiotensin-converting enzyme inhibitors (ACEi), beta-blockers (BB), and mineralocorticoid receptor antagonists (MRA) and diuretics, reduce these NP levels. This observation has led to the concept of biomarker-guided HF management using BNP or NT-proBNP. However, there is inconsistent data regarding the benefit of natriuretic peptide-guided therapy to reduce the mortality and cardiovascular outcomes. Because of this, serial measurement of NPs during treatment of HF did not find a high level of recommendation in the guidelines. Despite this lack of evidence, serial measurement of NPs, at least one at admission and one at predischarge, was used during management of hospitalized patients.

And, the best outcomes for these patients were seen when NP levels decreased by >30% [11]. This predischarge NP level may also be used as a point of reference (i.e., optivolemic NP level) when the patient presents to the emergency department again to aid the clinician for the judgment of hospitalizing the patient later. As a result, in patients admitted with acute decompensated HF, both absolute NT-proBNP discharge levels and a relative reduction of >30% in NT-proBNP levels from admission are significant predictors of readmissions and mortality [12]. However, in the setting of chronic HF patients, the gain that is made by NP-guided treatment has been modest [13].

3.1.2. *Myocardial injury*

Beyond their ability to diagnose myocardial infarction, troponin T (TnT) and troponin I (TnI) are frequently detectable in HF without obvious cause of ischemia. Elevations in either troponin I or troponin T levels in the setting of acute HF are of prognostic significance and must be interpreted in the clinical context [14]. In the ADHERE registry, 6.2% of patients with acute decompensated HF had an elevated troponin which was associated with worse in-hospital mortality [15]. As ischemia or myocardial infarction may be the precipitating cause of acute decompensation of HF, new HF guidelines recommend troponin measurement in all patients presenting acutely, in order to exclude or diagnose ischemia as a cause and also to assess prognosis as well [16]. In patients with chronic HF, 92% of patients were found to have measurable or elevated hsTnT (detection limit ≤0.001 ng/mL), and hsTnT >0.012 ng/mL was closely linked with poor clinical outcomes [17].

3.2. Neurohormonal activation

Serum aldosterone levels are increased in severe HF patients (New York Heart Association (NYHA) classes III and IV HF). In mild HF (NYHA classes I and II), serum aldosterone levels are not increased unless RAAS is activated by the excessive use of diuretics, leading to renal hypoperfusion [18]. Serum aldosterone measurement identifies not only HF patients likely to respond mineralocorticoid receptor antagonists but also severe HF patients who will benefit from interventions directed for advanced HF.

The second important response to cardiac dysfunction is the activation of the sympathetic nervous system. Chromogranin A (CgA) is a peptide found in adrenal medulla and a multiple number of endocrine cells. It is an important predictor of sympathetic system activation. CgA is a prohormone and needs to be metabolized in order to become biologically active. Its serum level is associated with HF severity, and it predicts mortality in acute HF. The highest mortality occurs when both CgA and NT-proBNP rise together [19].

Adrenomedullin (ADM) is a peptide hormone with strong hypotensive, natriuretic, and positive inotropic effect. It is secreted from the adrenal medulla and kidney upon pressure and volume overload. ADM causes vasodilation via production of nitric oxide (NO), and its level rises in HF as a compensatory mechanism. Due to its short half-life and circulating in the plasma as protein-bound, measurement of ADM is difficult. Alternatively, measurement of mid-regional proadrenomedullin (MR-proADM) is possible. MR-proADM is a precursor molecule of adrenomedullin; MR-proADM is elevated in patients with acute and chronic HF and is a strong predictor of mortality and HF hospitalization in addition to BNP or NT-proBNP [20]. The data, up to date, are promising, but the implementation of this biomarker into the clinical practice needs more evidence.

Arginine vasopressin (AVP) is an antidiuretic and vasoconstrictor hormone released from posterior hypophysis upon stimulation by change in plasma osmolality and hypovolemia. Production of AVP increases as a compensatory mechanism in HF. AVP is centrally involved in the regulation of free water clearance and plasma osmolality by regulating absorption of water from the collecting tubules of the kidney. AVP plays a role in HF, particularly in the context of hyponatremia which indicates poor prognosis in HF. Due to its short half-life and instability in laboratory circumstances, measurement of AVP is not practical. Copeptin is a stable C-terminal pro-peptide fragment of AVP. In the Biomarkers in Acute Heart Failure (BACH) trial, the elevated copeptin level strongly predicted mortality, and in those with hyponatremia, the elevated copeptin level was more predictive, even after adjusting for NT-proBNP and traditional variables [21]. In the future copeptin values may be used to guide therapy with vasopressin receptor antagonists; however, such data are not available yet.

Endothelin-1(ET-1) is a hormone released from the endothelium via stimulation by angiotensin II, inflammation, and vascular shear stress. It is responsible for profound vasoconstriction, production of reactive oxygen radicals, and ventricular remodeling. Its relation with pulmonary hypertension has been well known, and now its relation to HF has been suggested [22]. Specific treatment of HF patients with ET-1 antagonists yielded nothing. ET-1 may be used to identify HF patients who will benefit from these specific treatments.

Parathyroid hormone (PTH) is a peptide of 84 amino acids (1–84 PTH). PTH is recognized as a key regulator of mineral metabolism and bone health. Together, in association with vitamin D (vit D), PTH regulates homeostasis of calcium, phosphate, and bone turnover. In the parathyroid gland, PTH is secreted by the chief cells in response to decreased ionized calcium concentration in the blood. The increased PTH level is a well-known condition in patients with chronic renal failure. A growing body of evidence indicates that the progression of HF also leads to secondary hyperparathyroidism (SHPT). Secondary hyperaldosteronism and increased amounts of diuretics used for the relief of the patient in advanced stage of HF bring about secondary hyperparathyroidism, assumed to be caused by increased calcium and magnesium excretion in the urine and feces [23]. Measurement of serum PTH could provide complementary information and a simple biomarker strategy to categorize patients with advanced HF based on increased PTH levels, allowing rapid risk stratification in these patients [24].

3.3. Remodeling

Myocardial remodeling is the pivotal process leading to progressive myocardial dysfunction and risk in HF. While BNP, NT-proBNP, and troponin are all also linked to remodeling risk, other biomarkers are worth mention.

3.3.1. *Inflammation*

Apart from neuroendocrine and sympathetic nervous system, the immune system, via its pro-inflammatory pathways, has been shown to play a role in the development of adverse remodeling and progression of HF [25]. Therefore, inflammatory mediators have been the center of interest for potential biomarkers in HF. Although they have a prognostic importance, they have shortcomings as well. They are not specific to HF.

C-reactive protein (CRP) is the mostly studied inflammatory mediator in HF. It has been shown to be associated with severity of HF [26]. Although recent studies have confirmed the prognostic value of CRP in HF, because of its increased level in a multiple of conditions and not needing specific treatment makes its use in HF impractical. And, it lost its prognostic significance in models where multiple biomarkers were involved [27].

TNF-alfa increases oxidative stress, hence reduces pumping function of the heart, and is associated with the progression of HF [28]. Interleukin-6 (IL-6) affects the intercellular communication between cardiomyocyte and fibroblasts, and change in IL-6 levels causes cardiac dysfunction by changing the cardiac extracellular matrix. IL-6 has been shown to predict adverse events in HF, but due to the lack of diagnostic specificity, it has not been used generally in clinical practice. Pentraxin-3 is a novel promising inflammatory biomarker. It has been shown to predict adverse events in HF better than CRP [29].

Beta-blockers, RAS antagonists, statins, and immunosuppressants have been found to decrease the levels of cytokines in small clinical studies of patients with HF. However, "immunomodulatory" approaches applied in the double-blind, placebo-controlled studies had neutral or negative effects on hard clinical outcomes of patients with HF [30].

3.3.2. *Hypertrophy/fibrosis*

ST2 is a member of IL-1 receptor family. It could also be classified under inflammation subtitle. Production of ST2 is strongly induced in the setting of cardiomyocyte or cardiac fibroblast stretch. ST2 is closely involved in LV hypertrophy, fibrosis, and remodeling via its interaction with interleukin (IL)-33, a protein with anti-fibrotic and anti-remodeling properties [31]. Soluble form of ST, designated as sST2, neutralizes protective effects of ST2. Increasing ST2 concentrations (e.g., >35 ng/mL) are powerfully associated with adverse clinical outcomes in HF, and compared with BNP or NT-proBNP, ST2 is not as affected by age, renal function, atrial fibrillation, body mass index (BMI), or etiology of cardiomyopathy (ischemic or not) [32]. In a multivariable model that included traditional markers of risk in acute HF patients, ST2 had independent and additive prognostic information beyond NT-proBNP regardless of left ventricular ejection fraction (LVEF) [33]. In addition, serial measurement of ST2 after acute HF therapy provided incremental information beyond a single value and was superior to that provided by NT-proBNP [34]. sST2 levels may change with specific HF therapies. It was shown that beta-blockers reduce ST2 values, giving the promise of the future use of guided HF therapy using serial measurement of ST2 [35].

Galectin-3 (Gal-3) represents the interconnection between inflammation and fibrosis. It is secreted by activated macrophages and located in the vicinity of fibroblasts. Galectin-3 is involved in the inflammatory pathway following injury and ventricular remodeling via tissue repair, myofibroblast proliferation, and fibrogenesis. Its level starts to increase in the very early stages of HF, and this feature of Gal-3 may be used for the early diagnosis of HF before symptoms occur in the future [36]. Galectin-3 is elevated in patients with acute or chronic HF [37]. Gal-3 predicted mortality better than apelin and NT-proBNp in acute HF, especially in patients with HFpEF [38]. Although Gal-3 is frequently associated with HF risk in univariate analyses, it loses its prognostic significance in multivariate analyses after adjustment for renal function or other biomarkers. Serial measurement of galectin-3 in chronic HF patients may add to a single measurement, but to date, there are no known therapies that can alter Gal-3 values [39].

3.4. Comorbidities

Comorbidities often complicate the natural course of HF with deleterious impact on clinical status, symptoms, and HF progression. Therefore, comorbidities including renal dysfunction, hematologic abnormalities, and liver dysfunction are important markers of poor prognosis in HF.

3.4.1. Renal biomarkers

Renal dysfunction (RD) is a common finding in heart failure (HF) and has emerged as one of the most potent prognostic indicators in these patients [40]. Serum creatinine, estimated glomerular filtration rate (eGFR), and blood urea nitrogen (BUN) are important markers of renal function and provide prognostic information about HF [41]. An elevated admission blood urea nitrogen/creatinine (BUN/Cr) identifies acute HF patients likely to experience improvement in renal function with treatment. However, this improvement seems to be largely transient, and RD, in the setting of an elevated BUN/Cr, remains strongly associated with death [42]. In acute HF, prognosis is worse when both NT-proBNP and low eGFR levels rise.

Cystatin-C and β-trace protein (BTP) performed better than traditional renal markers for determining prognosis in HF, presumably due to an enhanced ability to gauge renal function at milder levels of abnormality [43]. Cystatin-C is a cysteine proteinase inhibitor produced by almost every human cell and secreted into circulation. Its removal occurs only by glomerular filtration, and because of this, it is a prototype indicator of renal function. It is not affected by age, gender, and muscle mass. Although cystatin-C was a bit more superior to eGFR for showing renal function, it is far more superior than eGFR for predicting prognosis in HF. Cystatin-C shows not only abnormal renal function but also inflammation and severity of HF as well as predicts mortality and morbidity in acute HF [44].

β-trace protein (BTP) is a novel indicator of renal function. Like cystatin-C, it is also found to be a better predictor of prognosis in HF [43]. It is a low molecular weight protein produced by a wide array of tissue, and it indicates worsening of kidney function. It gives additional prognostic information on top of NT-proBNP in acute HF [45]. Although both cystatin-C and BTP give promise for the guidance of HF management, they have not been used in clinical practice yet.

3.4.2. Hematologic biomarkers

Hematologic abnormalities including anemia, iron deficiency, and increased red blood cell distribution width (RDW) are rather frequent in HF patients and of importance in determining prognosis regardless of LVEF [46].

One of the largest HF registries has clearly demonstrated an independent association between lower hemoglobin values and mortality and morbidity in HF [47]. Although anemia is a common and ominous sign in HF, its treatment did not bring benefit in HF [48].

Iron deficiency (ID) is also a common comorbidity of patients with HF. It is the most frequent cause of anemia in patients with HF, but, most importantly, ID also occurs in non-anemic patients with HFrEF. The presence of ID, regardless of concomitant anemia, has been linked to high mortality and morbidity in HFrEF [49]. Unlike anemia, treatment of ID with intravenous iron therapy in HFrEF patients showed reduced hospitalization rates and improved HF symptoms, exercise capacity, and quality of life [50]. Ferritin and transferrin saturation may be used to identify iron-deficient patients with HFrEF likely to benefit from intravenous iron therapy.

Red blood cell distribution width (RDW) is another important hematologic biomarker in HF, and its prognostic significance is more than hemoglobin in chronic HF [51]. RDW had also been associated with an adverse outcome in acute HF [52]. Higher RDW was associated with HF hospitalizations in the general population as well [53]. RDW is believed to indicate combined inflammation and deranged iron metabolism in HF. Treatment response to high RDW has not been known yet; however, since being cheap and easily applicable, studies searching benefits of treatment targeting RDW should be focused.

3.4.3. Future directions

As discussed above, most of the features described for biomarkers in HF relates to prognostication. We have discussed that prognostic value of a biomarker is only useful if it shows specific change in clinical practice; such change should also translate into improvement in prognosis. This is somewhat accomplished for NT-proBNP and iron deficiency. However, for all other biomarkers, it remains unclear if specific therapy changes should be made in response to an abnormal result. The precision medicine will usher in the future based on the multiple biomarker strategy underpinning the diagnostic and prognostic certainty.

Author details

Hakan Altay

Address all correspondence to: sakaltay@yahoo.com

Department of Cardiology, Baskent University, Faculty of Medicine, Istanbul, Turkey

References

[1] Nieminen MS, Böhm M, Cowie MR, Drexler H, Filippatos GS, Jondeau G, et al. ESC committee for practice guideline (CPG). Executive summary of the guidelines on the diagnosis and treatment of acute heart failure: The task force on acute heart failure of the European Society of Cardiology. European Heart Journal. 2005;**26**(4):384-416

[2] McMurray JJ, Packer M, Desai AS, et al. Angiotensin-neprilysin inhibition versus enalapril in heart failure. The New England Journal of Medicine. 2014;**371**:993-1004

[3] Niederkofler EE, Kiernan UA, O'Rear J, Menon S, Saghir S, Protter AA, Nelson RW, Schellenberger U. Detection of endogenous B-type natriuretic peptide at very low concentrations in patients with heart failure. Circulation. Heart Failure. 2008 Nov;**1**(4): 258-264

[4] Boerrigter L, Lahr B, Heublein D, et al. Pro-B-type natriuretic peptide(1-108) circulates in the general community: Plasma determinants and detection of left ventricular dysfunction. Journal of the American College of Cardiology. 2011;**57**(12):1386-1395

[5] Maisel AS, Krishnaswamy P, Nowak RM, et al. Rapid measurement of B-type natriuretic peptide in the emergency diagnosis of heart failure. The New England Journal of Medicine. 2002;**347**:161-167

[6] Januzzi JL Jr, Camargo CA, Anwaruddin S, et al. The N-terminal pro-BNP. Investigation of Dyspnea in the emergency department (PRIDE) study. The American Journal of Cardiology. 2005;**95**:948-954

[7] Kim HN, Januzzi JL Jr. Natriuretic peptide testing in heart failure. Circulation. 2011; **123**(18):2015-2019

[8] Fuat A, Murphy JJ, Hungin AP, Curry J, Mehrzad AA, Hetherington A, Johnston JI, Smellie WS, Duffy V, Cawley P. The diagnostic accuracy and utility of a B-type natriuretic peptide test in a community population of patients with suspected heart failure. The British Journal of General Practice. 2006;**56**:327-333

[9] Maisel AS, McCord J, Nowak RM, et al. Bedside B-type natriuretic peptide in the emergency diagnosis of heart failure with reduced or preserved ejection fraction. Results from the breathing not properly multinational study. Journal of the American College of Cardiology. 2003;**41**:2010-2017

[10] Landsberg JW, Ponikowski P, et al. Mid-region pro-hormone markers for diagnosis and prognosis in acute dyspnea: Results from the BACH (biomarkers in acute heart failure) trial. Journal of the American College of Cardiology. 2010;**55**(19):2062-2076

[11] Michtalik HJ, Yeh HC, Campbell CY, et al. Acute changes in N-terminal pro-B-type natriuretic peptide during hospitalization and risk of readmission and mortality in patients with heart failure. The American Journal of Cardiology. 2011;**107**:1191-1195

[12] Bayes-Genis A, Lopez L, Zapico E, et al. NT-ProBNP reduction percentage during admission for acutely decompensated heart failure predicts long-term cardiovascular mortality. Journal of Cardiac Failure. 2005;**11**:S3-S8

[13] Eurlings LW, van Pol PE, Kok WE, et al. Management of chronic heart failure guided by individual N-terminal pro-B-type natriuretic peptide targets: Results of the PRIMA (can PRo-brain-natriuretic peptide guided therapy of chronic heart failure IMprove heart fAilure morbidity and mortality?) study. Journal of the American College of Cardiology. 2010;**56**:2090-2100

[14] Januzzi JL Jr, Filippatos G, Nieminen M, Gheorghiade M. Troponin elevation in patients with heart failure: On behalf of the third universal definition of myocardial infarction global task force: Heart failure section. European Heart Journal. 2012;**33**:2265-2271

[15] WFt P, De Marco T, Fonarow GC, et al. Cardiac troponin and outcome in acute heart failure. The New England Journal of Medicine. 2008;**358**:2117-2126

[16] Yancy CW, Jessup M, Bozkurt B, Butler J, Casey DE Jr, Colvin MM, Drazner MH, Filippatos GS, Fonarow GC, Givertz MM, Hollenberg SM, Lindenfeld J, Masoudi FA, McBride PE, Peterson PN, Stevenson LW, Westlake C. ACC/AHA/HFSA focused update of the 2013 ACCF/AHA guideline for the Management of Heart Failure: A report of the American College of Cardiology/American Heart Association Task Force on clinical practice guidelines and the Heart Failure Society of America. Journal of Cardiac Failure. 2017 Aug;**23**(8):628-651. DOI: 10.1016/j.cardfail.2017.04.014. Epub 2017 Apr 28, 2017

[17] Latini R, Masson S, Anand IS, et al. Prognostic value of very low plasma concentrations of troponin T in patients with stable chronic heart failure. Circulation. 2007;**116**:1242-1249

[18] Swedberg K, Eneroth P, Kjekshus J, Wilhelmsen L. Hormones regulating cardiovascular function in patients with severe congestive heart failure and their relation to mortality. CONSENSUS trial study group. Circulation. 1990;**82**:1730-1736

[19] Dieplinger B, Gegenhuber A, Struck J, Poelz W, Langsteger W, Haltmayer M, et al. Chromogranin a and C-terminal endothelin-1 precursor fragment add independent prognostic information to amino-terminal proBNP in patients with acute destabilized heart failure. Clinica Chimica Acta. 2009;**400**(1–2):91-96

[20] Shah RV, Truong QA, Gaggin HK, et al. Mid-regional pro-atrial natriuretic peptide and pro-adrenomedullin testing for the diagnostic and prognostic evaluation of patients with acute dyspnoea. European Heart Journal. 2012;**33**:2197-2205

[21] Maisel A, Xue Y, Shah K, et al. Increased 90-day mortality in patients with acute heart failure with elevated copeptin: Secondary results from the biomarkers in acute heart failure (BACH) study. Circulation. Heart Failure. 2011;**4**:613-620

[22] AG JS, Yandle TG, et al. Clinical significance of endogenous vasoactive neurohormones in chronic systolic heart failure. Journal of Cardiac Failure. 2010;**16**(8):635-640

[23] Alsafwah S, Laguardia SP, Arroyo M, Dockery BK, Bhattacharya SK, Ahokas RA, Newman KP. Congestive heart failure is a systemic illness: A role for minerals and micronutrients. Clinical Medicine & Research. 2007;**5**:238-243

[24] Altay H, Zorlu A, Binici S, Bilgi M, Yilmaz MB, Colkesen Y, Erol T, Muderrisoglu H. Relation of serum parathyroid hormone level to severity of heart failure. The American Journal of Cardiology. 2012;**109**(2):252-256

[25] Frangogiannis NG. Regulation of the inflammatory response in cardiac repair. Circulation Research. 2012;**110**(1):159-173

[26] lster SK, Braunwald E, Wood HF. A study of C-reactive protein in the serum of patients with congestive heart failure. American Heart Journal. 1956;**51**(4):533-541

[27] Matsubara J, Sugiyama J, Sugamura K, Konishi M, Ohba K, et al. Pentraxin 3 is a new inflammatory marker correlated with left ventricular diastolic dysfunction and heart failure with normal ejection fraction. Journal of the American College of Cardiology. 2011;**57**(7):861-869

[28] Moe GW, Marin-Garcia J, Konig A, Goldenthal M, Lu X, Feng Q. In vivo TNF-alpha inhibition ameliorates cardiac mitochondrial dysfunction, oxidative stress, and apoptosis in experimental heart failure. American Journal of Physiology. Heart and Circulatory Physiology. 2004;**287**(4):H1813-H1820

[29] Suzuki S, Takeishi Y, Niizeki T, Koyama Y, Ki-tahara T, Sasaki T, et al. Pentraxin 3, a new marker for vascular inflammation, predicts adverse clinical outcomes in patients with heart failure. American Heart Journal. 2008;**155**(1):75-81

[30] Hobbs FD, Roalfe AK, Davis RC, Davies MK, Hare R, Midlands Research Practices Consortium (MidReC). Prognosis of all-cause heart failure and borderline left ventricular systolic dysfunction: 5 year mortality follow-up of the echocardiographic heart of England screening study (ECHOES). European Heart Journal. 2007;**28**:1128-1134

[31] Sanada S, Hakuno D, Higgins LJ, et al. IL-33 and ST2 comprise a critical biomechanically induced and cardioprotective signaling system. The Journal of Clinical Investigation. 2007;**117**:1538-1549

[32] Rehman SU, Mueller T, Januzzi JL Jr. Characteristics of the novel interleukin family biomarker ST2 in patients with acute heart failure. Journal of the American College of Cardiology. 2008;**52**(18):1458-1465

[33] Januzzi JL Jr, Peacock WF, Maisel AS, et al. Measurement of the interleukin family member ST2 in patients with acute dyspnea: Results from the PRIDE (pro-brain natriuretic peptide investigation of Dyspnea in the emergency department) study. Journal of the American College of Cardiology. 2007;**50**:607-613

[34] Boisot S, Beede J, Isakson S, et al. Serial sampling of ST2 predicts 90-day mortality following destabilized heart failure. Journal of Cardiac Failure. 2008;**14**:732-738

[35] Gaggin HK, Motiwala S, Bhardwaj A, et al. Soluble concentrations of the interleukin receptor family member ST2 and β-blocker therapy in chronic heart failure. Circulation. Heart Failure. 2013;**6**:1206-1213

[36] Berlo JH, Cleutjens JP, Schroen B, et al. Galectin-3 marks activated macrophages in failure-prone hypertrophied cardiac dysfunction. Circulation. 2004;**110**(19):3121-3128

[37] Lok DJ, Van Der Meer P, de la Porte PW, et al. Prognostic value of galectin-3, a novel marker of fibrosis, in patients with chronic heart failure: Data from the DEAL-HF study. Clinical Research in Cardiology. 2010;**99**:323-328

[38] van Kimmenade RR, Januzzi JL Jr, Ellinor PT, et al. Utility of amino-terminal pro-brain natriuretic peptide, galectin-3, and apelin for the evaluation of patients with acute heart failure. Journal of the American College of Cardiology. 2006;**48**:1217-1224

[39] Motiwala SR, Szymonifka J, Belcher A, et al. Serial measurement of galectin-3 in patients with chronic heart failure: Results from the ProBNP outpatient tailored chronic heart failure therapy (PROTECT) study. European Journal of Heart Failure. 2013;**15**: 1157-1163

[40] Bock JS, Gottlieb SS. Cardiorenal syndrome: New perspectives. Circulation. 2010;**121**: 2592-2600

[41] Fonarow GC, Adams KF Jr, Abraham WT, et al. Risk stratification for in-hospital mortality in acutely decompensated heart failure: Classification and regression tree analysis. Journal of the American Medical Association. 2005;**293**:572-580

[42] Brisco MA, Coca SG, Chen J, Owens AT, McCauley BD, Kimmel SE, Testani JM. Blood urea nitrogen/creatinine ratio identifies a high-risk but potentially reversible form of renal dysfunction in patients with decompensated heart failure. Circulation. Heart Failure. 2013;**6**:233-239

[43] Manzano-Fernandez S, Januzzi JL Jr, Boronat-Garcia M, et al. β-trace protein and cystatin C as predictors of long-term outcomes in patients with acute heart failure. Journal of the American College of Cardiology. 2011;**57**:849-858

[44] Sarnak MJ, Katz R, Stehman-Breen CO, Fried LF, Jenny NS, Psaty BM, et al. Cystatin C concentration as a risk factor for heart failure in older adults. Annals of Internal Medicine. 2005;**142**(7):497-505

[45] Garcia M, Bonaque-González JC, Truong QA, Pastor-Pérez FJ, et al. β-trace protein and cystatin C as predictors of long-term outcomes in patients with acute heart failure. Journal of the American College of Cardiology. 2011;**57**(7):849-858

[46] Groenveld HF, Januzzi JL, Damman K, et al. Anemia and mortality in heart failure patients a systematic review and meta-analysis. Journal of the American College of Cardiology. 2008;**52**:818-827

[47] Young JB, Abraham WT, Albert NM, et al. Relation of low hemoglobin and anemia to morbidity and mortality in patients hospitalized with heart failure (insight from the OPTIMIZE-HF registry). The American Journal of Cardiology. 2008;**101**:223-230

[48] Swedberg K, Young JB, Anand IS, Cheng S, Desai AS, Diaz R, Maggioni AP, McMurray JJ, O'Connor C, Pfeffer MA, Solomon SD, Sun Y, Tendera M, van Veldhuisen DJ. RED-HF committees; RED-HF investigators. Treatment of anemia with darbepoetin alfa in systolic heart failure. The New England Journal of Medicine. 2013;**368**:1210-1219

[49] Jankowska EA, Rozentryt P, Witkowska A, Nowak J, Hartmann O, Ponikowska B, Borodulin-Nadzieja L, Banasiak W, Polonski L, Filippatos G, McMurray JJ, Anker SD, Ponikowski P. Iron deficiency: An ominous sign in patients with systolic chronic heart failure. European Heart Journal. 2010;**31**:1872-1880

[50] Jankowska EA, Tkaczyszyn M, Suchocki T, Drozd M, von Haehling S, Doehner W, Banasiak W, Filippatos G, Anker SD, Ponikowski P. Effects of intravenous iron therapy in iron-deficient patients with systolic heart failure: A meta-analysis of randomized controlled trials. European Journal of Heart Failure. 2016 Jul;**18**(7):786-795

[51] Felker GM, Allen LA, Pocock SJ, Shaw LK, Mc- Murray JJ, Pfeffer MA, et al. CHARM investigators. Red cell distribution width as a novel prognostic marker in heart failure: Data from the CHARM program and the Duke databank. Journal of the American College of Cardiology. 2007;**50**(1):40-47

[52] van Kimmenade RR, Mohammed AA, Uthamalingam S, van der Meer P, Felker GM, Januzzi JL Jr. Red blood cell distribution width and 1-year mortality in acute heart failure. European Journal of Heart Failure. 2010;**12**:129-136

[53] Borne Y, Smith JG, Melander O, Hedblad B, Engstrom G. Red cell distribution width and risk for first hospitalization due to heart failure: A population-based cohort study. European Journal of Heart Failure. 2011;**13**:1355-1361

3

Molecular Diagnostics of Pulmonary Diseases Based on Analysis of Exhaled Breath Condensate

Tereza Kačerová, Petr Novotný, Ján Boroň and Petr Kačer

Abstract

Measurements of biomarkers in exhaled breath condensate (EBC) extend a novel route for monitoring lung physiology and provide a beneficial insight into the pathophysiology of a specific disease. From the medicinal point of view, biomarkers present in EBC depict rather the processes occurring in lungs than those in the entire system. Therefore, particular profiles of exhaled biomarkers (e.g. cys-LTs, LTB_4, 8-isoprostane, etc.) apparently reveal information exclusively applicable to differential lung disease diagnoses. This chapter describes the developed analytical method being applied to a clinical study for differential diagnostics of various phenotypes of asthma, chronic obstructive pulmonary disease, lung cancer, etc. In particular, having determined cys-LTs and LXs by the described method, and having applied them as biomarkers of bronchial asthma, their distinctive potential was demonstrated to differentially diagnose the specific disease, clearly suggesting this method to be reckoned as a beneficial alternative to existing diagnostic methods. Consecutively, the developed method was expanded to other asthma markers as aldehydes, nitrotyrosine, 8-isoprostane, PGE_2, adenosine and finally, a supplementary study was carried out, engaging in detecting serotonin. The multi-marker screening and importance in the diagnostics of pulmonary diseases are referenced in the text as well.

Keywords: exhaled breath condensate, pulmonary diseases, leukotrienes, lipoxins

1. Introduction

From the very beginnings of civilizations, with tracks from Mesopotamia, Egypt, and ancient Greece, medical practitioners examined the potential of exhaled breath (EB) parameters as health-related signs usable for identifying various ailments and essentially mapping different physiological states. Via different odors, sounds, and breath dynamics often attributed to supernatural powers and superstitious believes, various lung diseases could be relatively well diagnosed and further progression could be predicted. For instance, the odors in EB as, for example, fruity traces of acetone aided to identify diabetes; a rather pungent characteristic odor was associated with a lung inflammation, while volatile vapors from urine revealed a kidney disease [1]. Modern investigations enlisted approx. 250 frequently detected volatile organic compounds (VOC's) in EB [2]. Early analyses did not incorporate sample pre-treatments as sample concentration and exclusively depended on relatively modest gas chromatography (GC) methods. The progress of technology, however, over the decades has permitted much more precise and sophisticated analyses of EB, some of which have been implemented to the clinical practice, as, for example, ethanol levels in blood or typical inflammations caused by common pathogens as *Helicobacter pylori* using 13/14C-urea [3]. As mentioned above, the prime advantage of EB analysis is the patient's comfort, especially eliminating the stressful intrusions to human organisms, yet there are challenges ahead. For instance, a breakthrough task is to find common internal standard reliably standardizing diagnoses for each pathological status. Furthermore, an opposite selection of multi-marker panel is to be conspicuously correlated to different health phenomena, providing the knowledge of characteristic concentrations. Moreover, it is often unclear which metabolic pathways in relation to different measured biomarkers are involved and some are probably yet to be discovered or decoded. Last but not the least, technological and procedural challenges include also the standardization in terms of the sample collection and treatment, and conceivably, endeavors to automatization of the complete process in the clinical practice.

2. Exhaled breath condensate

Compared to the currently widespread invasive and semi-invasive diagnostic methods, the analysis of exhaled breath condensate (EBC) is relatively new and has the first-rate potential to become a preferred and completely noninvasive alternative. EBC is a biological matrix reflecting the composition of the bronchoalveolar extra-cellular lung fluid. The main advantage of EBC as of a matrix is its specificity for the respiratory tract (the liquid is not influenced by process occurring in other parts of human organism). Many important biomolecules are present in exhaled breath in the form of an aerosol [4, 5] (**Figure 1**) which is condensed by cooling during the collection, forming the EBC matrix.

The collection of EBC is performed while using the condenser, which is currently available at a specialized clinical facility. During the collection, the exhaled air is led through the condenser into the cooling box that is pre-cooled to the temperature −20°C. In the cooling box, the aerosol particles are obtained and the gaseous phase is liquidized.

In the obtained liquid, typically known as EBC, more than 2000 compounds [6] have been identified so far and many of them are considered to represent sensitive biomarkers of lung diseases [7, 8]. The determination of the concentration of these molecules in EBC allows

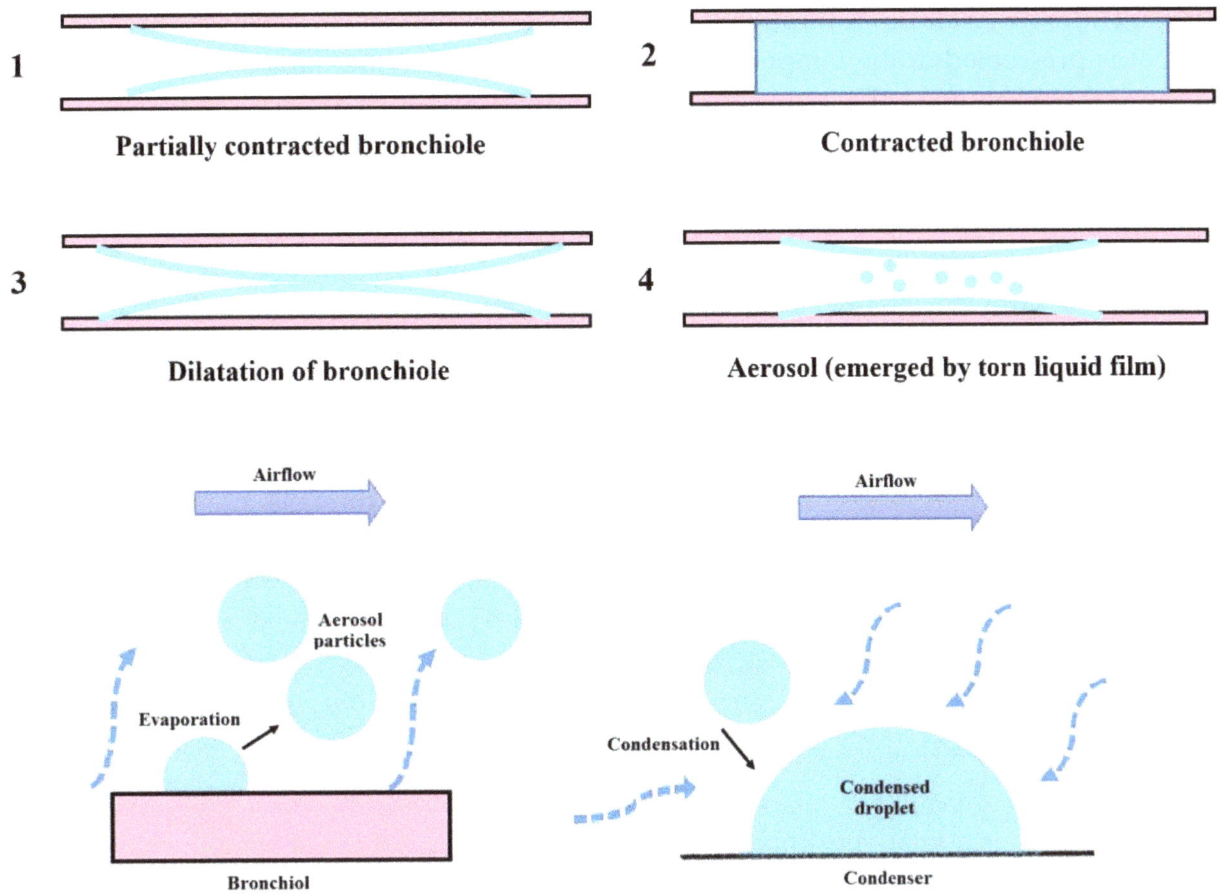

Figure 1. Formation of exhaled breath condensate.

assessing the type and severity of ongoing pathological process or even the efficiency of a therapeutic procedure, etc. In case of numerous pulmonary diseases, H_2O_2, cysteinyl leukotrienes (cys-LTs), lipoxins (LXs), malverines, resolvins, isoprostanes, prostaglandines, glutathione, adenosine, thiobarbituric acid, aldehydes, nitrotyrosine, cytokines represent a specific group of biomarkers and their concentration levels are elevated (eventually lowered) in airways and lungs as a result of an ongoing allergic reaction, inflammation, oxidative stress, and other processes [9–12].

The most significant advantage of EBC compared to other biological matrices (as are, for example, urine and blood) is the fact that EBC is a highly specific fluid for the respiratory system, so any other biochemical processes in human organism do not influence it.

3. The collection of EBC

During the collection of EBC, the exhaled air is led through the condenser, where some components are condensed. The patients should breath calmly and regularly during the whole process. The exhaled air flows through the mouthpiece and the one-way valve into the cooling cuff that is pre-cooled at the temperature of −20°C. In the cooling cuff, the aerosol particles and the obtained gaseous phase are condensed. This liquid is then gathered in the sample collection vial (the temperature remains the same) [13]. The whole process lasts approximately 7–12 min. It is necessary to obtain 120 l of EB in total, which corresponds to 1–2 ml of the condensate. The obtained condensate is then conserved in a micro-test-tube. In order to monitor the degrading process, the samples were labeled by deuterium-labeled internal standards. The prepared samples are then subsequently frozen and stored for a period not exceeding 6 months (−80°C).

As the collection of EBC is a noninvasive diagnostic method that does not burden the patient, it can be used in several different clinical studies. A regular collection of EBC enables, for example, monitoring of the impact of climate conditions on the patients. Globally, collection of EBC is a method that is suitable for clinical studies that are trying to understand the process in the organism which corresponds to some external impulses (physical activity, air quality, allergens, etc.)

4. Bronchial asthma

Bronchial asthma is a relatively common pulmonary disease, which is usually characterized by dyspnoea combined with intervals of a normal breathing [14–19]. Typical symptoms of asthma include constricted bronchial tubes and an increased secretion of sputum, which is abnormally dense and viscous [16]. Various sources agree that on the global scale, the asthma incidence accounts for around 300 million people, while the prognoses that are negative in the sense of the future number will keep rising. On the other hand, wide ranges of relatively efficient anti-asthmatic therapies are available (e.g., glucocorticoid therapy, β_2-receptors agonists, etc.) [17] enabling the majority of patients to live normal lives. However, there is still a small group of patients, who do not respond to any kind of current therapy. These patients are usually diagnosed as sever refractory asthmatics (SRA) [6], whose common feature is a lack of any response to any contemporarily available pharmacotherapy. SRA accounts for approximately 5% of all asthmatics, which represents 10 million of people [6].

Figure 2 describes the immunopathogenesis of asthma [20]. The asthma attack starts by exposure to an allergen, which causes synthesis of immunoglobulin E (IgE). IgE then binds to the surface of mast cells. As there occurs a re-exposure to the same allergen, the interaction between allergen and antibody triggers the release of mediators as are prostaglandins (PGDs), cys-LTs, LTB_4 and platelet-activating factor (PAF). These mediators cause bronchoconstriction that is connected to an immediate drop in FEV1 (= forced expiratory volume in 1 s; the FEV1 is the volume exhaled during the first second of a forced expiratory maneuver started from the level of total lung capacity). The allergen-antibody interaction also causes production of a wide range of cytokines (e.g., interleukin 4 and 5 (IL-4 and IL-5), tumor necrosis factor (TNF) and tissue growth factor (TGF)). These cytokines then activate neutrophils and eosinophils. Neutrophils produce proteases and PAF, and at the same time, eosinophils produce eosinophil cationic protein (ECP) and major basic protein (MBP). These

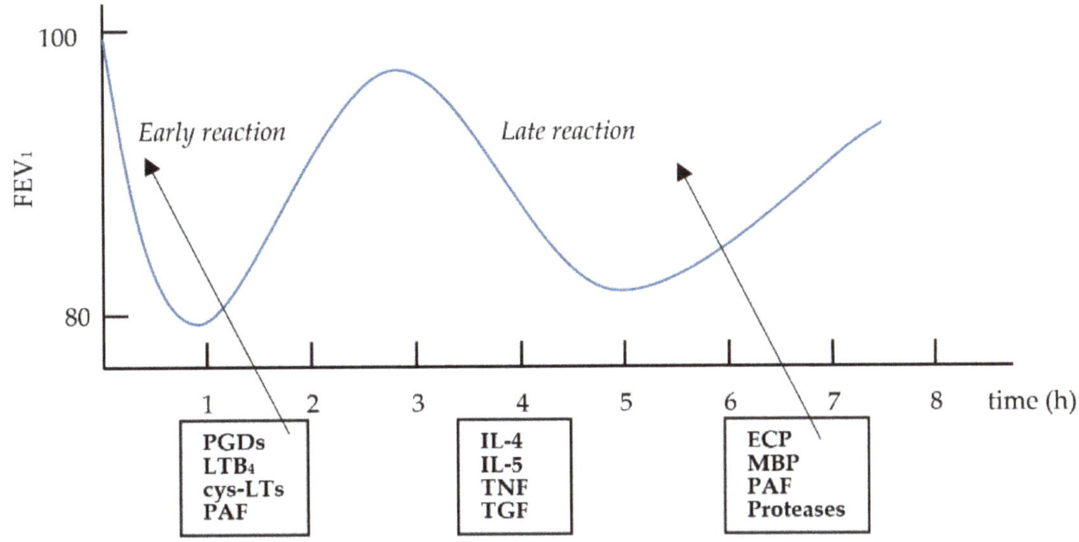

Figure 2. Immunopathogenesis of asthma [20].

products, eosinophils and neutrophils, cause mucus hypersecretion, edema, and constriction of smooth muscles. This is usually associated with the late asthma phase and it causes the second drop in FEV1.

4.1. The diagnostics of asthma

There are several options for the diagnostics of asthma; however, only an early and correct diagnosis of this life-threatening disease permits the physician to timely initiate an effective therapy and minimize the harm to the patient [18]. Several noninvasive methods are already in clinical use (e.g., spirometry, bronchomotoric tests, etc.). In some cases, invasive and *semi*-invasive methods appear to be an inevitable option to gain the correct diagnosis (e.g., open-lung biopsy and bronchoalveolar lavage) [21], yet it is to an unambiguous expense of the patient and often the health cost as well as a demanding laboratory examination.

Currently, a significant part of the relevant research centers focuses on methods of the so-called personalized diagnostics (or methods of personalized medicine), with the aim to stratify patients to characteristic groups (e.g., phenotypes) and thus achieve a more efficient therapy reflecting an individual phenotypic disposition (inclusive of genomic, proteomic and metabolomic profiles) [22, 23]. One of the examples of these endeavors (particularly for diagnostics of pulmonary diseases) is the measurement of a fractional exhaled nitric oxide (FeNO) [24–26] in EBC, helping to distinguish asthma from other pathogenetic processes diagnosed as chronic cough, gastroesophageal reflux disease (GERD), vocal cord dysfunction, bronchitis, chronic obstructive pulmonary disease (COPD), etc.

4.2. Asthma phenotypes

As asthma is a disease affecting millions of people of all ages worldwide, many criteria can be used for its classification. Nevertheless, the predominantly used criterion is the severity of the disease, as is presented in **Figure 3**, followed by the age of the first exacerbation [9, 26].

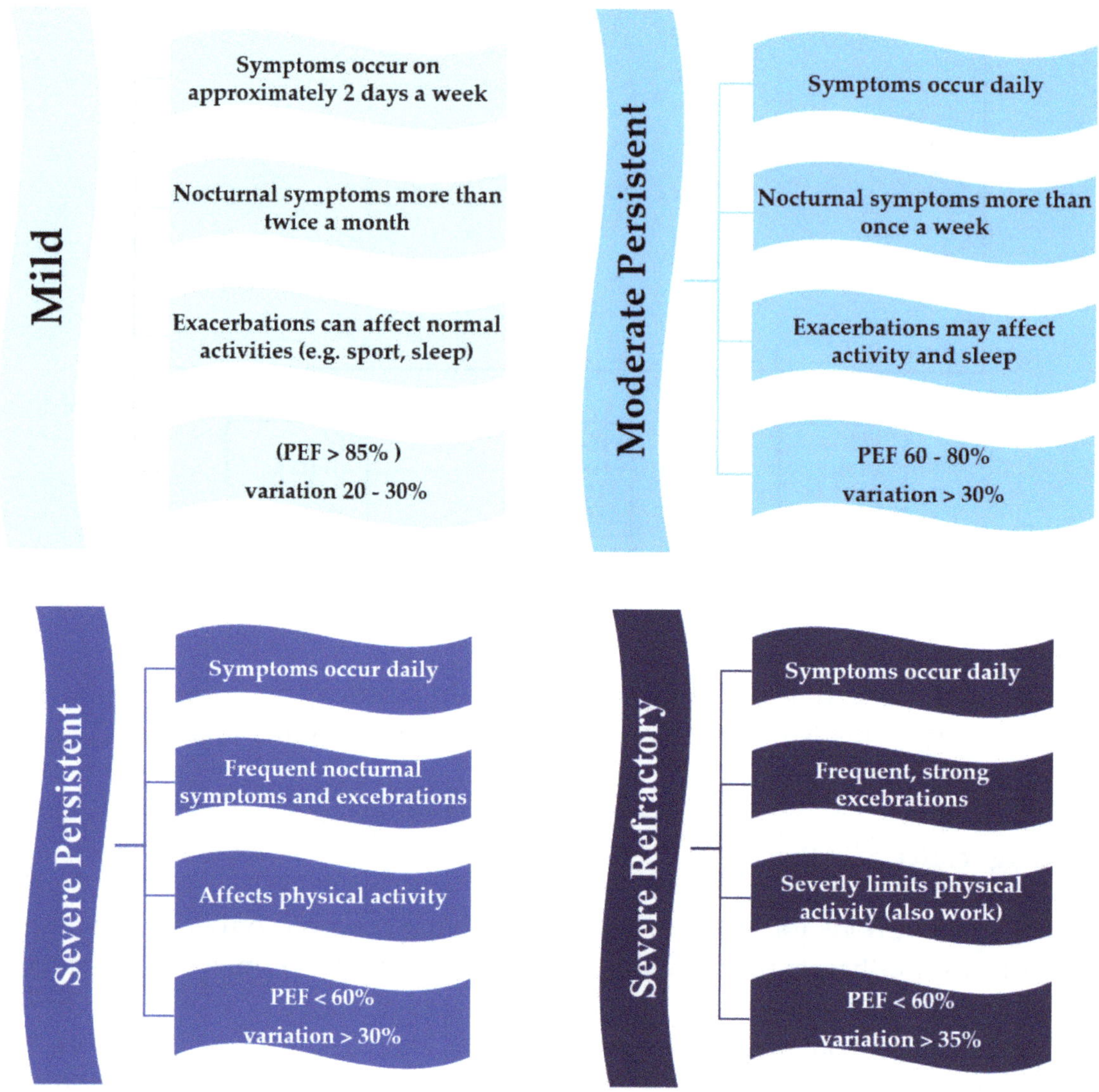

Figure 3. Asthma phenotypes.

5. Chronical obstructive pulmonary disease (COPD)

Chronical obstructive pulmonary disease (COPD) is a chronical inflammatory pulmonary disease [27–29]. The development of COPD usually lasts many years. During these years, bronchial tubes of COPD patients are getting more and more narrowed. COPD is also characterized by attacks of dyspnoea and persistent dry cough. The cough is often accompanied by expectorated mucus. In a late stage, it can cause obstructive, effortful, and painful breathing. These complications can be a hindrance also during simple physical activity. COPD patients are also prone to pneumonia. The main cause of COPD is often smoking. Other contributing factors include the genetic inheritance, a long exposition to dust particles, or a regular and frequent lung infection.

COPD is often divided into two main groups (phenotypes): chronic bronchitis and emphysema.

5.1. Chronic bronchitis

In chronic bronchitis [28], a typical symptom is a permanent constriction of bronchial tubes. Furthermore, an inhalation of harmful substances cause impairment of the respiratory mucous membrane, while a repeated damage to the membrane makes it thicker and lowers the tissue transparency. As a result, the affected cells increase the production of mucus, leading to the characteristic cough.

5.2. Emphysema

Emphysema is characterized by a loss of the pulmonary tissue, while the respiratory ways are abnormally widened distantly from terminal bronchioles [28].

The main cause of emphysema is smoking. The substances that are inhaled during smoking are led through the respiratory ways to bronchioles. In bronchioles, the substances provoke a local immune reaction, which is linked with the production of aggressive compounds via leucocytes (mainly free radicals responsible for oxidative stress). This reaction thus initiates a degradation of bronchioles. The afflicted bronchioles merge into huge lung sacs. These sacs have a smaller surface of the pulmonary tissue and thus the gas exchange between lungs and blood is limited.

The second cause of this disease can be disequilibrium between proteases and their inhibitors—anti-proteases. Some COPD patients suffer from the lack of alfa-1-tripsin (an anti-protease), which is the reason for a higher number of proteases in the respiratory ways, which damage the pulmonary tissue [29].

5.3. Asthma and COPD

Similar to asthma, COPD is a pulmonary disease and shares many similar symptoms (e.g., pulmonary obstruction, over-production of mucus, attacks of cough and dyspnoea, etc.).

Parameter	Asthma	COPD
Age (origin of the disease)	Childhood, anytime	40+
Development of the disease	Abrupt attack	Slower
Dyspnoea	Rather abrupt, variable	Often, rather permanent
Pulmonary obstruction	Mainly reversible	Often irreversible
Smoking	Not very common	80% of cases
Allergy	Often (or parents)	Rarely
Inflammation (can differ)	Rather eosinophil	Rather neutrophil
Bronchial hyperreactivity	Distinct	Less common
Glucocorticoid therapy	Mainly efficient	Rather inefficient
Mortality (inhabitants per year (world))	300 million (decreases)	600 million (increases)

Table 1. Asthma and COPD comparison.

Especially, these common characteristics cause that asthma and COPD are sometimes misdiagnosed [30–32]. This can cause an incorrect pharmacotherapy administration, followed by their health state not (or just slightly) improving.

However, several factors can be used to distinguish asthma from COPD (**Table 1**).

6. Biomarkers of pulmonary diseases present in EBC

The term biomarker herein refers to a measurable biomolecular factor applicable for the measurement of a disease progression or treatment-related biomolecular changes in the human organism. On a molecular scale, biomarker refers to "a subset of markers that might be discovered using metabolomics, proteomics, genomics and other -omics technologies or imaging technologies." Biomarkers play a major role in medicinal biology. Biomarkers may be foreseen as a promising tool in the near future due to their unique potential for early diagnoses, which obviously permit disease prevention, a drug target identification, a drug response monitoring, etc. The collection and analyses of substances present in EBC provide a simple, noninvasive, real-time, point-of-care clinical and research tool for the evaluation of lung pathophysiology.

Very significant role is played by some biomarkers that are produced from the arachidonic acid (some of them were already mentioned above). Arachidonic acid ((5Z,8Z,11Z,14Z)Eicosa-5,8,11,14-tetraenoic acid) is a polyunsaturated omega-6 fatty acid present in phospholipid cell membranes [11, 12]. The products of the metabolism of arachidonic acid are called eicosanoids. These molecules are characterized by the 20C chain. The production of eicosanoids is enabled by different enzymes (**Figure 4**), the only exception are isoprostanes which emerge through oxidation of arachidonic acid (non-enzymatic pathway).

6.1. Arachidonic acid metabolites

Arachidonic acid is a polyunsaturated fatty acid present in phospholipid bilayer. In human organism, arachidonic acid acts as a vasodilator or regulates inflammation as a key intermediate. There are several pathways which allow transformation of the arachidonic acid in a number of different metabolites (**Figure 4**). Among the most significant products of its metabolism can be classified leukotrienes, lipoxins, isoprostanes, and prostanoids [6, 33].

6.1.1. Leukotrienes

Leukotrienes (LTs) [6, 33] represent a group of biologically active molecules. LTs are produced by various tissue cells (e.g., leukocytes, macrophages, mastocytoma cells) as a response to both immunological and non-immunological stimuli. LTs are potent pro-inflammatory [33] mediators and their release is usually triggered by the organism coming in contact with an allergen. The interaction between LTs and their receptors can lead to a wide range of biological effects: leukocytes activation, bronchial smooth muscles contraction, vascular permeability stimulation and increased mucus production, etc. All of the described symptoms are typically connected not only to pathophysiology of bronchial obstruction, especially to asthma, but also to other lung inflammatory disorders.

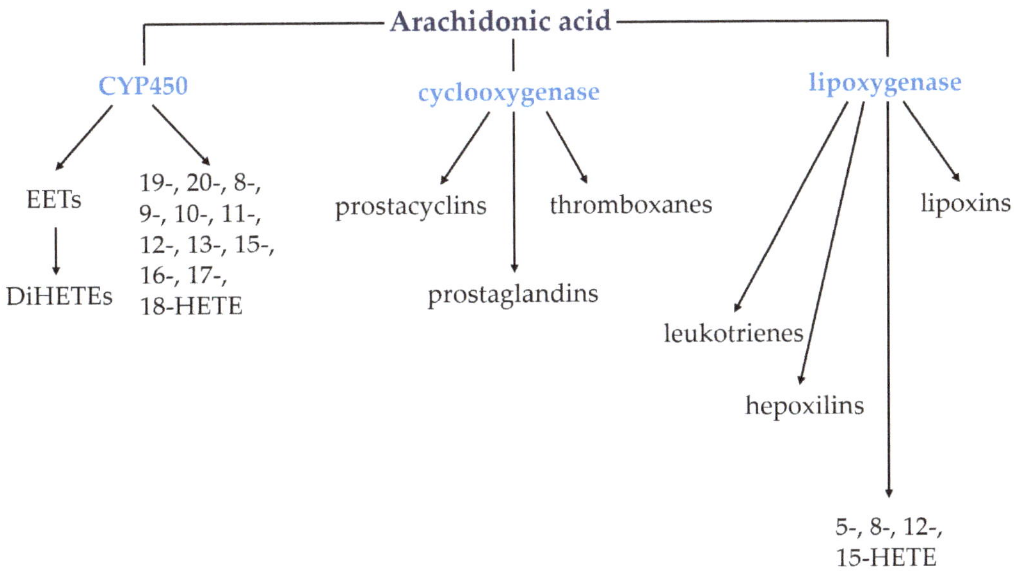

Figure 4. Biomarkers generated from arachidonic acid.

LTs are derivatives of arachidonic acid that are synthetized *via* the 5-lipoxygenase pathway (**Figure 5**). The major problem in the determination of LTs in body matrices is their low stability due to their sensitivity toward oxidation. This explains challenging analytical determination of the used assays and to a relatively high variability of the published data.

6.1.2. Lipoxins

Lipoxins (LXs) function in our organism as "natural antiasthmatics" as they are the anti-inflammatory mediators. Binding of LXs to their receptors also support the reconstructive process that is initiated in lungs immediately after the asthma attack.

LXs and LTs are derivatives of arachidonic acid and they are generated in three different metabolic pathways [34] . The first one is enabled by acetylsalicylic acid (ASA, in aspirin induced

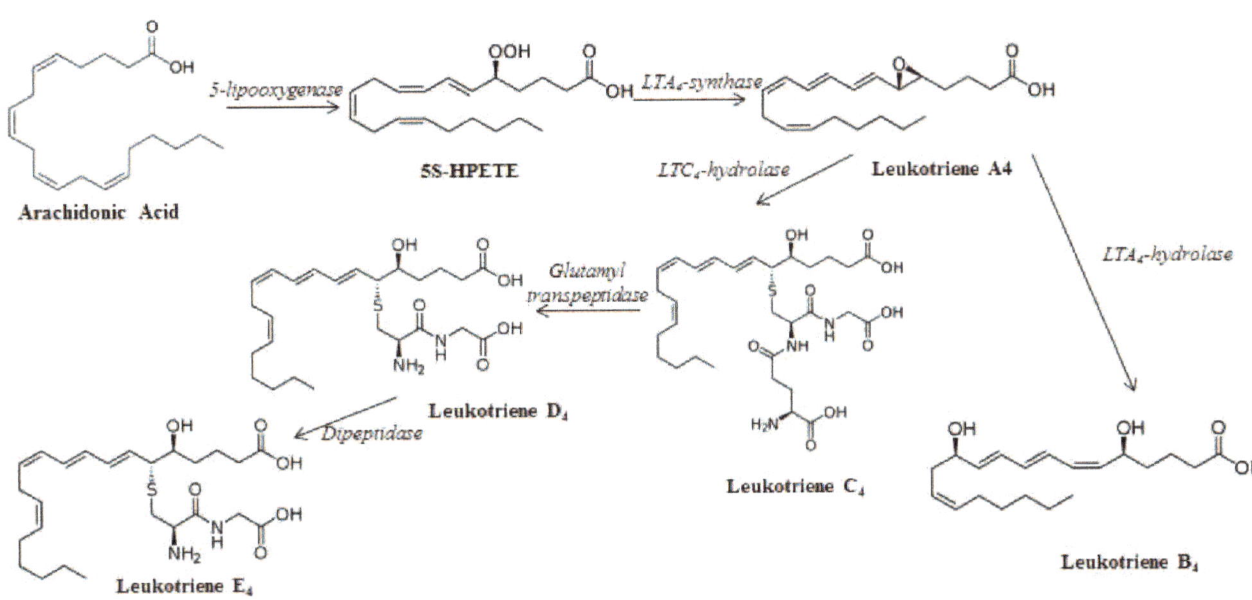

Figure 5. Biosynthesis of leukotrienes.

asthma), the second one by the enzyme 15-lipoxygenase, and the last one by 5-lipoxygenase which transforms arachidonic acid into LTA_4 and then into LXA_4 eventually into LXB_4 (**Figure 6**). On the other hand, the levels of LXs are usually lowered during inflammation.

6.1.3. Prostanoids

Prostanoids represent another group of biomarkers that are generated from the arachidonic acid. The synthesis is enabled by the enzyme cyclooxygensases (COX_1, COX_2) [6, 33]. Three major groups of biomarkers belong to the prostanoid family: prostacyclins, prostaglandins (PGD_2, PGE_2, and PGF_2), and thromboxanes (TXA_2, TXB_2). All of them represent significant participants in the inflammatory response. Thromboxanes are mainly responsible for vasoconstriction, while prostaglandins play an important role in the inflammatory and anaphylactic reactions. Another important function of thromboxanes and prostaglandins is their ability to adapt the inflammatory response and affect symptoms, such as fever, pain, or swelling.

The effect of prostanoids can be both pro- and anti-inflammatory with regard to the type of the inflammatory stimulus. Increased levels of some prostanoids with brocnhoconstrictive effects (PGE_2, PGD_2, PGF_2, and TBX_2) have been detected in EBC; however, the significance of their presence has not been sufficiently explained yet.

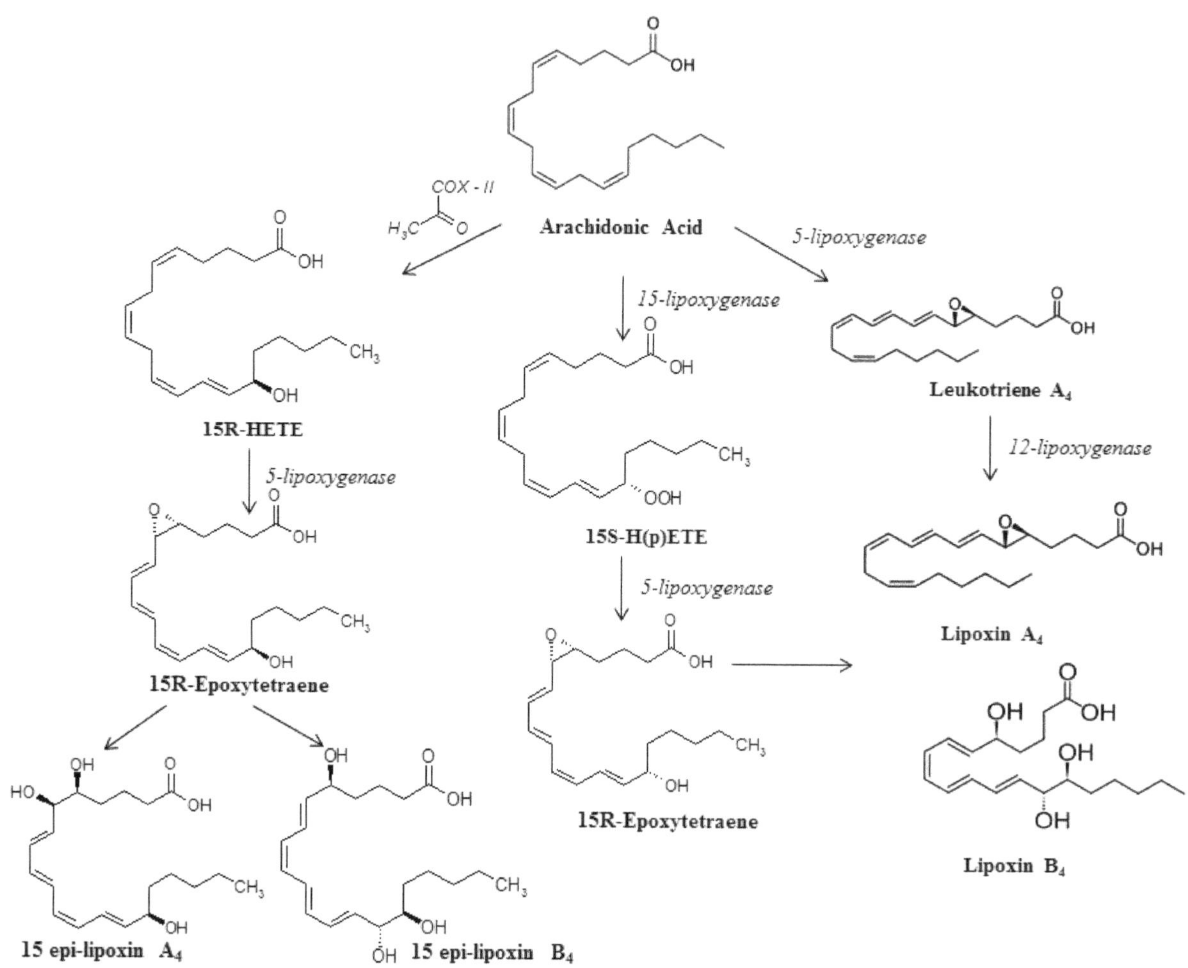

Figure 6. Biosynthesis of lipoxins.

6.2. Resolvins and protectins

Although the resolution of inflammation may have been regarded as a passive process, it has been proved that it can be actually described also as an active process in which numerous chemical mediators are involved. An example of these molecules may be resolvins and protectins. Both of them are synthetized from ω-3-PUFA precursors. Based on the model systems, it has been proved that resolvins and protectins participate in the anti-inflammatory response. In connection, the disproportion in their molecular levels can lead to diseases that are characterized by prolonged inflammation [33, 35]. At the same time, resolvin receptors may represent interesting targets for the future pharmacotherapies.

6.3. Oxidative stress biomarkers

6.3.1. Biomarkers of lipid peroxidation

6.3.1.1. Isoprostanes; 8-iso-prostaglandin F2α (8-iso-PGF2α or 8-isoprostane)

Isoprostanes are prostaglandin-like compounds formed *in vivo* from the free radical-catalyzed peroxidation of essential fatty acids (primarily arachidonic acid) without the direct action of cyclooxygenase (COX) enzymes [6, 8, 9, 33]. These non-classical eicosanoids possess potent biological activity as inflammatory mediators that augment the perception of pain. These compounds are accurate markers of lipid peroxidation in both animal and human models of oxidative stress.

8-iso-prostaglandin F2α (also known as 8-epi-PGF2α or 8-isoprostane) is a biomarker that has been shown to be useful for the assessment of oxidative stress *in vivo*. It is produced in the phospholipid membranes from the non-cyclooxygenase peroxidation pathways derived from arachidonic acid. It is present in EBC in physiological concentration levels which grows in the course of lifetime as a consequence of aging. Pathological levels in EBC are reasonably increased as a result of several lung diseases and disorders that are induced by oxidative stress (asbestosis, silicosis, lung cancer, COPD, etc.).

6.3.2. Biomarkers of nucleic acids damage

6.3.2.1. 8-hydroxy-2′-deoxyguanosine, 8-hydroxyguanosine, and 5-hydroxymethyl uracil

The steady-state levels of nucleic acids damage biomarkers represent the balance between formation and repair. As reviewed by Valavanidis et al. [36], increased levels of 8-hydroxy-2′-deoxyguanosine (8-OHdG), the principal product of DNA oxidation, represent a valuable biomarker of DNA damage by oxidative stress.

8-Hydroxyguanosine (8-OHG) is a nucleoside that is an oxidative derivative of guanosine. Measurement of the levels of 8-OHG is used as a biomarker of RNA damage by oxidative stress.

In a rat model, 8-OHdG was found to have anti-inflammatory effect. Rats treated with lipopolysaccharide (LPS) exhibited inflammatory lung injury dependent on neutrophils with an increase in pro-inflammatory cytokines such as interleukins 6 and 18 (IL-6, IL-18) and tumor necrosis factor α (TNF-α). Rats pre-treated with 8-OHdG prior to LPS treatment showed inhibited LPS-induced inflammatory responses. 8-OHdG anti-inflammatory action was found to be higher than for aspirin and other nucleosides (8-OHG, deoxyguanosine, guanosine, adenosine). 8-OHG and adenosine also exhibited anti-inflammatory activity, but it was much lower than for 8-OHdG. Deoxyguanosine was found to be almost ineffective. Compared to aspirin, which acts through cyclooxygenase (COX) inhibition, 8-OHdG seems to be more versatile and, therefore, more effective as it was found that 8-OHdG suppresses ROS formation in human neutrophils. However, in human organism, 8-OHdG is excreted in much lower concentrations than in rats and, therefore, only exogenously administered 8-OHdG could have a therapeutic potential as an anti-inflammatory agent. 8-OHdG is also considered to be a potential biomarker of cancers related to smoking (e.g., lung cancer).

5-Hydroxymethyl uracil (5-OHMeU) is an example of oxidized-pyrimidines. Low levels of these molecules have been detected as a consequence of DNA oxidation initialized by oxidative stress. Oxidized-pyrimidines are more likely to be repaired than other relative molecules, which may represent an explanation of their low detected pathological concentration levels. As the excision rate from DNA is different for various bases, participation of specific excision-repair enzymes might occur.

6.3.3. Biomarkers of peptides damage

6.3.3.1. o-Tyrosine, 3-chlorotyrosine and 3-nitrotyrosine

o-Tyrosine (*o*-Tyr), 3-chlorotyrosine (3-ClTyr), and 3-nitrotyrosine (3-NOTyr) are among the most prominent biomarkers of oxidative protein damage and are present in the body fluids of patients with diseases related to oxidative stress [6].

Free radicals cause alterations in cellular protein structure and function. Oxidized, nitrated, and chlorinated modifications of aromatic amino acids including phenylalanine and tyrosine are reliable biomarkers of oxidative stress and inflammation in clinical conditions. In human organism, tyrosine is formed from phenylalanine. Physiological *p*-tyrosine (*p*-Tyr) occurs by enzymatic oxidation of phenylalanine by phenylalanine hydroxylase. Important derivatives of tyrosine are catecholamines (dopamine, adrenaline, and noradrenaline) or thyroid hormones. *o*-Tyr and *m*-tyrosine (*m*-Tyr) are formed by the attack of ROS on phenylalanine. Unlike *p*-Tyr, *o*-Tyr and *m*-Tyr are not natural amino acids and are considered to be oxidative stress biomarkers. The biomarkers that are formed during protein oxidative damage are amino acids *o*-Tyr, 3-ClTyr, and 3-NOTyr (**Figure 7**).

6.4. The other biomarkers

6.4.1. Cytokines

Cytokines are proteins secreted by immune cells (e.g., B lymphocytes, T lymphocytes, macrophages, and mast cells) or fibroblasts and endothelial cells. Cytokines are fundamental regulators of the immune system and they play various roles in human organism (not only in immune system), as they influence: regeneration of the tissue, embryonal development, carcinogenesis, angiogenesis, etc. The function of numerous cytokines can be triggered by oxidative stress. In

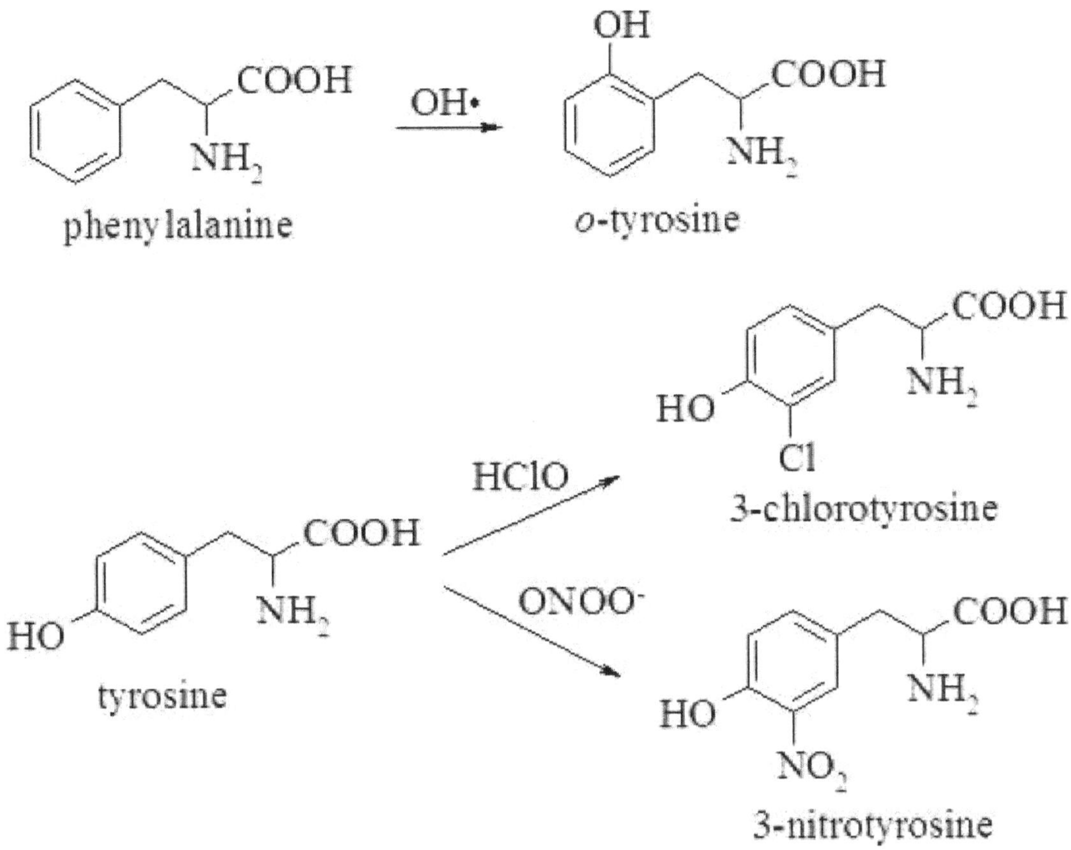

Figure 7. Formation of *o*-tyrosine, 3-chlorotyrosine, and 3-nitrotyrosine.

human organism, they can act as both inflammatory and anti-inflammatory molecules, however in the respiratory tract they are mainly considered to represent biomarkers of chronic inflammation.

A wide range of cytokines has been detected in EBC so far. An example of such cytokine can be tumor necrosis factor (TNF) or interferon (IFN). Low concentration levels [37–40] of both of these biomarkers have been detected in EBC. Specifically, TNF represents a biomarker of oncological diseases as its increased levels have been mainly described among lung cancer patients [41, 42]. Other cytokines that are detectable in EBC are various members of the interleukin family (IL-1, IL-2, IL-4, IL-5, IL-6, IL-8, IL-10 and IL-13).

6.4.2. Glutathione

Glutathione (GSH) is a tripeptide that functions in organism as an endogenous antioxidant. The main task of GSH is to prevent the cells to be damaged by free radicals and reactive oxygen species and thus protect the organism from oxidative stress. An important part of this process is the oxidation of GSH to glutathione disulfide (GSSG). This process occurs, for example, in the airway cells, where it is essential to protect the lungs and airways tissue which are exposed to the effect of external oxidants. Simultaneously, GSH is one of the regulators of the NO cycle. Decreased levels of GSH and proportionally increased levels of GSSG, which are mainly connected to the disproportion in the redox balance, represent a reliable biomarker of oxidative stress, usually coupled with inflammation [43]. Decreased levels of GSH in EBC have been mainly monitored in case of patients suffering from bronchial asthma. The results of another conducted study showed that significantly increased levels of GSSG occur in EBC of alcoholics [44].

6.5. Other molecules determined in EBC

6.5.1. Proteins and metabolites

The majority of pulmonary diseases is also characterized by alternations in the protein profile of the patients. Many of these changes are measurable in EBC and can be used for monitoring of pathological process occurring (mainly) in the respiratory tract. The changes in the structure and concentration levels of various proteins have recently become a popular and reliable tool for monitoring of the process and molecular alterations in lungs and airways. Based on the proteomic analysis of EBC, 44 unique proteins [45, 46] have been detected so far. Many of these proteins might become steady biomarkers of inflammation or oxidative stress, when scanning of the differences between the proteome profiles of healthy control subjects and subjects with various pulmonary diseases may represent a significant shift toward detecting new prognostic and/or diagnostic biomarkers.

6.5.2. Serotonin

Serotonin (5-hydroxytryptamin (5-HT)) is a neurotransmitter that is predominantly located in central nervous system and gastrointestinal tract (GIT). In GIT, 5-HT regulates bowel movements. In CNS, it is responsible for the regulation of mood, sleep, muscle contraction, and some cognitive functions (involving memory and learning abilities). It is also present in thrombocytes, where it is involved in the regulation of homeostasis and coagulation [47].

5-HT plays a significant role in many pathological and neuropsychiatric diseases [47, 48]. The serotonergic substances are also important in pharmacology. The genes that code various components of 5-HT system are the subject of the study as they could be factors of depression, schizophrenia, obsessive–compulsive disorder, aggression, alcoholism, migraine, and autism [49].

7. Experimental part

7.1. Analytical method for multi-marker screening

The following analytical methods combined with various pre-treatment methods are currently referenced in the literature for the determination of biomarkers present in EBC: HPLC-MS, GC-MS and EIA (ELISA). Based on validation parameters (e.g., accuracy, precision, limit of quantification (LOQ), limit of detection (LOD), linearity, selectivity, etc.) the methods described above can be compared.

LC-MS method in a highly selective and accurate SRM mode affords both quantitative and qualitative information about the monitored biomarkers and today seems to be method of the first choice. Liquid chromatography can be used in UHPLC, which is characterized by the fact that the separation of substances occurs at higher flow rate of the mobile phase (1 mL/min) on LC columns with smaller average particle size of the stationary phase (diameter of particles

<2 μm) and by shortening the time of LC-MS analysis. When using the so-called "stable-isotope-dilution assay," the accuracy and precision of the LC-MS method can be increased by suitable deuterated internal standards. However, the main disadvantage of the LC-MS analysis is the inclusion of the pre-treatment step (SPE, immunoaffinity extraction, etc.), when the EBC sample is recommended to exclude a contact to room temperature, ideally temperature above 0°C. This problem can be prevented by using the 2D technology for liquid chromatography. In the first dimension, an on-line SPE is carried out and the subsequent dimension uses the UHPLC. For detection of selected biomarkers, 2D UHPLC-MS method was developed and because of the sensitivity of biomarkers mentioned above, it is highly recommended.

Analysis of substances were realized on the LC-MS system consisting of quaternary pump and mass spectrometer operating on the principle of triple quadrupole equipped with electrospray ionization (ESI). To implement multimarker screening, it was necessary to carry out two types of analyses. The first one were determined substances containing amino group in its structure. The second one serves to determine substances with aldehyde and carboxylic groups. These two analyses were necessary because of the different conditions of derivatization reactions (acid vs. alkaline environment) and the resulting liquid chromatography at different conditions (different composition of the mobile phase used on different chromatographic columns).

7.1.1. Determination of the amino compounds

For the derivatization of compounds containing an amino group in its structure (*o*-tyrosine (*o*-Tyr), 3-nitrotyrosine (3-NO_2-Tyr), 3-chlorotyrosine (3-Cl-Tyr), hydroxyguanosin (8-OHG) and 8-hydroxy-2′-deoxyguanosine (8-OHdG) were used as derivatization reagent 3-aminopyridyl-N-hydroxysukcinimidyl carbamate (= APDS). To 500 μl of the EBC sample-containing deuterium labeled analyte analogues was added to 450 μl of borate buffer (pH 8.5) and 50 μl of APDS derivatization agent (concentration of 1 mg/ml of acetonitrile). Derivatization reactions were carried out for 10 min at 4°C. Thus prepared sample was subjected to LC-ESI-MS/MS analysis on chromatographic column XTerra MS (C18 50 × 1 mm × 3.5 μm) (Waters, Republic of Ireland). The substances were subjected to analysis where isocratic elution method with a mobile phase composed of acetonitrile: water (60:40—v/v) (water = 0.1% formic acid) was used. The column was tempered to 25°C. Mobile phase flow rate was 150 μl/min. The volume of the analyzed samples was 10 μl. Mass spectrometer parameters were optimized to the following values: capillary voltage −2500 V, the inlet capillary temperature 300°C, the temperature of the evaporator HESI 300°C, sheath gas (nitrogen) pressure 45 psi, auxiliary gas (nitrogen) 10 ArbU. Measurement parameters were optimized for use in neutral loss mode in the interval 250–500 Da (Q1) → 130–380 Da (Q3) with CID energy 15 eV in the negative electrospray ionization (ESI-).

7.1.2. Determination of aldehydes and carboxylic acids

Derivatization of aldehydes (n-aliphatic aldehydes (C6–C12), malondialdehyde (MDA), 4-hydroxynonenal (4-HNE), 4-hydroxyhexenal (4-HHE) and substances with a carboxyl group in its structure 8-isoprostane (8-iso-PGF2α), cys-LTs, LTB_4 was carried out using derivatization with Girard's reagent T (GirT) in the presence of N-(3-dimethylaminopropyl)-N′-ethylkarbodiimide hydrochloride (EDC) and N-hydroxysuccinimide. To the sample containing 100 μl of EBC with deuterium-labeled internal standards were added 10 μl of each derivatization reagent GirT (c = 100 μl/ml), reagent EDC together with 10 μl of sulfo-N-hydroxysuccinimide, 10 μl of 1% hydrochloric acid and 270 μl of propan-2-ol. Derivatization proceeded for 30 minutes and in such way prepared sample was immediately analyzed by LC-ESI-MS/MS. Chromatographic column used was a Thermo Hypercarb (100 × 21 mm × 5 μm) with pre-column Hypercarb (Thermo Electron Corporation, USA). For separation of substances, was used the isocratic elution method with a mobile phase composed of methanol: water (40:60—v/v) (pH adjusted with ammonium hydroxide to 9). Flow rate of mobile phase was 150 μl/min. Chromatographic column temperature was 30°C and the sample volume was 10 μl. Mass spectrometer parameters were optimized to the following values: capillary voltage 3000 V, capillary inlet temperature 300°C; HESI evaporator temperature 300°C, sheath gas (nitrogen) pressure 45 psi and auxiliary gas (nitrogen) 10 ArbU. Measurement parameters were optimized for use in neutral loss mode in the interval 150–750 Da (Q1) → 91–691 Da (Q3) with CID energy − 16.5 eV in the positive electrospray ionization (ESI+).

8. Case studies

8.1. Asthma phenotyping

The first aim of the study was to determine levels of the pro-inflammatory cys-LTs and levels of the anti-inflammatory LXs in EBC of patients suffering from different asthma phenotypes (including also SRA), compare the obtained data between the groups of asthmatics, and make the comparisons with healthy control subjects.

As is presented in **Figure 8**, the study showed that both levels of cys-LTs and LXs were changing among different asthma phenotypes. According to the results, EBC of SRA patients contained the highest levels of the pro-inflammatory cys-LTs but at the same time the lowest levels of the anti-inflammatory LXs. The results of the analysis of EBC of healthy control subjects were inverse to these (i.e., EBC of health controls contained the highest levels of LXs but on the contrary the lowest levels of cys-LTs).

The remaining groups have spread in the interval from healthy control subjects to SRA. The order of these groups was based on the raising severity of the asthma phenotype (mild asthma → moderate persistent asthma → difficult asthma) (**Figure 8**).

According to the results (**Figure 15**), it is possible to use cys-LTs and LXs for the differential diagnostics of asthma and identify various asthma phenotypes. The diagnosis can be assessed on the phenomenon that the concentration levels of LXs and cys-LTs are complementary and connected by dynamic equilibrium (i.e., increasing levels of the inflammatory LTs lead to a corresponding decrease in the levels of the anti-inflammatory LXs). This occurs due to the fact that biochemical synthesis (both cys-LTs and LXs are generated from LTA_4) enhancing the production of LXs simultaneously lower the generation of LTs. Combining cys-LTs with LXs offers an interesting alternative to the currently used methods of molecular diagnostics of bronchial asthma. **Figure 8** describes the principle of equilibrium between the pro-inflammatory LTs and the anti-inflammatory LXs. The developed method represents a potential tool for asthma phenotyping accuracy improvement, which was proved in a clinical study, which enabled the separation of patients into five groups:

a. Severe refractory asthma.

b. Severe asthma.

c. Moderate persistent asthma.

d. Mild asthma.

e. Non-asthmatics—healthy control subjects.

8.2. Monitoring of efficacy of the used pharmacotherapy

The developed method was used in a parallel study. The study was conducted to prove whether the method could be applied for monitoring of efficacy of the used pharmacotherapy. In this case, *per oral* and inhaled glucocorticoid treatments have been compared. Results of the study are present in **Figure 9**. In the clinical study of 35 patients with *per oral* glucocorticoid therapy, 35 patients with inhaled glucocorticoid therapy and 32 people from the healthy control group were involved.

From the results, it is obvious that the PCA analysis divided the subjects into three groups. The first group contained only healthy control subjects; however, the two remaining have

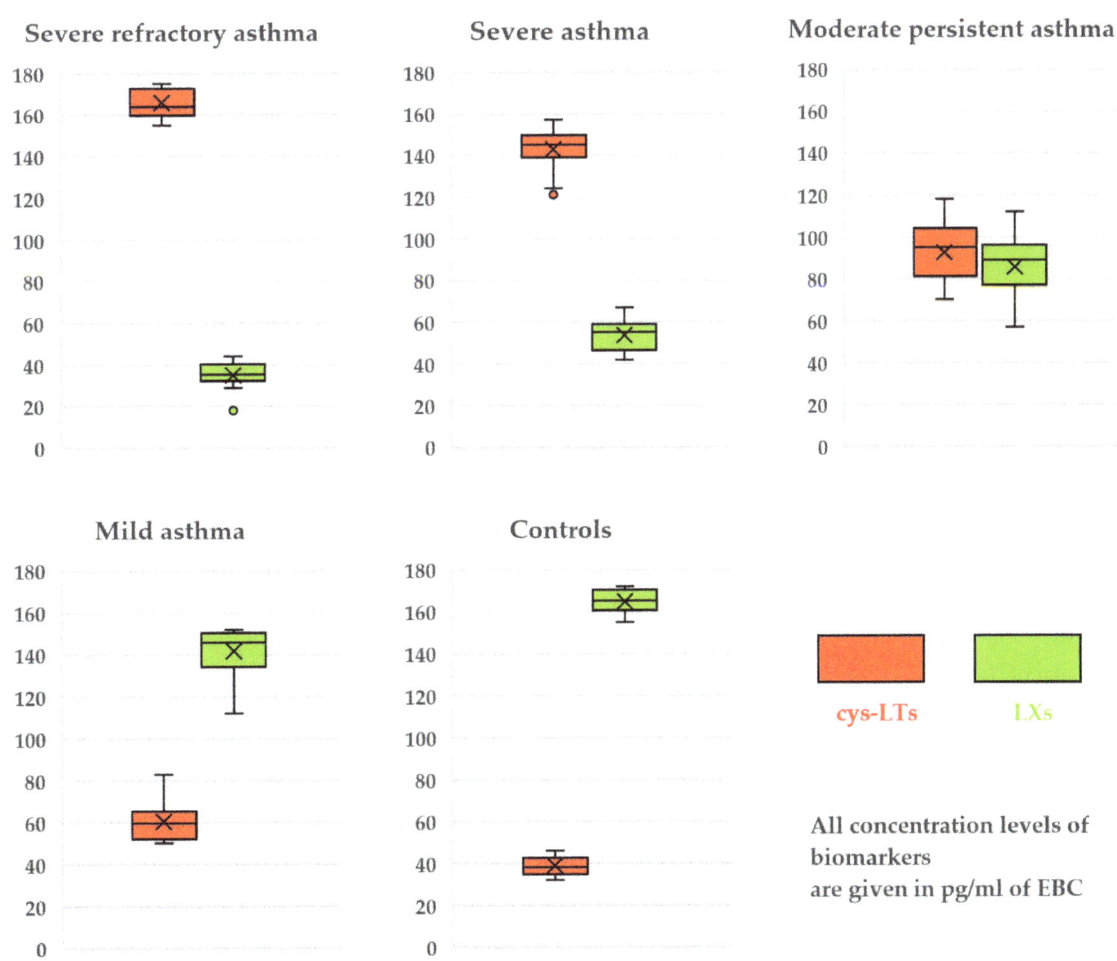

Figure 8. Statistically evaluated clinical results: levels of cys-LTs and LXs in different asthma phenotypes.

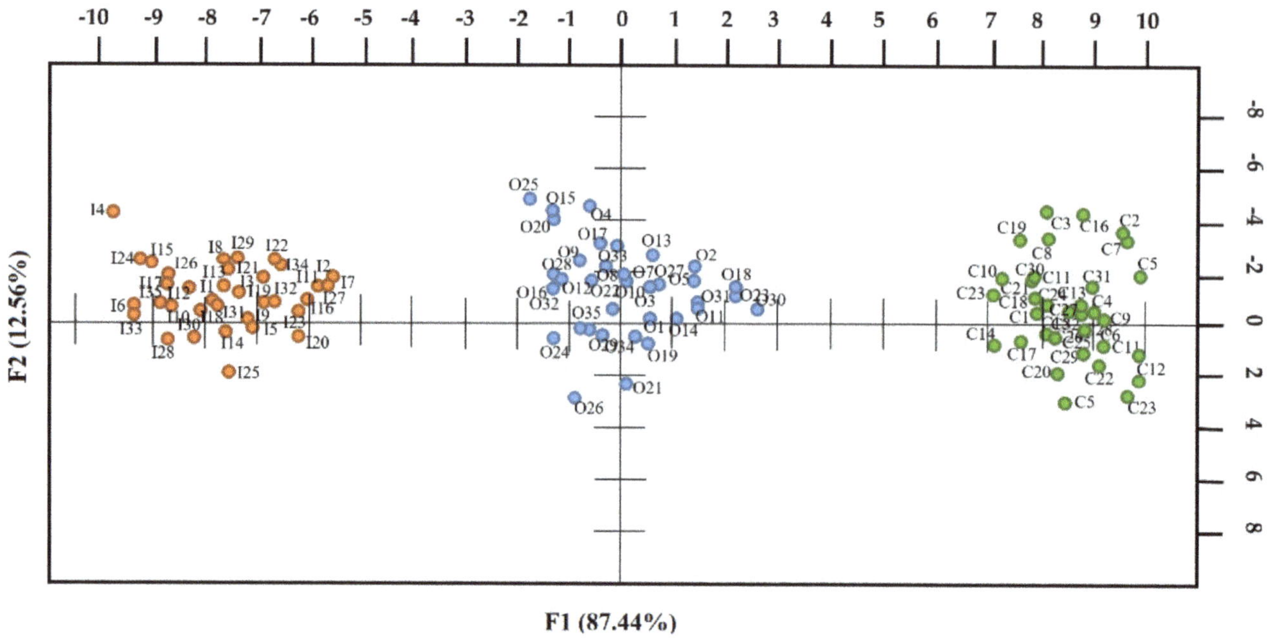

Figure 9. Monitoring of efficacy of the used pharmacotherapy.

been separated according to the type of glucocorticoid application. The results also show that on these terms more efficient was the *per oral* glucocorticoid therapy, as the cluster representing patients with *per oral* treatment is in the spectrum closer to the controls.

The study has also confirmed that the developed method can be used for such monitoring, which could in the future make the asthma pharmacotherapy more accurate. Furthermore, the method could also enable controlling of dosing and comparing of the efficacy of different anti-asthmatic drugs, which would globally improve asthma treatment.

8.3. Asthma and COPD separation

Apart from cys-LTs and LXs, EBC contains a wide range of other different biomarkers. The research has shown that biomarkers of oxidative stress play a significant role in the development of some pulmonary diseases. Examples of such biomarkers can be 8-isoprostan, MDA, HHE, HNE and other aldehydes and biomarkers connected to damage of proteins (*o*-Tyr, 3-ClTyr and 3-NOTyr) or nucleic acids (8-OHdG, 8-OHG and 5-OHMeU).

These biomarkers allowed extension of the developed method, which was originally based on the detection of levels of cys-LTs and LXs. An example of such extensions can be separation of asthma and COPD on molecular level.

The metabolic fingerprinting of EBC of patients suffering from COPD showed a significant increase of biomarkers of neutrophil inflammation—LTB_4 and also biomarkers of oxidative stress (mainly *o*-Tyr and 8-isoprostane). The developed method was used in a clinical study that was aimed at detection and description of differences between COPD patients and SRA (SRA were chosen because their profile is quite similar to the profile of COPD patients and thus their diagnosis is often altered). The obtained results were compared to the analysis of EBC of healthy control subjects (two control groups were chosen—one for COPD patients and one for SRA).

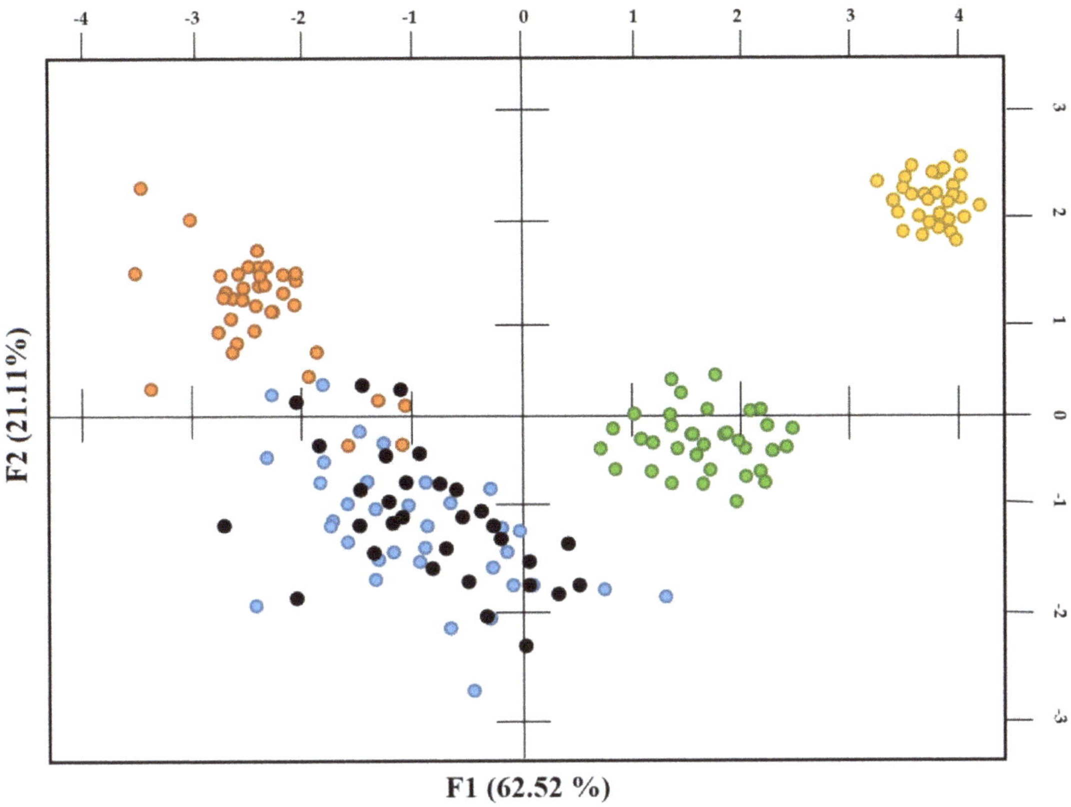

Figure 10. Results of clinical study: separation of COPD patients (light blue—bronchitis, dark blue—emphysema) and SRA patients (orange); control groups: green—COPD controls; yellow—SRA controls.

According to the results (**Figure 10**), the PCA analysis has divided the patients into four groups based on their biomarker profiles. The results show that profiles of SRA and COPD patients were different, which allows an accurate separation of these two diseases. The figure also shows that the control groups were separated. Further, the results show that it is not possible with this method to separate (on the molecular level) the two phenotypes of COPD—chronical bronchitis and emphysema.

8.4. Biomarker panel for monitoring of pathogenesis of pulmonary diseases

As a significant part of the study, a panel of biomarkers that can be used for differentiation of various pulmonary diseases was designed. The analyzed biomarkers are divided into two main groups. The first group contained biomarkers of eosinophil inflammation—cys-LTs (ΣLTC$_4$, LTD$_4$, LTE$_4$), the anti-inflammatory eicosanoids—LXs (Σ LXA$_4$, LXB$_4$) and anti-inflammatory resolvins (RvD1). The second group contained biomarker of neutrophil inflammation—LTB$_4$, 8-isoprostane which is biomarker of oxidative stress connected to damage of phospholipid membrane, biomarkers of damage of proteins (Σ *o*-tyrosin, NO-tyrosin and Cl-tyrosin) and biomarkers of damage of nucleic acids (Σ 5-OHMeU, 8-OHG and 8-OHdG).

The first two graphs show results of the analysis of EBC of patients suffering from SRA and moderate persistent asthma. The results are compared with the analysis of EBC of healthy control subjects.

According to the graph (**Figure 11**), it is obvious that EBC of patients who suffer from asthma contained increased levels of cys-LTs (the highest levels—SRA, this confirms the study mentioned above). On the contrary, EBC of asthmatics contained lowered levels of the anti-inflammatory LXs and resolvins. Considering the asthma-phenotyping-study, it can be also said that the results of analysis of EBC of SRA and controls were inverse.

Figure 12 shows the results of the monitoring of LTB_4, 8-isoprostane, biomarkers of damage of proteins and nucleic acids. Levels of LTB_4 showed the same trend as cys-LTs, for example, the highest levels were detected in EBC of SRA and the lowest in EBC of healthy controls. At the same time, levels of 8-isoprostane were slightly elevated among the group of patients with moderate persistent asthma and even more among SRA. The differences in levels of biomarkers responsible for damage of proteins and nucleic acids were slightly higher in EBC of asthmatics, but the differences were not so significant, which means that these biomarkers are not so specific and influential in case of bronchial asthma.

Figures 13 and **14** show same biomarkers as the previous **Figures 11** and **12**, but in EBC of patients who suffer from COPD, asbestosis and lung cancer.

From **Figure 13**, it is quite obvious that biomarkers cys-LTs, LXs and resolvins do not play a significant role in pathogenesis of these diseases, as their levels are comparable to those detected among healthy control subjects (the levels are just slightly elevated and only COPD patients show some more noticeable deviations).

Figure 14 shows that illnesses characterized by damage of the pulmonary tissue are usually connected to increased levels of biomarkers of oxidative stress. One of these significant

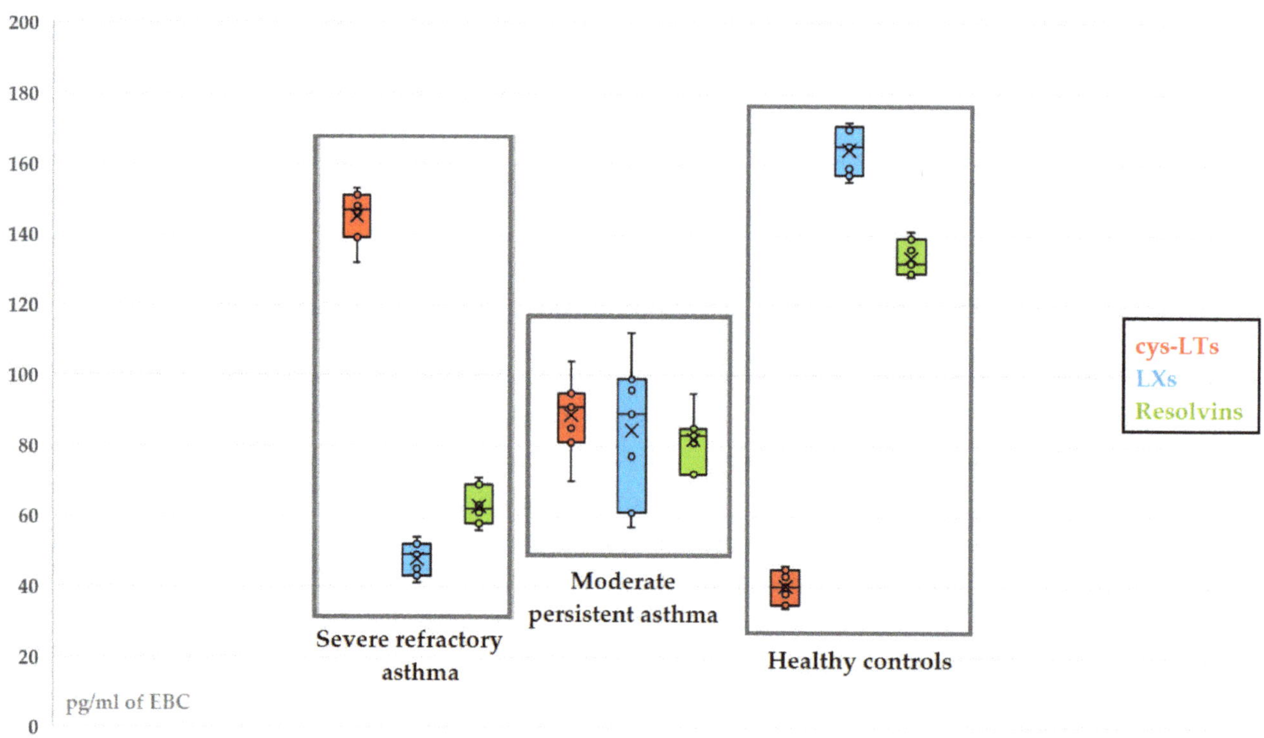

Figure 11. Evaluated clinical results: levels of cys-LTs, LXs and resolvins in EBC of SRA, moderate persistent asthma and healthy controls.

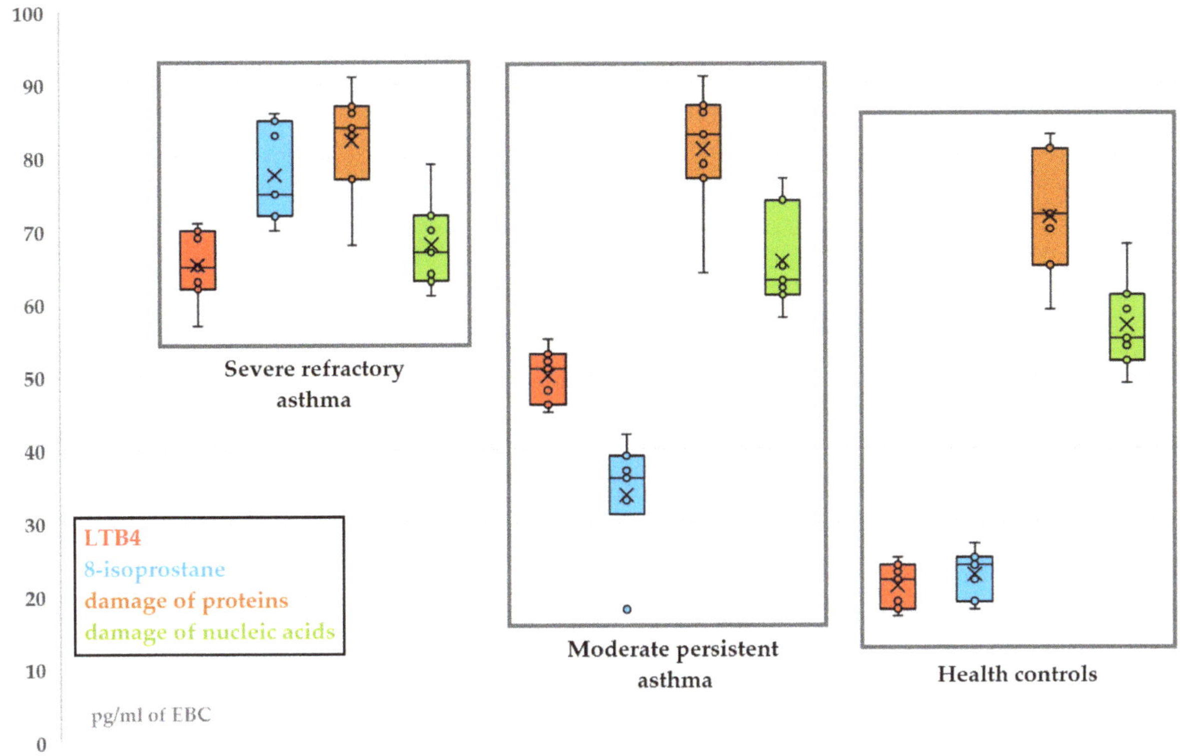

Figure 12. Evaluated clinical results: levels of LTB_4, 8-isoprostane, biomarkers of proteins and nucleic acids damage in EBC of SRA, moderate persistent asthma and healthy controls.

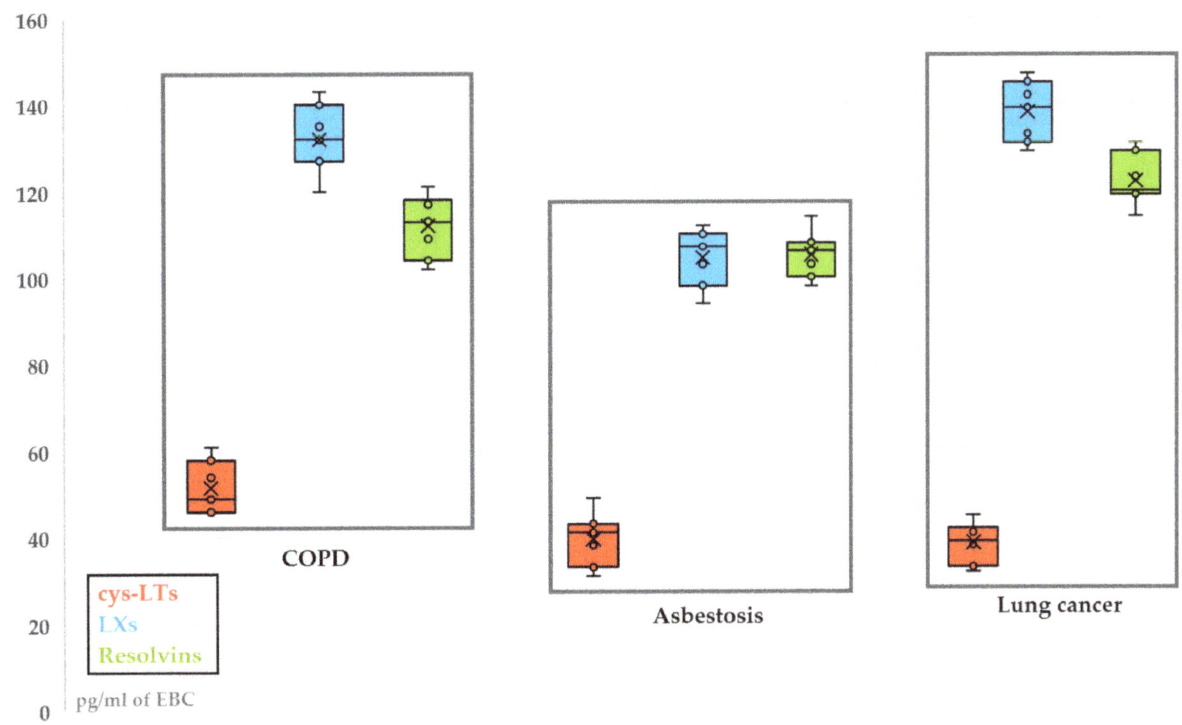

Figure 13. Evaluated clinical results: levels of cys-LTs, LXs, and resolvins in EBC of COPD, asbestosis, and lung cancer patients.

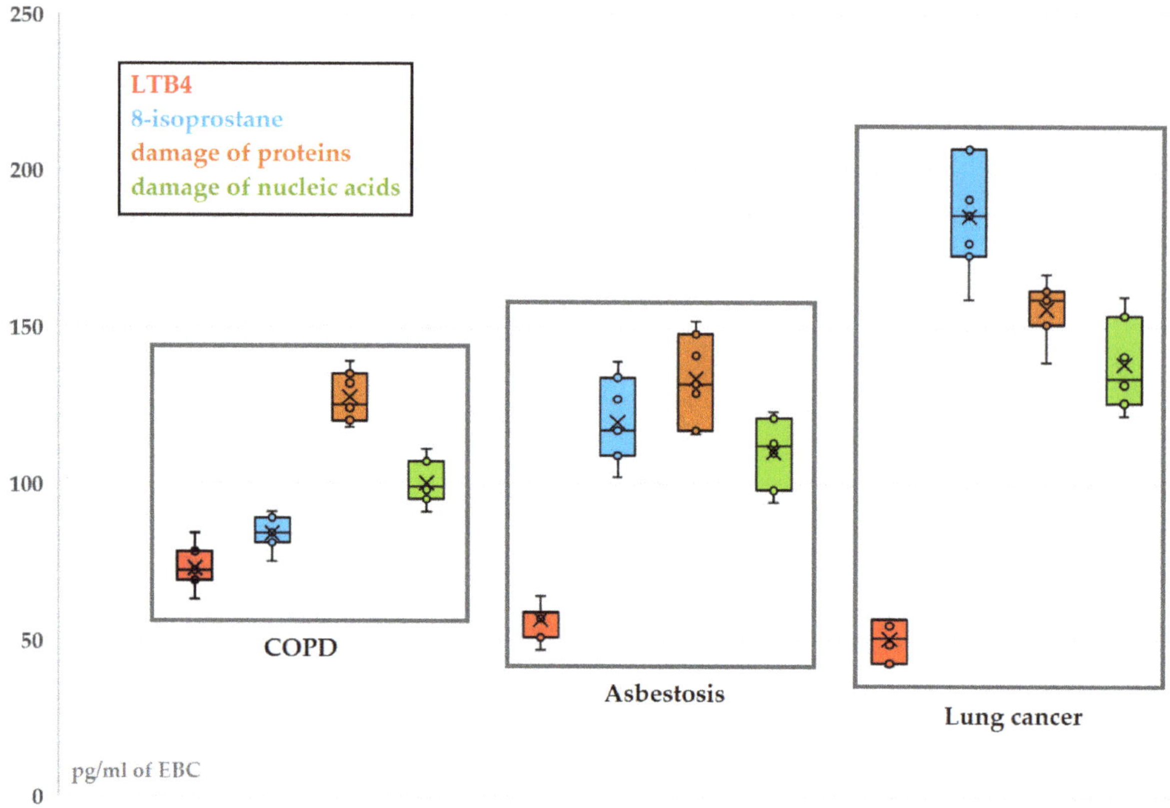

Figure 14. Evaluated clinical results: levels of LTB_4, 8-isoprostane, biomarkers of proteins and nucleic acids damage in EBC of COPD, asbestosis, and lung cancer patients.

indicators of ongoing tissue necrosis processes is 8-isoprostane. The analysis of EBC showed that the levels of this biomarker are increased among COPD and asbestosis patients and even more among people suffering from lung cancer. Similar information is provided by the biomarkers of proteins damage (tyrosines) and nucleic acids damage (5-OHMeU, 8-OHG, and 8-OHdG). The levels of these molecules were elevated in EBC of patients with COPD and asbestosis and it can be said that the highest levels are specific for lung cancer (average concentration of tyrosines is approximately 75 pg/ml of EBC for healthy controls and 160 pg/ml of EBC for patients with lung cancer).

8.5. Serotonin in EBC of SRA

Based on the clinical experience, it is proved that SRA patients positively respond to SSRI (selective serotonin reuptake inhibitors) antidepressants therapy. SSRI antidepressants usually improve physical state of patients, which may seem as a quite logical coincidence. However, much more surprising is the fact that when SRA patients are prescribed SSRI antidepressants, their breath functions improve significantly. This phenomenon prompted to performed research aimed at the detection of serotonin in EBC of SRA. The obtained results were compared with serotonin levels in EBC of other asthma phenotypes and healthy control subjects.

According to the results (**Figure 15**), it is obvious that the levels of serotonin in EBC of SRA are different as compared to other asthma phenotypes and healthy control subjects. However,

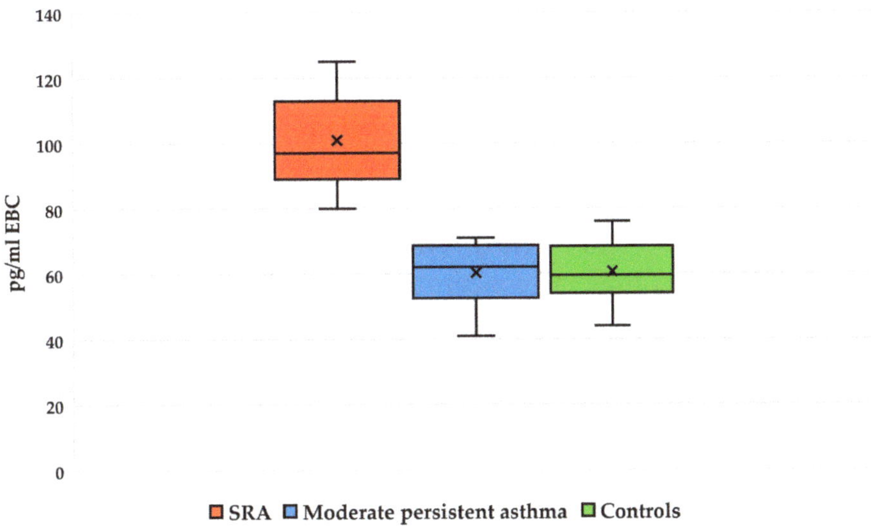

Figure 15. Evaluated clinical results: levels of 5-HT in EBC of SRA, moderate persistent asthma and healthy controls.

surprisingly, the levels were significantly elevated (in case of SRA patients) which is against all expectations (it was expected to detect lower levels of serotonin, which would provide a possible explanation of positive SRA's responsiveness to SSRI antidepressants therapy). Probably, even more interesting is the fact the levels of serotonin of other asthma phenotypes and health controls were the same, which indicates that the deviation appears only among SRA.

The interpretation of these results is quite complicated. One of the possible hypotheses is that SRA could be a different disease that would only demonstrate itself as asthma (i.e., patients have similar symptoms as asthmatics, but the cause of the disease could be different). However, this theory will require further research in the future. One of the possible extensions could be monitoring of levels of serotonin in cerebrospinal fluid, which would provide information about the process behind the blood-brain barrier. On the other hand, the study proved that there many significant physiological differences between SRA and other asthmatics, which could be used in the future for the development of a possible drug against SRA.

9. Conclusions

Measurements of biomarkers in EBC offer a novel way of monitoring lung inflammation, damage by oxidation stress with an insight into the pathophysiology of different diseases. The described diagnostic method was based on the detection and quantification of biomarkers in a matrix specific for the respiratory tract—EBC. As the collection of EBC is completely noninvasive, the method offers a broad spectrum of application. The method is applicable to children as well as to senior people and it is appropriate also in case of longitudinal studies that are trying to precisely understand the processes occurring on the molecular level in the respiratory tract. The method can be easily repeated which proves its suitability for regular monitoring of the pharmacotherapy efficiency or the impact of various allergens. The results obtained from the EBC analysis represent reliable characterization of the exhaled biomarkers profile (LXs, cys-LTs, LTB_4, 8-isoprostane, tyrosines, etc.), which is relevant for diagnostics, separation, and phenotyping of different respiratory diseases. Nevertheless, EBC analysis requires standardization and validation including sample collection and sample pre-analysis treatment (e.g., internal standardization, storing, pre-treatment method application, etc.).

Model clinical studies were carried out as a part of the work, which applied a methodology based on the molecular diagnostics of EBC. The method allowed an asthma phenotyping, which was founded on the fact that the concentration levels of cys-LTs and LXs are not only complementary but also intra-related by a dynamic equilibrium. This phenomenon, however, affords not only asthma phenotyping but also other diagnostics as, for example, monitoring of efficacy of the used pharmacotherapy. The analysis of EBC also showed that the detected biomarkers can be used for the differentiation of various pulmonary diseases (more specifically (apart from asthma) COPD, asbestosis, and lung cancer). Increased (or decreased) levels of some biomarkers are specific only for some diseases and thus these can be selectively differentiated as much as, for example, asthma from COPD.

Additionally, an experiment was conducted and focused on determining serotonin in EBC. The aim of this study was to assess the positive effects of the SSRI (selective serotonin re-uptake inhibitors) antidepressants on SRA. High levels of serotonin were detected in EBC of SRA patients, which was in contradiction to the initial assumption. Simultaneously, a hypothesis was formulated stating that SRA probably functions on different molecular principles. This could have probably been the reason for SRA inefficiency with the commonly used drugs.

For the future research, one can only recommend focusing on large longitudinal studies to ascertain whether sequential measurements in individual patients reflect asthma severity and the degree of a lung inflammation, and on studies engaged to the relationships between the concentrations of asthma biomarkers and its symptoms. In order to implement the EBC analysis to the clinical practice as well as reliably guiding the pharmacological treatment of asthma and the effect of drugs on asthma markers present in EBC, further controlled studies are required to be conducted. In particular, studies are recommended determining the expediency of the EBC analysis for predicting a treatment response, and assessing new therapies. Obviously, this outlines a great deal of work to be done. The fact that EBC analyses are currently used in various clinical trials and studies corroborates the above arguments. On the other hand, it is important to proclaim that the fact whether and when EBC analyses will become applicable to the clinical settings is still difficult to predict.

Acknowledgements

The work was supported from The Ministry of Education, Youth and Sports of the Czech Republic under the NPU I (LQ1604) National Sustainability Program II (Project BIOCEV-FAR) and by the project "BIOCEV" (CZ.1.05/1.1.00/02.0109). European Regional Development Fund-Project "PharmaBrain" (No. CZ. CZ.02.1.01/0.0/0.0/16_025/0007444), project AZV MZ 17-31852A and by the "Sustainability for the National Institute of Mental Health (LO1611).

Author details

Tereza Kačerová[1,2], Petr Novotný[3], Ján Boroň[3] and Petr Kačer[1, 4*]

*Address all correspondence to: petr.kacer@1lf.cuni.cz

1 BIOCEV, 1st Medicinal Faculty Charles University, Vestec, Czech Republic

2 Grammar School Nad Štolou 1, Prague 7, Czech Republic

3 ESSENCE LINE, s.r.o., Prague 5, Czech Republic

4 National Institute of Mental Health, Klecany, Czech Republic

References

[1] Cserhati E. The history of bronchial asthma from the ancient times till the Middle Ages. Acta Physiologica Hungarica. 2004;**91**(3-4):243-261. DOI: 10.1556/APhysiol.91.2004.3-4.8

[2] Pauling L, Robinson AB, Teranish R, Cary P. Quantitative analysis of urine vapor and breath by gas-liquid partition chromatography. Proceedings of the National Academy of Sciences of the United States of America. 1971;**68**(10):2374

[3] Gisbert JP. Breath test with C-13-urea for *H. pylori* infection diagnosis by means of mass spectrometry and infrared spectrophotometry. Salud I Ciencia. 2006;**15**(1):461-463

[4] Johnson GR, Morawska L. The mechanism of breath aerosol formation. Journal of Aerosol Medicine and Pulmonary Drug Delivery. 2009;**22**(3):229-237

[5] Schwarz K, Biller H, Windt H, Koch W, Hohlfeld JM. Characterization of exhaled particles from the healthy human lung: A systematic analysis in relation to pulmonary function variables. Journal of Aerosol Medicine and Pulmonary Drug Delivery. 2010;**23**(6):371-379

[6] Hammarström S. Leukotrienes. Annual Review of Biochemistry. 1983;**52**:355-377

[7] Montuschi P, Mores N, Trové A, Mondino C, Barnes PJ. The electronic nose in respiratory medicine. Respiration. 2013;**85**(1):72-84

[8] Sapey E, editor. Bronchial Asthma: Emerging Therapeutic Strategies. Rijeka: InTech; 2012

[9] Montuschi P. New Perspectives in Monitoring Lung Inflammation. Analysis of Exhaled Breath Condensate. Vol. 11. Boca Raton: CRC Press; 2005

[10] Cap P, Pehal F, Chladek J, Maly M. Analysis of exhaled leukotrienes in nonasthmatic adult patients with seasonal allergic rhinitis. Allergy (Oxford, United Kingdom). 2005; **60**(2):171-176

[11] Effros RM. Dilution of respiratory solutes in exhaled condensates—From the authors. American Journal of Respiratory and Critical Care Medicine. 2003;**167**(5):802

[12] Kharitonov SA, Chung KF, Evans D, OConnor BJ, Barnes PJ. Increased exhaled nitric oxide in asthma is mainly derived from the lower respiratory tract. American Journal of Respiratory and Critical Care Medicine. 1996;**153**(6):1773-1780

[13] Papineri R. Journal of aerosol medicine: Deposition, clearance, and effects in the. Lung. 1997;**10**(2):105-116

[14] Chapman EA, Thomas PS, Stone E, Lewis C, Yates DH. A breath test for malignant mesothelioma using an electronic nose. European Respiratory Journal. 2012;**40**:448-454

[15] Vyas A, Zhang Q, Gunaratne S, Lee W, Lin JL, Lin JS, Warwick G, Thomas PS. The effect of temperature on exhaled breath condensate collection. Journal of Breath Research. 2012;**6**(3):7

[16] Koczulla AR, Noeske S, Herr C, De e F, Pinkenburg O, Schmid S, Örres RA, Vogelmeier C, Bals R. Ambient temperature impacts on pH of exhaled breath condensate. Respirology. 2010;**15**(1):155-159

[17] Vestbo J, Hurd S, Agustí AG, Jones PW, Vogelmeier C, Anzueto A, Barnes PJ, Fabbri LM, Martinez FJ, Nishimura M, Stckley RA. Global strategy for the diagnosis, management, and prevention of chronic obstructive pulmonary disease. American Journal of Respiratory and Critical Care Medicine. 2013;**187**(4):347-365

[18] Ćalušić AL, Varnai VM, Macan J. Acute effects of smoking and food consumption on breath condensate pH in healthy adults. Experimental Lung Research. 2011;**37**(2):92-100

[19] Kazani S, Planaguma A, Ono E, Bonini M, Zahid M, Marigowda G, Wechsler ME, Levy BD, Israel E. Exhaled breath condensate eicosanoid levels associate with asthma and its severity. Journal of Allergy and Clinical Immunology. 2013;**132**(3):547-553

[20] Lincova D, Farghali H. Základní a aplikovaná farmakologie. 2nd ed. Praha: Galén; 2007. 672 p. ISBN: 9788072623730.

[21] Nicolaou NC, Lowe LA, Murray CS, Woodcock A, Simpson A, Custovic A. Exhaled breath condensate pH and childhood asthma: Unselected birth cohort study. American Journal of Respiratory and Critical Care Medicine. 2006;**174**(3):254-259

[22] Malinovschi A, Pizzimenti S, Sciascia S, Heffler E, Badiu I, Rolla G. Exhaled breath condensate nitrates, but not nitrites or FENO, relate to asthma control. Respiratory Medicine. 2011;**105**(7):1007-1013

[23] Kačerová T, Kuzma M, Kačer P. Molecular diagnosis of bronchial asthma based on the content of cysteinyl leukotrienes and lipoxines in exhaled breath condensate. Chemicke Listy. 2017;**111**:50-55

[24] Čáp P, Benčová A, Jeseňák M. Vyšetřování vydechovaného oxidu dusnatého u asthma bronchiale. 1st ed. Praha: Mladá fronta; 2014. ISBN 978-80-204-3363-3.

[25] Collins D, Lomíček J, Lomíčková Z. Diferenciální diagnostika prvního kontaktu. 1st ed. Praha: Grada; 2007. ISBN 978-80-247-0897-3.

[26] Sedlák V. kol., a., Doporučený diagnostiky a léčby otížně léčitelného bronchiálního astmatu. 2011.

[27] Koblížek V, Chlumský J, Zindr V, Neumannová K, Zatloukal J, Sedlák V. Doporučený postup ČPFS pro diagnostiku a léčbu stabilní CHOPN. 2012.

[28] Di Stefano A, Capelli A, Lusuardi M, Balbo P, Vecchio C, Maestrelli P, Mapp CE, Fabbri LM, Donner CF, Sae a M. Severity of airflow limitation is associated with severity of airway inflammation in smokers. American Journal of Respiratory and Critical Care Medicine. 1998;**158**(4):1277-1285

[29] Retamales I, Ellio WM, Meshi B, Coxson HO, Pare PD, Sciurba FC, Rogers RM, Hayashi S, Hogg JC. Amplification of inflammation in emphysema and its association with latent adenoviral infection. American Journal of Respiratory and Critical Care Medicine. 2001;**164**(3):469-473

[30] Fattahi F, ten Hacken NHT, Löfdahl CG, Hylkema MN, Timens W, Postma DS, Vonk JM. Atopy is a risk factor for respiratory symptoms in COPD patients: Results from the EUROSCOP study. Respiratory Research. 2013;**14**(1):10-10

[31] Hardin M, Silverman EK, Barr RG, Hansel NN, Schroeder JD, Make BJ, Crapo JD, Hersh CP. The clinical features of the overlap between COPD and asthma. Respiratory Research. 2011;**12**(1):127-127

[32] Barnes PJ. Mediators of chronic obstructive pulmonary disease. Pharmacological Reviews. 2004;**56**(4):515-548

[33] Kuban P, Foret F. Exhaled breath condensate: Determination of nonvolatile compounds and their potential for clinical diagnosis and monitoring. Analytica Chimica Acta. 2013;**805**:1-18

[34] Serhan CN, Hamberg M, Samuelsson B. Lipoxins: Novel series of biologically active compounds formed from arachidonic acid in human leukocytes. Biochemical and Biophysical Research Communications. 1984;**118**(3):943-949

[35] Ariel A, Serhan CN. Resolvins and protectins in the termination program of acute inflammation. Trends in Immunology. 2007;**28**(4):176. DOI: 10.1016/j.it.2007.02.007

[36] Valavanidis A, Vlachogianni T, Fiotakis K, Loridas S. Pulmonary oxidative stress, inflammation and cancer: Respirable particulate matter, fibrous dusts and ozone as major causes of lung carcinogenesis through reactive oxygen species mechanisms. International Journal of Environmental Research and Public Health. 2013;**10**(9):3886-3907. DOI:10.3390/ ijerph10093886

[37] Bucchioni E, Kharitonov SA, Allegra L, Barnes PJ. High levels of interleukin-6 in the exhaled breath condensate of patients with COPD. Respiratory Medicine. 2003;**97**: 1299-1302

[38] Carpagnano GE, Barnes PJ, Geddes DM, Hodson ME, Kharitonov SA. Increased leukotrience B4 and interleukin-6 in exhaled breath condensate in cystic fibrosis. American Journal of Respiratory and Critical Care Medicine. 2003;**167**:1109-1112

[39] Carpagnano GE, Resta O, Foschino-Barbaro MP, Gramiccioni E, Carpagnano F. Interleukin-6 is increased in breath condensate of patients with non-small cell lung cancer. International Journal of Biological Markers. 2002;**17**:141-145

[40] Shahid SK, Kharitonov SA, Wilson NM, Bush A, Barnes PJ. Increased interleukin-4 and decreased interferon-γ in exhaled breath condensate of children with asthma. American Journal of Respiratory and Critical Care Medicine. 2002;**165**:1290-1293

[41] Carpagnano GE, Spanevello A, Curci C, Salerno F, Palladino GP, Resta O, Di Gioia G, Carpagnano F, Foschino Barbaro MP. IL-2, TNF-alpha, and leptin: Local versus systemic concentrations in NSCLC patients. Oncology Research. 2007;**16**:375-381

[42] Dalaveris E, Kerenidi T, Katsabeki-Katsafli A, Kiropoulos T, Tanou K, Gourgoulianis KI, Kostikas K. VEGF, TNF-alpha and 8-isoprostane levels in exhaled breath condensate and serum of patients with lung cancer. Lung Cancer. 2009;**64**:219-225

[43] Corradi M, Folesani G, Andreoli R, Manini P, Bodini A, Piacentini G, Carraro S, Zanconato S, Baraldi E. Aldehydes and glutathione in exhaled breath condensate of children with asthma exacerbation. American Journal of Respiratory and Critical Care Medicine. 2003;**167**:395-399

[44] Yeh MY, Burnhamc EL, Moss M, Brown LAS. Non-invasive evaluation of pulmonary glutathione in the exhaled breath condensate of otherwise healthy alcoholics burnham. Respiratory Medicine. 2008;**102**:248-255

[45] Cheng Z, Chan AK, Lewis CR, Thomas PS, Raftery MJ. Comparative Proteomics Analysis of Exhaled Breath Condensate in Lung Cancer Patients. Journal of Cancer Therapy. 2011;**2**:1-8

[46] Fumagalli M, Ferrari F, Luise i M, Stolk J, Hiemstra PS, Capuano D, Viglio S, Fregonese L, Cerveri I, Corana F, Tinelli C, Iadarola P. Profiling the proteome of exhaled breath condensate in healthy smokers and COPD patients by LCMS/MS. International Journal of Molecular Sciences. 2012;**13**:13894-13910

[47] Nishizawa S, Benkelfat C, Leyton M. Differences between males and females in ratesof serotonin synthesis in human brain. Medical Science. 1997;**94**(10):5308-5313

[48] Blenau W, Baumann A, editors. Serotonin Receptor Technologies. Vol. 1. Berlin: Humana Press; 2015

[49] Holmgren H, Gerth E, Ljungström E, Larsson P, Almstrand AC, Bake B, Olin AC. Effects of breath holding at low and high lung volumes on amount of exhaled particles. Respiratory Physiology & Neurobiology. 2013;**185**(2):228-234

4

Biomarkers in Leishmaniasis: From Basic Research to Clinical Application

Sofia Esteves, Inês Costa, Célia Amorim,
Nuno Santarem and Anabela Cordeiro-da-Silva

Abstract

Leishmania is an intracellular protozoan parasite and the etiological agent of a vector-borne disease known as leishmaniasis. This neglected tropical disease exhibits high morbidity and mortality putting at risk people from multiple countries worldwide. It is endemic in 97 countries and 700,000–1 million new cases are estimated to occur each year. Leishmaniasis management is very challenging, the symptoms are non-pathognomonic (in both human and canine populations) and the treatments are associated with significant toxicity. Therefore, the need for detection in symptomatic and asymptomatic hosts is important to tackle the dissemination of infection, increasing the need for highly specific biomarkers. In this complex the available disease biomarkers will be addressed in a retrospective manner, focusing on their development from laboratory to their direct use in clinical settings.

Keywords: leishmaniasis, biomarkers, diagnosis techniques

1. Introduction

1.1. Leishmaniasis as a neglected tropical disease

Neglected tropical diseases are a diverse group of diseases that prevail in tropical and subtropical countries. The geographical distribution of these diseases associated with lack of sanitation, close contact with domestic animals, livestock and infectious vectors contributes to disease dissemination, affecting more than 1 billion people and costs billions each year in developing economies.

Leishmaniasis is a devastating and significantly under-recognized vector-borne disease that causes serious global health burden. After malaria, it is the second parasitic disease with the highest mortality rate [1]. It mainly affects populations in Africa, Asia and Latin America, and is associated with malnutrition, population displacement, poor housing, weak immune system and lack of resources [1].

Although this disease was initially limited to the tropics and subtropics, several factors lead to the spread of leishmaniasis to new locations [2]. Perturbations of the natural vector ecosystem caused by urbanization, deforestation, global warming and natural disasters have a serious impact in disease dissemination. Increased people and animal migration, traveling and military operations contribute to disease spreading. Organ transplantation, lack of *Leishmania* screening in the blood bank or immune suppressive therapies can also contribute to disease perpetuation [2, 3].

This disease can be presented in several ways, the most common ones being: Cutaneous Leishmaniasis (CL), Mucocutaneous Leishmaniasis (MCL) and Visceral Leishmaniasis (VL), also known as kala-azar. Depending on the specific clinic-pathological form of the disease, symptoms range from cutaneous and mucosal tissue lesions to vital visceral organ damage [4, 5].

1.2. Epidemiology

Out of 200 countries and territories reporting to WHO, 97 are endemic for leishmaniasis (**Figure 1**). This includes 65 countries endemic for both VL and CL, 10 countries endemic only for VL and 22 endemic only for CL (**Figure 1**) [1].

Ninety percent of global VL cases were reported from seven countries: Brazil, Ethiopia, India, Kenya, Somalia, South Sudan and Sudan. About 95% of CL cases occur in the Americas, the

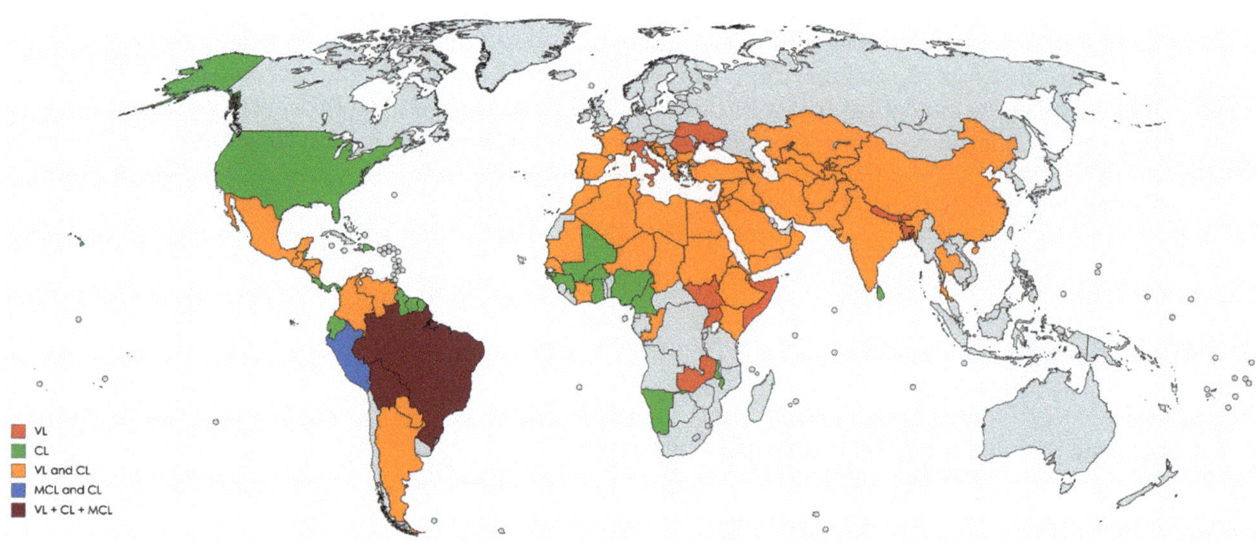

Figure 1. World map: Human leishmaniasis distribution. VL, Visceral Leishmaniasis; CL, Cutaneous Leishmaniasis; MCL, Mucocutaneous Leishmaniasis. Status of endemicity of the different forms of leishmaniasis in 2016, according to the World Health Organization.

Mediterranean basin, Middle East and Central Asia. An estimated 0.6–1 million new cases occur worldwide annually. Over 90% of MCL cases occur in Bolivia, Brazil, Ethiopia and Peru [1].

1.3. Clinical forms of the disease

CL is the most common form of leishmaniasis affecting humans. It is a skin infection that develops as a nodule in the site of inoculation, consequence of macrophage infection in the dermis. This may progress to a dermal granuloma, an ulcer that heals spontaneously or several inflamed ulcers, on the exposed parts of the body, such as the face, arms and legs [1, 5, 6]. These lesions can take months or years to heal and may leave behind atrophic scars with a hyperpigmented halo [2]. The incubation period ranges from 1 week to several months [1].

MCL is less common than CL. Unlike CL, which is confined to small areas of the skin, MCL aggressively spreads to the oral and nasal mucosa and is characterized by progressive ulcers and lesions of the face leading to significant disfiguration. The lesions can lead to partial or total destruction of the mucous membranes of the nose, mouth, throat cavities and surrounding tissues [1]. These progressively destructive ulcers, unlike CL, are not self-healing and can appear months or years after the first episode of CL. The dynamic and evolution of MCL is not completely understood [4, 7]. In endemic areas, it has been noted that in 1–10% of patients, the CL form evolves into MCL 5 years after healing [3].

VL, also known as kala-azar, is the most severe form of leishmaniasis and is fatal if left untreated in over 95% of cases [1, 8]. An incubation period (from 1 month to 2 years) is followed by clinical manifestations such as fever, splenomegaly, hepatomegaly, weight loss, progressive anemia and pancytopenia. These systemic infection symptoms are associated to the dissemination of parasites throughout the blood and reticuloendothelial system and lead to enlarged lymph nodes, spleen and liver [5].

Post-kala-azar Dermal Leishmaniasis (PKDL) is a complication of VL in areas where *Leishmania donovani* (*L. donovani*) is endemic. It is characterized by a hypopigmented macular, maculopapular, and nodular rash in a patient suffering a sequel of VL where the skin is the main focus of the infection. It usually appears 6 months to 1 or more years after apparent cure of the disease but may occur earlier or even simultaneously with visceral leishmaniasis [1, 9]. PKDL is confined to two geographically distinct zones, South Asia (India, Nepal, and Bangladesh) and East Africa (Sudan). In the South Asian variant, polymorphic lesions (macules/patches with papulonodules) are frequent, while the Sudanese variant has papular or nodular lesions. Lesions, especially the papulonodules, are parasite-rich, driving speculation that PKDL plays an important role in anthroponotic transmission of VL [10].

1.4. The vector

Leishmania protozoan parasites are transmitted by the bite of a very small (2–3 mm long) insect vector, known as the phlebotomine sandfly. Solely the female sandfly transmits the parasites, and only 30 from the 500 species of phlebotomine transmit this disease [1]. Female sandflies become infected with *Leishmania* parasites upon a blood meal from an infected person or animal which they need for egg development. Over a period between 4 and 25 days, the parasites develop in the sandfly. This development period can be extended at low temperatures or shortened at high temperatures [3]. The transmission cycle is completed when the infectious female sandfly feeds and inoculates a host with the parasite [1].

1.5. Life cycle

The parasite life cycle requires the transmission of infectious protozoan between sandflies and a mammalian host. *Leishmania* parasites present two distinct forms: promastigotes and amastigotes. Promastigotes are the flagellated, motile forms of the parasites that develop and morphologically differentiate in the sandfly midgut to an infectious metacyclic form that is transmitted to the mammalian host when the sandfly takes a blood meal. These metacyclic promastigotes are phagocytosed by mono and polymorphonuclear cells and transformed into the ovoid shape with short flagellum known as amastigote. Upon differentiation, they replicate within the host cells. The replication may lead to the rupture of these cells, allowing infection of other phagocytes. The life cycle becomes complete when the sandfly takes another blood meal with amastigotes [11, 12].

Different *Leishmania* species are capable of causing disease and, depending on the species, the mammalian host presents different symptomatology. Although being divided by clinical symptoms, these species can also be divided by their geographical distribution in two main groups: Old World (the Eastern Hemisphere) species and New World species (caused by *Leishmania* species found in Central and South America) [2] (**Table 1**).

Location	Complex	Species	Clinical forms of the disease
Old World	*Leishmania donovani*	*L. donovani*	CL, VL, PKDL, MCL (rare)
		L. infantum	CL, VL (children), PKDL, MCL (rare)
	Leishmania tropica	*L. tropica*	CL, MCL (rare), VL (rare)
		L. major	CL, MCL (rare)
		L. aethiopica	CL, DCL
New World	*Leishmania mexicana*	*L. mexicana*	CL, DCL (rare)
		L. amazonensis	CL, DCL, MCL, VL (rare), PKLD (rare)
		L. venezuelensis	CL, DCL (rare)
	Leishmania (Viannia) braziliensis	*L. braziliensis*	CL, MCL, VL
		L. panamensis	CL, MCL
		L. guyanensis	CL, MCL
		L. peruviana	CL
	Leishmania donovani	*L. infantum*	CL, VL (children), PKDL, MCL (rare)

VL, Visceral Leishmaniasis; CL, Cutaneous Leishmaniasis; MCL, Mucocutaneous Leishmaniasis; PKDL, Post-Kala-azar Dermal Leishmaniasis; DCL, Diffused Cutaneous Leishmaniasis. Adapted from Kevric et al. [2].

Table 1. Geodistribution of the organisms prevalent and disease patterns.

VL form, the most severe form of leishmaniasis, is caused by *L. donovani* (East Africa and the Indian subcontinent) and *L. infantum* (Europe, North Africa, Latin America). While *L. donovani* infects all age groups, *L. infantum* infects mostly children and immunosuppressed individuals. However, due to increasing prevalence of Human Immunodeficiency Virus (HIV) infection in the Mediterranean basin, HIV-VL coinfection in the adult population is reported frequently [13].

1.6. Transmission pattern

There are two types of disease transmission: zoonotic, where the disease is transmitted from animal to vector and then to human; and anthroponotic, transmitted from human to vector to human. Transmission also varies according to geographical regions, where *L. donovani* is responsible for anthroponotic transmission and *L. infantum* for zoonotic transmission. Traditionally, anthroponotic transmission occurs in the Indian subcontinent and East Africa, and zoonotic transmission is mostly restricted to the Mediterranean basin and South America regions.

L. donovani is found only in the Old World (except for transmission in patients that have traveled), where it is notoriously associated with VL of the rural poor areas in the northeast of the Indian subcontinent and with VL in East Africa [8, 14]. *L. infantum* is mostly associated to the zoonotic disease with the dog as a natural reservoir.

Domestic animals play a role as new opportunistic hosts, in vector adaptation to urban environments [3]. Animals such as the wild canid, marsupials and rodents have been described as reservoirs of human VL [15]. However, zoonotic VL epidemics have been associated only in areas where Canine Leishmaniasis (CanL) is endemic (**Figure 2**), indicating that dogs are the main reservoir in this type of transmission [16]. Due to the proximity of domestic dogs and human populations, CanL control is more than a veterinary concern, it is also a public health issue due to the zoonotic potential of the disease.

1.7. Canine leishmaniasis

CanL is a major concern for the veterinary community, having high mortality and morbidity rates. Moreover, in endemic areas, domestic dogs are the primary target of infection allowing perpetuation of the life cycle [17].

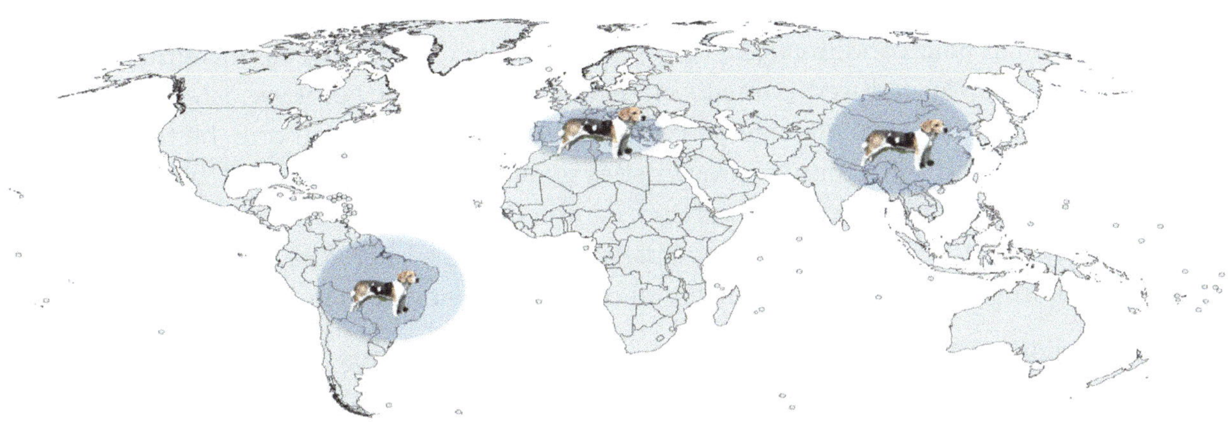

Figure 2. World map: Regions with higher canine leishmaniasis incidence – Brazil, Mediterranean basin and China.

After an incubation period that can range from 3 months to several years, dogs may start presenting clinical signs. However, some dogs remain asymptomatic and never develop any signs [17]. Therefore, dogs can present different forms of the disease: symptomatic, oligosymptomatic and asymptomatic. Dogs that develop few mild symptoms are classified as oligosymptomatic. Even so, it is relevant to mention that it is not consensual that all forms of the disease enable the transmission of the parasite. Infected dogs present non-specific cutaneous alterations such as alopecia, onychogryposis, dermatitis, skin ulceration, anorexia, weight loss and visceral manifestations with splenic, renal and hepatic disorders [18], making an accurate diagnosis impossible.

Given that canine disease usually precedes the appearance of human cases and a clear correlation between canine and human infection rates has been demonstrated, CanL must be considered as a risk for human health [3].

2. Importance of diagnosis

The available therapies for leishmaniasis are far from optimal due to their toxicity, high costs, lack of efficacy, lack of access in certain areas, and emerging drug resistance. Treatment efficacy depends on strains and species and there are currently no effective vaccines available for any form of human leishmaniasis [2].

Some vaccines exist for veterinary use. Being launched in Portugal in 2011, CaniLeish® was the first vaccine for CanL in the European Union. In Brazil, LeishTec® vaccine was also registered but only offers about 40% of protection against infection. LetiFend® has recently been registered in Europe, but there is limited information available [19]. Despite the efforts, *Leishmania* vaccinology still has a lot to improve till an effective and universal vaccine is developed [20].

In the absence of human vaccines and due to the zoonotic character of the disease, accurate detection of infection in humans and dogs is crucial for the control of leishmaniasis [21].

Several specific challenges associated to *Leishmania* infection and leishmaniasis must be overcome. As for any disease, the diagnostic process should be simple, robust, automated, requiring inexpensive reagents and minimal operator intervention without diminishing the fidelity of the results. Notwithstanding, considering that this disease affects mostly poor people in countries with undeveloped and underfinanced health systems, the tests should be cheap and easy to perform in field conditions [22, 23]. Moreover, the detection of asymptomatic infection, often characterized by reduced parasite loads and low specific serology, is essential. In fact, clinical and epidemiological management of *Leishmania* infections can only be fully successful once a diagnostic test with these characteristics is available [24]. The available tools are adequate for detection of disease, (in conjunction with clinical evaluation) but present limitations for diagnosis of infection in asymptomatic patients and dogs. Therefore, the information of real prevalence of infection and overall burden of disease is believed to be underestimated [22].

Coinfection with HIV is common in VL cases and has a disastrous impact since immunocompromised individuals have more severe manifestations and atypical symptoms that complicate treatment [2]. Pregnant women can be considered a risk population, as HIV-infected patients, being more susceptible to *Leishmania* relapse and changes in immune response. Immunosuppression by HIV had an enormous impact and highly contributed to the increased number of leishmaniasis cases [3]. Coinfection of *L. donovani* and *L. infantum* with HIV has been identified as a meaningful clinical problem, and presents higher mortality rates. Up to 70% of VL cases in southern Europe are associated with HIV infection. VL is the third most frequent opportunistic infection in many parts of the world, and the coinfection with HIV is now reported in 35 countries [25].

3. Biomarkers to use in diagnosis

Every methodology has a detection limit associated but the specificity of the diagnosis platform is mostly influenced by the antigen used, relying on it to produce high confidence results.

Several antigens were proposed overtime but the most common one is crude soluble antigen (CSA) [13, 26]. Although the sensitivity of CSA in Enzyme-Linked Immunosorbent Assay (ELISA) is high, cross-reactivity with other diseases (trypanosomiasis, toxoplasmosis and tuberculosis) occurs frequently, leading to false positive results [27, 28]. Therefore specificity can be low due to cross-reactivity and is not suitable in detecting seropositivity in asymptomatic dogs [29–31]. This is transversal to other serological techniques like Direct Agglutination Test (DAT) or Indirect Fluorescent Antibody Technique (IFAT) which are based on the recognition of the parasite total antigens. The specificity and sensitivity problems associated to conventional assays (such as IFAT, DAT, and CSA ELISA) may be overcome using recombinant polypeptides containing specific epitopes that are able to induce an immune response in most dogs and humans with VL. Hence, there has been a focus on expressing and purifying *Leishmania* proteins that elicit an immune response in dogs and humans and analyze them and their potential for serological tests [32–34].

The evolution of molecular technology (immunoproteomics) and sequencing of the *Leishmania* genome in 2005 have been powerful tools for the discovery of recombinant *Leishmania* proteins to use in the serodiagnosis of human and canine leishmaniasis [35, 36]. Variability in the humoral response concerning different parasite antigens observed in infection suggests that a combination of recombinant proteins can improve the diagnosis efficiency [37]. In fact, each antigen carries often both specific immune-dominant epitopes and other regions that are not important for serological recognition [38]. Therefore, an ideal test would contain a combination of relevant epitopes in a single recombinant antigen, more specific than crude antigen preparation and more sensitive than single epitope-based ELISA [39]. In fact, chimeric multi-epitope proteins are part of the future strategy to look for novel high specific antigens [40]. Several recombinant proteins with high efficacy have reasonable results for the diagnosis of human and canine VL, but development of suitable antigens for diagnosis is still necessary [34].

The most common used antigens belong to different protein families, such as the kinesin-related proteins, heat shock proteins, acidic ribosomal proteins, nuclear proteins, enzymes and other antigens which are associated with parasite function [41].

3.1. Kinesin-related proteins

Kinesins are a family of motor proteins in eukaryotic cells, and constitute part of the microtubule cytoskeleton in *Leishmania* parasites, important in its growth and differentiation [42–44].

Several *Leishmania* antigens have been characterized, as the recombinant K39 antigen (rK39), a 39-aminoacid-repetitive B-cell epitope of the kinesin-related protein of *L. infantum*. The rK39 ELISA has shown to be capable of detecting human and canine VL.

The K9 and K26 are two other hydrophilic antigens of *L. infantum*, and their recombinant antigens (rK9 and rK26) have been used to diagnose VL. The rK28 is a recombinant fusion protein with tandem repeats of K39 kinesin regions and K26, and has been used to detect high levels of antibody responses in infected patients, using ELISA [13, 37].

The rK39, an antigen used for VL diagnosis, is highly conserved among VL species [15]. Several studies carried out in VL endemic areas have demonstrated that the rK39 ELISA is a sensitive and a specific method for the serodiagnosis of human VL [34, 45–47]. An important aspect of the anti-rK39 antibody is that the titer correlates directly with the disease activity, indicating its potential for use in predicting response to therapy [48]. The rk39 has also been tested for ELISA and Flow Cytometry (FC) assays showing high sensitivity and specificity in detecting clinical forms of CanL [49]. rK39 is further addressed in Section 5—Successful diagnosis approaches—from laboratory to field conditions.

VL patients also have a strong antibody response to K26, which can complement rK39 in a better and more accurately diagnosis of human VL [50]. Specific and independent antibody reactivity to each of these antigens (rK9, rK26 and rK39) have been studied and tested in serodiagnosis of canine VL [31, 51].

Another antigen that has been successfully used in the diagnosis of human VL is rK28. This recombinant fusion antigen was used for ELISA and has shown sensitivity and specificity values similar or higher than those obtained for rK39. Therefore, this antigen has been proposed as a new choice, especially regarding regions where rK39 has shown low levels of sensitivity [52]. In Sudan and in India [53], human serological surveys using rK28 antigen have shown good performance with high sensitivity and specificity [54]. ELISA with rK28 antigen was 100% sensitive and specific in serological diagnosis of CanL [54]. The sensitivity of rK28 was slightly higher than rK39, although no significant differences in the detection of positive dogs were observed, indicating that both antigens may be useful for diagnosing CanL, as previously observed in VL in human [54, 55].

KE16 is another kinesin gene derived from the C-terminus of the kinesin protein from an isolate of *L. donovani* [56] that has been successfully cloned and expressed. It is used in the rKE16 dipstick test, a one-step rapid immunochromatographic test. Results showed that this antigen can be used as a highly specific and sensitive tool for VL diagnosis, although, in dogs, the average of positive cases among asymptomatic dogs was low [34, 56, 57].

3.2. Heat shock proteins

Heat Shock Proteins (HSPs) are a family of proteins that are produced by cells in response to stressful conditions. They are highly conserved molecules that play important roles in protein folding, assembly of protein complexes, and translocation of proteins across cellular compartments.

The *L. donovani* HSP70 was identified after screening of a cDNA library with serum from a patient with VL [58]. It is found in prokaryotic and eukaryotic cells and is a highly conserved protein. HSP70s from other *Leishmania* species (*L. infantum* and *L. braziliensis* [59]) have also been characterized.

rHSP70 had high sensitivity and specificity values, being superior to CSA in the diagnosis of CL [60]. The antigenicity of heat shock proteins in general and of HSP70 specifically is not unexpected, since antibodies against the parasite recombinant HSPs have been found in sera of patients with different parasitic diseases [61, 62]. Other authors have described rHSP70 as a preeminent antigen present in *Leishmania* [63]. Specific antibodies against *L. braziliensis* rHSP70 or rHSP83 were found in 95% of sera from ML or CL patients and a high recognition of rHSP70 by sera from the same patients has been detailed [59].

L. infantum-rHSP83 is a possible antigen to be used in the serodiagnosis of leishmaniasis, due to its high specificity and sensitivity and insignificant cross-reactivity with other infectious diseases [48]. Members of the HSP83/90 family have also been described as immunodominant antigens during infections caused by *L. donovani*, *L. braziliensis* and *L. infantum* [64].

Another gene, *LmSti1*, encoding a stress-inducible protein STI1 [65] was strongly recognized in sera from human patients with CL, VL and post-kala azar CL [48].

3.3. Ribosomal proteins

Ribosomal proteins have been described to induce antibodies in animal and humans infected with the parasite, making them a favorable candidate to assess its diagnosis potential.

Studies have described some *Leishmania* ribosomal proteins function as immunoregulatory molecules [41, 59]. As a matter of fact, the eukaryotic ribosome is composed of four RNA molecules and more than 70 ribosomal proteins [66]. Furthermore, the acidic ribosomal proteins (P-proteins) have been detailed as prominent antigens during *Leishmania* infections [41, 67].

The large subunit of ribosomes contains various copies of a protein called P protein. P1, P2 and P0 form a complex notorious for having an essential role in protein synthesis. Three *L. infantum* antigens (LiP2a, LiP2b and LiP0), homologous to acidic ribosomal proteins, were identified after immunoscreening of a cDNA expression library with CanL serum [68]. They are also recognized by sera from patients with either VL or MCL [41, 69].

The ribosomal proteins LiP2a, LIP2b, LiP0/LcP0 and LeIF, all conserved antigens of *Leishmania*, have been shown to be recognized by the immune system of the host [70].

The *L. infantum* acidic ribosomal proteins, LiP2a and LiP2b, have disease-specific antigenic determinants identified by more than 80% of canine VL [70]. Engineered LiP2a and LiP2b recombinant proteins are shown to be useful as tools to discriminate between VL and Chagas disease [71]. *L. infantum* P0 ribosomal protein is also recognized by a high percentage of the sera from dogs with VL [70].

The acidic ribosomal proteins (P1, P2 and P0) are recognized by antibodies frequently found in sera from systemic lupus erythematosus (SLE) patients. These autoantibodies recognize an amino acid sequence located at the C-terminal ends of the three P proteins [72]. Furthermore, patients with chronic Chagas heart disease produce a strong humoral response against the C-terminal of *Trypanosoma cruzi* ribosomal P proteins. *Leishmania* ribosomal P2a and P2b C-terminal end of the proteins is also well conserved and these proteins are recognized by sera from both SLE and Chagas disease patients [69]. The anti-P antibodies produced during the *Leishmania* infection do not recognize the conserved C-terminal domain of the P proteins. Therefore, to avoid cross-reactivity, engineered versions of the recombinant proteins LiP2a and LiP2b, without the C-terminal ends, have been found to be useful for the diagnosis of MCL and VL [69].

3.4. Peroxiredoxins

Tryparedoxins belong to a particular class of oxidoreductases related to thioredoxins and found in trypanosomatids. They bear oxidoreductase activity toward disulfide bridges and are crucial to the parasite, as they are expressed in all stages of development [73]. These proteins are believed to be involved in *Leishmania* detoxification of peroxides.

LiTXN1 protein is present in the cytosol and upregulated in the infectious forms of the parasite, indicating that it plays an important role during infection. LiTXN1 preferentially reduces the cytosolic *L. infantum* peroxiredoxins, LicTXNPx1 and LicTXNPx2 [73].

LicTXNPx antigen is highly immunogenic during both human and canine infections [74]. High antibody titers are found during the *Leishmania* infection and these decrease after its resolution [75].

Anti-LicTXNPx antibodies are present in both symptomatic and asymptomatic experimental canine infections, making this antigen a good candidate marker and a prognostic indicator for monitoring the response to CanL treatment [75]. An ELISA with both LicTXNPx and rK39 antigens (LAM-ELISA) was performed to improve specificity and sensitivity of this methodology and presented promising results. This test associated with DAT may be a valuable tool for screening CanL [22, 30].

3.5. Cysteine proteinases

This family of proteins is associated to disease progression. Activity of cysteine proteases can be found in parasite surface or inside the macrophage endoplasmatic reticulum. Domains of cysteine proteinases (CP), type I (CPB) and type II (CPA), were used to diagnose active and recovered cases of VL in both humans and dogs. *Leishmania* cysteine proteinases had already been used as vaccines targets and in chemotherapy [76].

A recombinant cysteine proteinase from *L. chagasi*, rLdccys1, has shown to be a good biomarker for the different stages of both human and CanL. ELISA assays showed high sensitivity and specificity. Moreover, the fact that it is possible to detect clinical and subclinical forms of the disease in canines indicates that this biomarker is important in the control of CanL in endemic areas [77, 78].

3.6. Nuclear proteins

Histones are structural proteins involved in the organization and function of DNA within the eukaryotic nucleus. There are four main classes of histones: H2A, H2B, H3 and H4 which form the nucleosomal core unit of chromatin. These proteins are among the most conserved proteins in eukaryotic organisms, maintaining sequence and function in trypanosomatids. Histones are prominent antigens found in animals during *Leishmania* infection that trigger a specific immune response and antibody production [39]. Also, sera from children infected with VL specifically recognize the *L. infantum* H2A and H2B histones, with high specificity and sensitivity in ELISA assays.

3.7. A2 proteins

A2 proteins of *L. donovani* are only present in the amastigote stage, and help visceralization of parasites in the mammalian host. They are overexpressed in the amastigote stage in *L. donovani* as well as *L. mexicana* species complex, including *L. amazonensis*, but not in *L. tropica* or *L. braziliensis* species complexes. Anti-A2 antibodies were detected in human and dog sera suffering from active VL [79, 80]. Also, it was found that rA2 is more sensitive when compared to the rK39 and rK26 antigens, for serological detection of asymptomatic infection in dogs [34].

3.8. *Leishmania* homolog of receptors for activated C kinase

Leishmania homolog of receptors for activated C Kinase (LACK) was identified after a search for parasite antigens recognized by a protective Th1 clone derived from the spleen of BALB/c mice that had been vaccinated with a soluble extract of *L. major* promastigotes. It has been proposed that the LACK protein contains an immunodominant epitope that acts as a target of early immune responses [41, 81].

3.9. rKLO8

Sudan has the highest number of reported cases in East Africa [82], in particular in eastern and central regions. Field tests based on rK39 commonly have a high reliability in various countries [83, 84]; however, the low sensitivity in Sudan limits its use in this region. A novel *L. donovani*-derived recombinant immunodominant protein (rKLO8) was tested for detection of VL in Sudan.

The results presented with rKLO8 show increased reactivity with patient sera as compared to rK39 ELISA [85]. The rKLO8 ELISA is more sensitive than the DAT and rK39 strip test, and VL patients from Sudan were tested and have decreased immune responses to rK39, confirming the low sensitivity of rK39 strip test in Sudan. Malaria is common in VL endemic regions of Africa and Asia [86] and is known to be a major cause of cross reactivity to rK39 [84]. Sera of malaria patients were tested and did not give a signal in the rKLO8 ELISA. In conclusion, rKLO8 is a novel recombinant protein of *L. donovani* with increased reactivity to VL sera from Sudan and a valuable candidate to be used in diagnosis in this area [84].

3.10. Secreted proteins

Traditionally the intrinsic intracellular and surface proteins of the parasites were targeted as primary source of antigens. Recently, secreted proteins are considered an untapped source of possible antigens and are being exploited using combinations of bioinformatic and immunoproteomic approaches [87, 88] .

3.11. Lipids

Lipid levels are known to vary in acute and chronic infections. In these infections, there is typically a decrease of total cholesterol levels and an increase in the concentration of triglyceride-rich lipoproteins; mainly very low-density lipoproteins. Moreover, apolipoprotein A1, apolipoprotein B and low-density lipoprotein cholesterol levels decrease. In leishmaniasis, this lipid concentration difference may have a prognostic and diagnostic role, as lipids play an important role in the innate and adaptive immune response. Although these have potential as clinical markers, several factors have to be taken into account when interpreting lipids values, such as: genetic and environmental factors, malnutrition, reduced food intake during acute infection, and acute kidney injury and/or acute liver failure (many times associated with this neglected disease), all which influence lipids parameters. More efforts have to be put in the study of these molecules as disease markers [89].

4. Diagnosis approaches

Due to its wide range of manifestations, leishmaniasis diagnosis can be difficult [90]. Clinical manifestations can also be confused with other illnesses, often common in *Leishmania* endemic areas, such as malaria, toxoplasmosis and tuberculosis [91]. Age, medical history and host immune system response are crucial parameters for diagnosis.

Diagnosis of diseased patients and animals can be confirmed with conventional laboratorial techniques, such as visualization of the parasite in tissues by microscopic examination of a stained specimen, or *in vitro* culture of the parasite from biopsies or aspirates from lesions, lymph nodes, spleen and bone marrow. Other diagnosis methods include molecular detection of parasitic DNA in tissue samples and serological tests that detect anti-*Leishmania* antibodies [6]. Overall, the available techniques can detect active disease. Still, leishmaniasis has intrinsic particularities that require not only the detection of symptomatic (diseased) conditions but also asymptomatic (infected, not diseased). This control is important, especially in the context of CanL, as the asymptomatic animals act as reservoirs, and as mentioned above, increase the risk for the human variant of the disease. An already complex scenario rendered more complicated by the need to distinguish treated, exposed and vaccinated. Therefore, leishmaniasis is a very particular disease and one of the many examples where ongoing research for a new and affordable diagnosis approaches is necessary.

4.1. Parasitological diagnosis

The gold standard for diagnosis is the microscopic observation of parasites in tissue samples. Parasite rich localizations like bone marrow, skin lesions, liver, lymph nodes and spleen are preferred. Identification of amastigotes by direct examination of aspirates is also possible but must be done by experts since the results are often dependent on the observer [6]. It can also originate false negative results due to the low number of parasites in some samples, particularly in asymptomatic cases. Most often, diagnostic is obtained by observation of the *Leishmania* amastigote forms in stained microscopic preparations with Giemsa [8]. The best results are obtained with parasite rich regions like spleen aspirates. With bone marrow aspirates, the sensitivity decreases considerably and lymph nodes aspirates have the worst sensitivity ranges [4]. This method requires trained personnel and involves invasive sampling, a risky procedure that can lead to fatal hemorrhage, which can only be performed in a place with access to appropriate medical facilities. Lymph node and bone marrow aspirates are safer; however, material obtained is less concentrated and therefore less sensitive, elevating the risk of false negatives [92]. All these methods include invasive sampling, are time-consuming and impracticable to be performed on a large scale [3].

The culture of infected tissues is another classical diagnostic test, although the major problem with this technique is that different species of *Leishmania* can have different growth requirements and contaminations are recurrent. The culture is performed through the inoculation of the triturated tissue in adequate media. Both techniques (microscopic exam and culture) have an overall sensitivity of around 85% [3]. The best results are obtained with spleen aspirates (93–98% of sensitivity). When it comes to bone marrow aspirates, the sensitivity comes down to 60 to 85% and worse results are obtained with lymph nodes aspirates (sensitivity ranges between 52 to 58%) [4]. Despite being more sensitive than microscopic examination, it is time consuming and expensive, therefore rarely used for clinical diagnosis [93].

4.1.1. *Xenodiagnosis*

A positive serological test result is not enough to prove that an infected dog is capable of transmitting the pathogen to the vector. Lack of sensitivity contributes to the lack of diagnostic control efficiency. The only technique that evaluates if an infected mammalian host can transmit the parasite by natural means to the vector is xenodiagnosis [94–96]. Sandflies are placed inside specific containers and placed in contact with dogs for a certain period of time for a blood meal to occur. After the feeding, the sandflies are separated and the feeding rate is calculated. The presence of parasites in the sandfly can be evaluated by direct observation of the promastigote forms by optical microscopy or Polymerase Chain Reaction (PCR). This test can be highly specific and sensitive, depending on parasite load and procedure implementation [96].

4.1.2. Montenegro skin test

The Montenegro Skin Test evaluates the late cellular hypersensitivity response. A solution with promastigotes is injected intradermally, and a positive result consists in the appearance of a hardened papule, equal or greater than 5 mm after 48 hours of injection. The test is low cost and highly sensitive (can reach over 90%). A positive result is possible within 3 months after infection, and relates to the disease evolution. Specificity is low (around 75%) due to the overall large number of false positive results in cases of unapparent infection and cross-reactivity with some pathologies, as well as technical problems [97].

4.2. Molecular methodologies

PCR technology has become an indispensable tool for the diagnosis of many parasitic diseases, including leishmaniasis. It suffers similar limitations to the parasitological tests, where the success is limited by the quality of the sample (parasite rich specific locations), as these techniques are based on the amplification of specific parasitic DNA sequences. Although several DNA targets exist, like rRNA or ITS-1 gene, the most common DNA target is the *Leishmania* kinetoplast (kDNA) present in the minicircles of the parasite [98]. The diagnostic sensitivity of these approaches is above 95% [99, 100] . In asymptomatic dogs the reported efficacy is lower, less than 70% [100]. *Leishmania* DNA has been found to be present in the canine oral mucosa, and can possibly be used for diagnostic. Oral swabs have shown positive results in molecular diagnosis of infected dogs. Although, in samples from asymptomatic dogs, the diagnosis test showed lack of sensitivity. Oral swabs combined with conjunctival ones can be used for detection of *L. infantum* in asymptomatic dogs. The big advantage of this test is that the sample collection is non-invasive, and combining this two swab methods, can significantly contribute for detecting different stages of the infection [101]. The sensitivity of a PCR assay depends on three factors: the physicochemical conditions of the reaction, the concentration of the DNA target and the selected PCR primers [38, 102, 103]. Amplification-based methods include the conventional PCR and qPCR (quantitative polymerase chain reaction) [104]. Real-time PCR (qPCR) is an innovative approach of target DNA quantification, faster than conventional PCR [102].

Although these techniques have a higher sensitivity for asymptomatic cases and early-stage infections when compared to serological methods, they imply high costs due to sophisticated equipment, reagents and specialized personnel [103, 105, 106].

4.3. Serological diagnosis

Serological tests are based on the screening of antigen or antibodies. Antigen detection should be more specific for diagnosis that antibody-based immunodiagnostic tests. Thus, antigen levels are expected to correlate with parasite burden, being useful when antibody prediction is deficient. This approach should avoid cross-reactivity and distinguish active from past infections [8]. However, this technique is still unreliable (lack of specificity and variable sensitivity). Efforts are being made to improve this tool, as it stands as a promising approach.

Currently, most clinical and surveillance laboratories use serological techniques to detect pathogen-specific antibodies, since direct methods are often either invasive, potentially fatal or expensive. *Leishmania* infection is characterized by the presence of a significant humoral response, leading to the production of antibodies against *Leishmania* species. Serological methods to detect these anti-*Leishmania* antibodies are useful as alternative diagnosis tests for both human and canine *Leishmania* infections [107]. The presence of anti-*Leishmania* antigens/antibodies in both asymptomatic and symptomatic infected dogs has allowed the development of agglutination tests, immunofluorescent serologic tests (such as Western blotting), immunochromatographic tests, and enzyme-linked immunosorbent assays (ELISAs). The sensitivity depends on the methodology but the specificity will depend on the antigen used. Serological tests are the current tests of choice to diagnose CanL. Although, these tests often lack sensitivity and specificity due to dog low specific antibody titers in the early stages of infection. Significant cross-reactivity has also been reported [108]. Additionally, after a successful treatment, antibody levels take a while to decrease. This can mask a relapse, making it impossible to diagnose it. The introduction of commercial vaccines against CanL raised concerns since it can lead to antibody production and might prevent accurate results in serological tests for the diagnosis. This may not allow differentiating between Infected and Vaccinated Animals (DIVA) [19]. Most commercially available vaccines against CanL are not DIVA. This difficults the serological identification of animals that become sick or infected in the future [19].

4.3.1. Direct agglutination test

Originally created as an alternative to the risky procedure of splenic aspirates, the Direct Agglutination Test (DAT) was the first antibody detection test used in VL diagnosis and has been used for more than 25 years. DAT is a simple semi-quantitative diagnostic tool, with a high sensitivity (91–100%), specificity (72–100%), accuracy, reliability and inexpensiveness [4, 109].

DAT detects parasite antibodies in infected blood or serum through direct agglutination. It is a semi-quantitative method based on visual agglutinations obtained by the increased dilution of blood or serum mixed with stained, killed parasites in V-shaped wells [110]. If the result is negative (absence of anti-*Leishmania* antibodies) DAT antigen accumulates at the bottom of the plate. If there are anti-*Leishmania* antibodies present, the antigens form a film over the well (positive result) [6, 111]. DAT has some disadvantages; it requires moderate technical expertise (the interpretation of the results depend on the person analyzing the results, creating inter-observer discrepancy) [112], serial dilutions must be done (requiring a considerable volume of antigen) and has a relatively long incubation time [112]. DAT results remain positive long after the patient is cured (anti-*Leishmania* antibodies can persist for years as a result of a VL infection), making this test inappropriate for detecting relapses [8].

4.3.2. Enzyme-linked immunosorbent assay

Enzyme-linked immunosorbent assay (ELISA) is an important serodiagnosis technique used in almost all infectious diseases, including VL. ELISA assays are based on the detection of antibodies present in blood or serum. An antigen/recombinant protein is used to coat the plate and samples are added and incubated. A secondary antibody conjugated with an enzyme recognizes and binds to the primary antibody. After adding a substrate, product susceptible to colorimetric determination is developed and the results can be measured by optical density techniques.

This tool is frequently used to detect anti-*Leishmania* antibodies due to its high sensitive and specificity as well as good reproducibility and high throughput screening of large number of samples, at an affordable expense. However, the specificity of this technique depends on the antigen used. ELISA's major disadvantage is its inadaptability in poor-resource field conditions and requiring specialized operators.

4.3.3. Indirect fluorescent antibody technique

Indirect Fluorescent Antibody Technique (IFAT) is an extremely valuable tool that allows assessment of anti-*Leishmania* antibody titers produced by infected individuals. It is a quite useful method in epidemiological studies and in clinical practice [113]. Promastigote or amastigote forms have been used as a source for antigens used by IFAT [25]. IFAT is based on the use of fluorophores to detect antibodies that recognize the parasites. It involves the use of a primary antibody that binds to the antigen and allows the formation of an antigen-antibody complex. Posteriorly, the binding of a fluorophore-conjugated secondary antibody results in an amplified signal that can be examined by fluorescence microscopy. IFAT is the serological gold standard for diagnosis of CanL in most countries. This analytical methodology differs from ELISA as it resorts to the whole body parasite as antigen [113]. Although having a high specificity and sensitivity (100% and 90%, respectively), IFAT sensitivity is lower for asymptomatic infections when compared to ELISA [29, 114].

4.3.4. Immunochromatographic tests

Immunochromatographic (IC) tests are recurrently used in large-scale screenings. The results obtained from IC tests consider the epidemiological context and do not require antibody titration [115]. IC test is based on chromatographic and relies on capillary action. An antigen-antibody complex is formed and entrapped on the membrane. The sample migrates across this membrane, the antibodies present in the blood recognize the antigen and the labeled antibody present in the membrane resulting in the formation of a colored product. IC tests are inexpensive, practical, rapid and suitable for field use. However, these tests frequently lead to false positives with patients in endemic regions that have already been infected in the past. Resultantly, this technique does not work in the diagnosis of relapsed patients [115]. Much like ELISA, the specificity and sensitivity of IC test is dependent on the antigen used.

4.3.5. Flow cytometry

Flow Cytometry (FC) is an emerging technique for the diagnostic of several infectious diseases [116]. It has a high throughput capacity, possibility of quantification, high reproducibility and sensitivity and potential for multiplexing [49]. This technique analyses and sorts cells or particle suspensions in a controlled fluid stream, through the measurement of fluorescence and scatter induced illumination, allowing the acquisition of structural and functional data.

The flow cytometry technique can quantify the antibodies against *Leishmania* surface antigens, restraining potential cross-reactivity against more conserved intracellular structures [117] and showing potential to monitor post chemotherapy VL, in order to evaluate the success of treatment [118].

As described before, every diagnosis technique has its downsides. Parasite demonstration in tissue smears and culture provide definitive diagnosis of VL, but generally have a lower sensitivity than serologic methods with a high risk associated. Microscopy techniques lacks sensitivity, whereas culture requires a longer time to obtain a result and is vulnerable to contamination [119].

Molecular diagnostic tools like PCR and real-time PCR are quite sensitive and specific although difficult to perform in field conditions and costly [8]. Its use remains largely restricted to some hospitals and research centers [90].

Serological tests are often not sensitive enough to detect asymptomatic individuals, having to be combined with classical methods of diagnosis to confirm. ELISA, IFAT, DAT and rK39 immunochromatographic strip test (ICT) are highly sensitive and specific when analyzing active VL in immunocompetent individuals. This does not happen when titers decline and parasite charge is lower. Due to this, false negative results frequently happen in immunocompromised patients and asymptomatic *Leishmania* infections [120].

In that way, the big challenge in the field is to isolate, recombine, produce and identify new proteins capable of detecting asymptomatic leishmaniasis cases and early stages of infection in VL endemic regions, using safe techniques that are easy, fast, sensitive and with a fair cost.

The importance of serological methods has been rising in vector-borne diseases, due to the low sensitivity associated to the microscopic methods [52]. Molecular biology developments over the years have led to advances in techniques that aided in VL control and had significant progress in surveillance and diagnosis of this disease [52].

The main problem with leishmaniasis diagnosis is the identification of markers that can detect the presence of low titres of antibodies. Thus, new markers are needed to contribute for a more accurate diagnosis capable of detecting asymptomatic cases and early stages of disease in large screening studies [38, 121].

5. Successful diagnosis approaches-from laboratory to field conditions

Currently, the scientific community is investing in developing VL tests based on antigen detection, such as rapid diagnostic tests.

Rapid diagnostic tests (RDTs) are equipment-free diagnostic devices that are adequate for field conditions. The results of this test can be read easily and in a short amount of time. Most RDTs work by capturing either an antigen or an antibody on a solid surface and then attaching molecules that allow detection by the naked eye.

5.1. Immunochromatographic Tests

These Immunochromatographic Tests (ICTs) usually based on immunochromatography with a dipstick, are used for VL diagnosis using protein from *Leishmania* as the antigen [110]. The RDTs for VL, above all but not exclusively the rK39-based ICTs, seem to be the present solution for field diagnosis in field settings due to their ease of use, convenience and cost, making them potentially favorable to increase patients' access to VL diagnosis and treatment [110]. There is a limited number of commercially available RDTs for VL [110] (**Table 2**).

The scientific technological advances in recombinant antigens as reagents for the serological diagnosis of VL have resulted in high sensitivity and specificity of the serological tests. Several recombinant proteins have been shown to be useful for the diagnosis of *Leishmania* infection both in humans and dogs [34]. Recombinant antigens such as the above mentioned rK9, rK16, rK26, rK28 and rk39 have been evaluated for its potential use in rapid diagnostic tests in field conditions.

Of all commercial RDTs, the rK39 is the most widely used. The rK39 rapid immune-chromatographic dipstick test was developed to meet the need for diagnosis in field conditions. Among the recombinant antigens, this one showed promising diagnosis and has been extensively tested in the last 5 years with IC tests in several leishmaniasis endemic areas [60, 122], being associated with several commercial applications (**Table 2**). It is an easy and qualitative test able to detect anti-*Leishmania* circulating antibodies, not requiring scientifically trained personnel. The test procedure involves adding the patient's blood or serum with diluent buffer on the strip [110]. These rK39 ICTs give an immediate result (typically between 10 and 20 minutes) and give a binary reading (positive or negative) [110]. This test has been approved by the Food and Drug Administration and tested by the World Health Organization in many endemic countries. The rapid rK39 immunochromatographic dipstick test is both

Application	Product name	Bound antigen	Manufacturer
Human	DiaMed-IT LEISH	rK39	Bio-Rad Laboratories
	OnSite *Leishmania* Ab Rapid Test	rK39	CTK Biotech, Inc
	Crystal KA (Kala azar)	rKE16	Span Diagnostics, Lda
	Kalazar Detect™	rK39	InBios International Inc
Dog	Canine Visceral Leishmaniasis Dipstick*	rK39	InBios International Inc
	Anigen Rapid *Leishmania* Ab Test Kit	Na	Vtrade
	Anigen Rapid *Leishmania* Ab Test Kit	Na	BIONOTE
	Speed Leish K	Kinesin Capture Complex	Virbac Animal Health
	DPP® Canine Leishmaniasis	rK39	Bio-Manguinhos/Fiocruz
	ImmunoRun	Na	Biogal, Galed Labs.
	Canine *Leishmania* Antibody Test	HRPO Conjugate	Quicking Biotech
	Leishmania Ab	na	EcoDiagnóstica

Data representative of available information in 2016.

Table 2. Immunochromatographic tests available for *Leishmania* diagnosis.

sensitive (67–100%) and specific (70–100%) [34]. In the Indian subcontinent (India and Nepal), the test proved to have a high sensitivity and specificity but in East Africa (Sudan, Kenya and Ethiopia) the results were not so remarkable [34, 123]. These results in East Africa are not entirely understood; however, lower antibody levels for rK39 in this region might be the reason for these decreased values of sensitivity and specificity [31]. Several studies have been carried out using the dipstick form of rK39 in dogs. The results revealed an overall good sensitivity in symptomatic dogs, although the number of studies for a proper analysis is too small for a detailed comparison [34, 124]. This recombinant antigen can also be used in a latex agglutination test, where latex is used for antigen absorption. The attachment of molecules to latex particles can be accomplished through either physical adsorption or covalent coupling. However, the sensitivity of this latex test is relatively low [34]. In comparison to DAT and ELISA, dipstick rK39 is a better choice for field conditions, sufficiently sensitive and highly specific method for the diagnosis of active VL in humans as well as in dogs [34].

The diagnosis of CanL remains a problem due to lack of sensitivity or specificity in the current diagnostic tests. Nevertheless, rapid tests like the immunochromatographic-dipstick test using rK39 and rK26 proteins of *L. infantum* [32] as antigens seem to be most appropriate for diagnosis of symptomatic cases of CanL but lack sensitivity for asymptomatic dogs. Research should continue in order to develop a more sensitive and specific recombinant assay able to detect asymptomatic cases [31].

5.2. Latex agglutination kit

Latex Agglutination Kit (KATex) is a simple, noninvasive, rapid, reliable and easily executable extensively used in diagnosis of *L. donovani* in endemic areas as Sudan, India and Nepal. It is not commonly used in *L. infantum* endemic areas [125]. Latex beads coated with anti-*Leishmania* antibodies detect the presence of a low molecular weight, heat-stable glycoconjugate antigen in urine [126]. This antigen is present in both promastigote and amastigote forms of VL patients with active infection. It has a high specificity (from 82 to 100%) and a sensitivity that varies from 47 to 95%. Although, for immunocompromised patients, the sensitivity and specificity have been reported at 85–100% and at 96–100%, respectively. The antigen may be detectable from one to 6 months after treatment. The method is appropriate for the diagnosis of primary VL, for monitoring the efficacy of treatment and for the detection of sub-clinical infection. KAtex test was also tested with oral fluids, which demonstrated the usefulness of oral-fluid collection in the detection of both *Leishmania* antibodies and DNA [125]. Sensitivity was higher in saliva that in urine, but specificity was lower. The immunoassay probably detects the same antigen present in urine [125].

6. Conclusion and remarks

Currently, several biomarkers for diagnosis are available in research laboratories, with expensive and sophisticated equipment requiring trained operators, precluding their direct application for field use.

Due to the specific characteristics associated to serological methodologies, they are accepted as the ideal diagnosis approach for both human and animal use, enabling epidemiological studies. Still, a significant limitation of serological tests is their capacity to detect asymptomatic cases. Further challenges associated to the advent of vaccination still need to be addressed.

Ultimately, the goal is to find biomarkers that detect different clinical forms of the disease that can be used universally in a rapid diagnosis kit.

Acknowledgements

This chapter is a review of results of the project NORTE-01-0145-FEDER-000012, supported by Norte Portugal Regional Operation Programme (NORTE 2020), under the Portugal 2020 Partnership Agreement, throught the European Regional Development Fund (FEDER).

Author details

Sofia Esteves[1,2†], Inês Costa[1,2†], Célia Amorim[1,2,4], Nuno Santarem[1,2*] and Anabela Cordeiro-da-Silva[1,2,3*]

*Address all correspondence to: santarem@ibmc.up.pt and cordeiro@ibmc.up.pt

1 Instituto de Investigação e Inovação em Saúde, Universidade do Porto, Porto, Portugal

2 Instituto de Biologia Molecular e Celular, Parasite Disease Group, Universidade do Porto, Porto, Portugal

3 Departamento de Ciências Biológicas, Faculdade de Farmácia da Universidade do Porto, Porto, Portugal

4 Departamento de Quimica, Faculdade de Farmácia da Universidade do Porto, Porto, Portugal

†Authors with equivalent contributions

References

[1] World Health Organization. Leishmaniasis. Available from: http://www.who.int/leishmaniasis/en/ [Accessed: 2017-11-30]

[2] Kevric I, Cappel MA, Keeling JH. New world and old world Leishmania infections: A practical review. Dermatologic Clinics. 2015;**33**:579-593

[3] Torres-Guerrero E, Quintanilla-Cedillo MR, Ruiz-Esmenjaud J, et al. Leishmaniasis: A review. F1000Research. 2017;**6**:750

[4] Chappuis F, Sundar S, Hailu A, et al. Visceral leishmaniasis: What are the needs for diagnosis, treatment and control? Nature Reviews. Microbiology. 2007;**5**:873-882

[5] Roberts MTM. Current understandings on the immunology of leishmaniasis and recent developments in prevention and treatment. British Medical Bulletin. 2005;**75–76**:115-130

[6] WHO. Technical Report of the TDR Disease Reference Group on Chagas Disease HT and L. Research Priorities for Chagas Disease, Human African Trypanosomiasis and Leishmaniasis; 2012. p. 100

[7] Strazzulla A, Cocuzza S, Pinzone MR, et al. Mucosal leishmaniasis: An underestimated presentation of a neglected disease. BioMed Research International. 2013. Epub ahead of print 2013. DOI: 10.1155/2013/805108

[8] Daniell H. NIH Public Access. 2012;**76**:211-220

[9] Murray HW, Berman JD, Davies CR, et al. Advances in leishmaniasis. [Review] [199 refs]. Lancet 9496;**366**:1561-1577

[10] Mukhopadhyay D, Dalton JE, Chatterjee M. Post kala-azar dermal leishmaniasis : An unresolved mystery PKDL: Current scenario a role for antimonial drugs. Trends in Parasitology. 2015;**2015**:11-14

[11] Bates PA. Transmission of Leishmania metacyclic promastigotes by phlebotomine sand flies. International Journal for Parasitology. 2007;**37**:1097-1106

[12] Kaye P, Scott P. Leishmaniasis: Complexity at the host–pathogen interface. Nature Reviews. Microbiology. 2011;**9**:604-615

[13] Gontijo CMF, Maria MN. Laboratory diagnosis of visceral leishmaniasis laboratory diagnosis of visceral leishmaniasis. Clinical and Diagnostic Laboratory Immunology. 2002;**9**:951-958

[14] Report WH. The Wo World rld Health Report 2004 Changing History

[15] Schallig HDFH, da Silva ES, van der Meide WF, et al. Didelphis marsupialis (common opossum): A potential reservoir host for zoonotic leishmaniasis in the metropolitan region of Belo Horizonte (Minas Gerais, Brazil). Vector Borne and Zoonotic Diseases 2007; 7: 387–393.

[16] Coelho EAF, Ramírez L, Costa MAF, et al. Specific serodiagnosis of canine visceral leishmaniasis using Leishmania species ribosomal protein extracts. Clinical and Vaccine Immunology. 2009;**16**:1774-1780

[17] Gomes YM, Paiva Cavalcanti M, Lira RA, et al. Diagnosis of canine visceral leishmaniasis: Biotechnological advances. Veterinary Journal. 2008;**175**:45-52

[18] Solcà MDS, Bastos LA, Guedes CES, et al. Evaluating the accuracy of molecular diagnostic testing for canine visceral leishmaniasis using latent class analysis. PLoS One;**9**. Epub ahead of print 2014. DOI: 10.1371/journal.pone.0103635

[19] Solano-Gallego L, Cardoso L, Pennisi MG, et al. Diagnostic challenges in the era of canine *Leishmania infantum* vaccines. Trends in Parasitology. 2017;**33**:706-717

[20] Gradoni L. Canine Leishmania vaccines: Still a long way to go. Veterinary Parasitology. 2015;**208**:94-100

[21] Pejcic B, Marco RD, Parkinson G. The role of biosensors in the detection of emerging infectious diseases. Analyst. 2006;**131**:1079

[22] Santarém N, Silvestre R, Cardoso L, et al. Application of an improved enzyme-linked immunosorbent assay method for serological diagnosis of canine leishmaniasis. Journal of Clinical Microbiology. 2010;**48**:1866-1874

[23] Soper SA, Brown K, Ellington A, et al. Point-of-care biosensor systems for cancer diagnostics/prognostics. Biosensors & Bioelectronics. 2006;**21**:1932-1942

[24] Jani IV, Janossy G, Brown DWG, et al. Multiplexed immunoassays by flow cytometry for diagnosis and surveillance of infectious diseases in resource-poor settings. The Lancet Infectious Diseases. 2002;**2**:243-250

[25] Sakkas H, Gartzonika C, Levidiotou S. Laboratory diagnosis of visceral leishmaniasis. Journal of Vector Borne Diseases. 2016;**53**:8-16

[26] Desjeux P. Leishmaniasis: Current situation and new perspectives. Comparative Immunology, Microbiology and Infectious Diseases. 2004;**27**:305-318

[27] Porrozzi R, Santos MV, Teva A, et al. Comparative evaluation of enzyme-linked immunosorbent assays based on crude and recombinant Leishmanial antigens for serodiagnosis of symptomatic and asymptomatic *Leishmania infantum* visceral infections in dogs. Clinical and vaccine immunology. . Epub ahead of print 2007. DOI: 10.1128/CVI.00420-06

[28] Kumar R, Pai K, Pathak K, et al. Enzyme-linked immunosorbent assay for recombinant K39 antigen in diagnosis and prognosis of Indian visceral leishmaniasis. Clinical and Diagnostic Laboratory Immunology. 2001;**8**:1220-1224

[29] Mettler M, Grimm F, Capelli G, et al. Evaluation of enzyme-linked immunosorbent assays, an immunofluorescent-antibody test, and two rapid tests and gel tests for serological diagnosis of symptomatic and asymptomatic Leishmania infections in dogs evaluation of enzyme-linked immunosorbent A. Journal of Clinical Microbiology. 2005;**43**:5515-5519

[30] Sousa S, Lopes AP, Cardoso L, et al. Seroepidemiological survey of *Leishmania infantum* infection in dogs from northeastern Portugal. Acta Tropica. 2011;**120**:82-87

[31] Pattabhi S, Whittle J, Mohamath R, et al. Design, development and evaluation of rK28-based point-of-care tests for improving rapid diagnosis of visceral leishmaniasis. PLoS Neglected Tropical Diseases;**4**. Epub ahead of print 2010. DOI: 10.1371/journal.pntd.0000822

[32] Burns JM, Shreffler WG, Benson DR, et al. Molecular characterization of a kinesin-related antigen of Leishmania chagasi that detects specific antibody in African and American visceral leishmaniasis. Proceedings of the National Academy of Sciences. 1993;**90**:775-779

[33] Carvalho FAA, Charest H, Tavares CAP, et al. Diagnosis of American visceral leishmaniasis in humans and dogs using the recombinant Leishmania donovani A2 antigen. Diagnostic Microbiology and Infectious Disease. 2002;**43**:289-295

[34] Farahmand M, Nahrevanian H. Application of recombinant proteins for serodiagnosis of visceral leishmaniasis in humans and dogs. Iranian Biomedical Journal. 2016;**20**:128-134

[35] Maia C, Campino L. Methods for diagnosis of canine leishmaniasis and immune response to infection. Veterinary Parasitology. 2008;**158**:274-287

[36] Ivens AC. The genome of the Kinetoplastid parasite, Leishmania major. Science (80-). 2005;**309**:436-442

[37] Boarino A, Scalone A, Gradoni L, et al. Development of recombinant chimeric antigen expressing immunodominant B epitopes of *Leishmania infantum* for serodiagnosis of visceral leishmaniasis. Clinical and Vaccine Immunology. 2005;**12**:647-653

[38] Porrozzi R, Santos Da Costa MV, Teva A, et al. Comparative evaluation of enzyme-linked immunosorbent assays based on crude and recombinant leishmanial antigens for serodiagnosis of symptomatic and asymptomatic *Leishmania infantum* visceral infections in dogs. Clinical and Vaccine Immunology. 2007;**14**:544-548

[39] Soto M, Requena JM, Quijada L, et al. Multicomponent chimeric antigen for serodiagnosis of canine visceral leishmaniasis. Journal of Clinical Microbiology. 1998;**36**:58-63

[40] Faria AR, de Castro Veloso L, Coura-Vital W, et al. Novel recombinant multiepitope proteins for the diagnosis of asymptomatic *Leishmania infantum*-infected dogs. PLoS Neglected Tropical Diseases. 2015;**9**:13-16

[41] Requena JM, Alonso C, Soto M. Evolutionarily conserved proteins as prominent immunogens during Leishmania infections. Parasitology Today. 2000;**16**:246-250

[42] Albers K, Fuchs E, Biol JC, et al. Frontiers in cell biology: Articles kinesin and dynein superfamily proteins and the mechanism of organelle transport. Science (80-). 2005;**279**: 519-526

[43] Lawrence CJ, Dawe RK, Christie KR, et al. A standardized kinesin nomenclature. The Journal of Cell Biology. 2004;**167**:19-22

[44] Gerald NJ, Coppens I, Dwyer DM. Molecular dissection and expression of the LdK39 kinesin in the human pathogen, Leishmania donovani. Molecular Microbiology. 2007;**63**: 962-979

[45] Zijlstra EE, Daifalla NS, Kager PA, et al. rK39 enzyme-linked immunosorbent assay for diagnosis of Leishmania donovani infection. Clinical and Diagnostic Laboratory Immunology. 1998;**5**:717-720

[46] Ozensoy S, Ozbel Y, Turgay N, et al. Serodiagnosis and epidemiology of visceral leishmaniasis in Turkey. The American Journal of Tropical Medicine and Hygiene. 1998;**59**: 363-369

[47] Zerpa O, Ulrich M, Benitez M, et al. Epidemiological and immunological aspects of human visceral leishmaniasis on Margarita Island, Venezuela. Memórias do Instituto Oswaldo Cruz. 2002;**97**:1079-1083

[48] Celeste BJ, Arroyo Sanchez MC, Ramos-Sanchez EM, et al. Recombinant *Leishmania infantum* heat shock protein 83 for the serodiagnosis of cutaneous mucosal, visceral leishmaniases. The American Journal of Tropical Medicine and Hygiene. 2014;**90**:860-865

[49] Sousa S, Cardoso L, Reed SG, et al. Development of a fluorescent based immunosensor for the serodiagnosis of canine leishmaniasis combining immunomagnetic separation and flow Cytometry. PLoS Neglected Tropical Diseases. 2013;**7**:1-7

[50] Bhatia A, Daifalla NS, Jen S, et al. Cloning, characterization and serological evaluation of K9 and K26: Two related hydrophilic antigens of *Leishmania chagasi*. Molecular and Biochemical Parasitology. 1999;**102**:249-261

[51] Rosati S, Ortoffi M, Profiti M, et al. Prokaryotic expression and antigenic characterization of three recombinant Leishmania antigens for serological diagnosis of canine leishmaniasis. Clinical and Diagnostic Laboratory Immunology. 2003;**10**(6):1153

[52] Negri V, Sinagra AJ, Romagosa CM, et al. An rK28-based immunoenzymatic assay for the diagnosis of canine visceral leishmaniasis in Latin America. The American Journal of Tropical Medicine and Hygiene. 2016;**95**:92-98

[53] Reithinger R, Quinnell RJ, Alexander B, et al. Rapid detection of *Leishmania infantum* infection in dogs: Comparative study using an immunochromatographic dipstick test, enzyme-linked immunosorbent assay, and PCR. Journal of Clinical Microbiology. 2002; **40**:2352-2356

[54] Venturin GL, Bragato JP, Silva KLO, et al. Recombinant K28 antigen in ELISA in the diagnosis of canine visceral leishmaniosis. Parasite Immunology. 2015;**37**:670-673

[55] Manuscript A, Blood W, Count C. NIH Public Access 2009;49:1841-1850

[56] Sivakumar R, Sharma P, Chang K-P, et al. Cloning, expression, and purification of a novel recombinant antigen from Leishmania donovani. Protein Expression and Purification. 2006;**46**:156-165

[57] Sivakumar R, Dey A, Sharma P, et al. Expression and characterization of a recombinant kinesin antigen from an old Indian strain (DD8) of Leishmania donovani and comparing it with a commercially available antigen from a newly isolated (KE16) strain of *L. donovani*. Infection, Genetics and Evolution. 2008;**8**:313-322

[58] MacFarlane J, Blaxter ML, Bishop RP, et al. Identification and characterisation of a Leishmania donovani antigen belonging to the 70-kDa heat-shock protein family. European Journal of Biochemistry. 1990;**190**:377-384

[59] Skeiky YAW, Benson DR, Guderian JA, et al. Immune responses of leishmaniasis patients to heat shock proteins of Leishmania species and humans. Infection and Immunity. 1995;**63**:4105-4114

[60] Mohammadiha A, Haghighi A, Mohebali M, et al. Canine visceral leishmaniasis: A comparative study of real-time PCR, conventional PCR, and direct agglutination on sera for the detection of *Leishmania infantum* infection. Veterinary Parasitology. 2013;**192**:83-90

[61] Hedstrom R, Culpepper J, Harrison RA, et al. A major immunogen in Schistosoma mansoni infections is homologous to the heat-shock protein Hsp70. The Journal of Experimental Medicine. 1987;**165**:1430-1435

[62] Zügeli U, Kaufmann SHE. Immune response against heat shock proteins in infectious diseases. Immunobiology. 1999;**201**:22-35

[63] De Andrade CR, Kirchhoff LV, Donelson JE, et al. Recombinant Leishmania Hsp90 and Hsp70 are recognized by sera from visceral leishmaniasis patients but not Chagas' disease patients. Journal of Clinical Microbiology. 1992;**30**:330-335

[64] Justicia J, Rosales A, Bañuel E, et al. To print this article, please use the print button in the bottom toolbar of the web reader. Journal of Clinical Nursing. 2004;**19**:3274-3290

[65] Romero GAS, Boelaert M. Control of visceral leishmaniasis in latin America - a systematic review. PLoS Neglected Tropical Diseases;**4**. Epub ahead of print 2010. DOI: 10.1371/journal.pntd.0000584

[66] Wilson DN, Cate JHD. The structure and function of the eukaryotic. Cold Spring Harbor perspectives in biology. 2012;**4**:1-18

[67] Cordeiro-da-silva A, Borges MC, Guilvard E, et al. Dual role of the Leishmania major ribosomal protein S3a homologue in regulation of T- and B-cell activation. Infection and Immunity. 2001;**69**:6588-6596

[68] Soto M, Requena JM, Garcia M, et al. Genomic organization and expression of two independent gene arrays coding for two antigenic acidic ribosomal proteins of Leishmania. The Journal of Biological Chemistry. 1993;**268**:21835-21843

[69] Soto M, Requena JM, Quijada L, et al. Specific serodiagnosis of human leishmaniasis with recombinant Leishmania P2 acidic ribosomal proteins. Clinical and Diagnostic Laboratory Immunology. 1996;**3**:387-391

[70] Wallace GR, Ball AE, MacFarlane J, et al. Mapping of a visceral leishmaniasis-specific immunodominant B-cell epitope of Leishmania donovani Hsp70. Infection and Immunity. 1992;**60**:2688-2693

[71] Quijada L, Requena JM, Soto M, et al. Mapping of the linear antigenic determinants of the *Leishmania infantum* Hsp70 recognized by leishmaniasis sera. Immunology Letters. 1996;**52**:73-79

[72] Elkon K, Bonfa E, Llovet R, et al. Properties of the ribosomal P2 protein autoantigen are similar to those of foreign protein antigens. Proceedings of the National Academy of Sciences of the United States of America. 1988;**85**:5186-5189

[73] Castro H, Sousa C, Novais M, et al. Two linked genes of *Leishmania infantum* encode tryparedoxins localised to cytosol and mitochondrion. Molecular and Biochemical Parasitology. 2004;**136**:137-147

[74] Santarém N, Silvestre R, Tavares J, et al. Immune response regulation by Leishmania secreted and nonsecreted antigens. Journal of Biomedicine & Biotechnology. 2007. Epub ahead of print 2007. DOI: 10.1155/2007/85154

[75] Santarém N, Tomás A, Ouaissi A, et al. Antibodies against a *Leishmania infantum* peroxiredoxin as a possible marker for diagnosis of visceral leishmaniasis and for monitoring the efficacy of treatment. Immunology Letters. 2005;**101**:18-23

[76] Rafati S, Nakhaee A, Taheri T, et al. Expression of cysteine proteinase type I and II of *Leishmania infantum* and their recognition by sera during canine and human visceral leishmaniasis. Experimental Parasitology. 2003;**103**:143-151

[77] De Souza Dias S, Da Costa Pinheiro PH, Katz S, et al. A recombinant cysteine proteinase from Leishmania (Leishmania) chagasi suitable for serodiagnosis of American visceral leishmaniasis. The American Journal of Tropical Medicine and Hygiene. 2005;**72**:126-132

[78] Henrique P, Nunes A, Hayde J, et al. A recombinant cysteine proteinase from Leishmania (Leishmania) chagasi as an antigen for delayed-type hypersensitivity assays and serodiagnosis of canine visceral leishmaniasis. Veterinary Parasitology. 2009;**162**:32-39

[79] Ghedin E, Zhang WW, Charest H, et al. Antibody response against a Leishmania donovani amastigote-stage-specific protein in patients with visceral leishmaniasis. Clinical and Diagnostic Laboratory Immunology. 1997;**4**:530-535

[80] Zhang WW, Charest H, Ghedin E, et al. Identification and overexpression of the A2 amastigote-specific protein in Leishmania donovani. Molecular and Biochemical Parasitology. 1996;**78**:79-90

[81] Mougneau E, Altare F, Wakil a E, et al. Expression cloning of a protective Leishmania antigen. Science. 1995;**268**:563-566

[82] Alvar J, Vélez ID, Bern C, et al. Leishmaniasis worldwide and global estimates of its incidence. PLoS One;**7**. Epub ahead of print 2012. DOI: 10.1371/journal.pone.0035671

[83] Maalej IA, Chenik M, Louzir H, et al. Comparative evaluation of ELISAs based on ten recombinant or purified Leishmania antigens for the serodiagnosis of Mediterranean visceral leishmaniasis. The American Journal of Tropical Medicine and Hygiene. 2003;**68**: 312-320

[84] Abass E, Bollig N, Reinhard K, et al. rKLO8, a novel Leishmania donovani - derived recombinant immunodominant protein for sensitive detection of visceral leishmaniasis in Sudan. PLoS Neglected Tropical Diseases;**7**. Epub ahead of print 2013. DOI: 10.1371/journal.pntd.0002322

[85] Abass E, Kang C, Martinkovic F, et al. Heterogeneity of Leishmania donovani parasites complicates diagnosis of visceral leishmaniasis: Comparison of different serological tests in three endemic regions. PLoS One. 2015;**10**:1-13

[86] van den Bogaart E, Berkhout MMZ, Adams ER, et al. Prevalence, features and risk factors for malaria co-infections amongst visceral leishmaniasis patients from Amudat hospital, Uganda. PLoS Neglected Tropical Diseases;**6**. Epub ahead of print 2012. DOI: 10.1371/journal.pntd.0001617

[87] Pinedo-Cancino V, Laurenti MD, Kesper N, et al. Evaluation of Leishmania (Leishmania) infantum excreted-secreted antigens for detection of canine leishmaniasis. Acta Tropica. 2016;**161**:41-43

[88] Lima BSS, Fialho LC, Pires SF, et al. Immunoproteomic and bioinformatic approaches to identify secreted *Leishmania amazonensis*, *L. braziliensis*, and *L. infantum* proteins with specific reactivity using canine serum. Veterinary Parasitology. 2016;**223**:115-119

[89] Filippas-Ntekouan S, Liberopoulos E, Elisaf M. Lipid testing in infectious diseases: Possible role in diagnosis and prognosis. Infection. 2017;**45**:575-588

[90] Reithinger R, Dujardin JC. Molecular diagnosis of leishmaniasis: Current status and future applications. Journal of Clinical Microbiology. 2007;**45**:21-25

[91] Silvestre R, Santarém N, Teixeira L, et al. Evaluation of Leishmania species reactivity in human serologic diagnosis of leishmaniasis. The American Journal of Tropical Medicine and Hygiene. 2009;**81**:202-208

[92] Srividya G, Kulshrestha A, Singh R, et al. Diagnosis of visceral leishmaniasis: Developments over the last decade. Parasitology Research. 2012;**110**:1065-1078

[93] Andrade RA, Reis AB, Gontijo CMF, et al. Clinical value of anti-Leishmania (Leishmania) chagasi IgG titers detected by flow cytometry to distinguish infected from vaccinated dogs. Veterinary Immunology and Immunopathology. 2007;**116**:85-97

[94] Courtenay O, Carson C, Calvo-Bado L, et al. Heterogeneities in *Leishmania infantum* infection: Using skin parasite burdens to identify highly infectious dogs. PLoS Neglected Tropical Diseases. 2014;**8**:26

[95] Courtenay O, Quinnell RJ, Garcez LM, et al. Infectiousness in a cohort of Brazilian dogs: Why culling fails to control visceral leishmaniasis in areas of high transmission. The Journal of Infectious Diseases. 2002;**186**:1314-1320

[96] Magalhães-Junior JT, Mota TF, Porfirio-Passos G, et al. Xenodiagnosis on dogs with visceral leishmaniasis: Canine and sand fly aspects related to the parasite transmission. Veterinary Parasitology. 2016;**223**:120-126

[97] Gomes CM, de Morais OO, Roselino AM, et al. Complementary exams in the diagnosis of American tegumentary leishmaniasis. Anais Brasileiros de Dermatologia. 2014;**89**:701-709

[98] Rodgers MR, Popper SJ, Wirth DF. Amplification of kinetoplast DNA as a tool in the detection and diagnosis of Leishmania. Experimental Parasitology. 1990;**71**(3):267-275

[99] Moreira MAB, Luvizotto MCR, Garcia JF, et al. Comparison of parasitological, immunological and molecular methods for the diagnosis of leishmaniasis in dogs with different clinical signs. Veterinary Parasitology. 2007;**145**:245-252

[100] Mohammadiha A, Mohebali M, Haghighi A, et al. Comparison of real-time PCR and conventional PCR with two DNA targets for detection of *Leishmania (Leishmania) infantum* infection in human and dog blood samples. Experimental Parasitology. 2013;**133**:89-94

[101] Aschar M, de Oliveira ETB, Laurenti MD, et al. Value of the oral swab for the molecular diagnosis of dogs in different stages of infection with *Leishmania infantum*. Veterinary Parasitology. 2016;**225**:108-113

[102] Carson C, Quinnell RJ, Holden J, et al. Comparison of Leishmania OligoC-TesT PCR with conventional and real-time PCR for diagnosis of canine Leishmania infection. Journal of Clinical Microbiology. 2010;**48**:3325-3330

[103] Bastien P, Procop GW, Reischl U. Quantitative real-time PCR is not more sensitive than ' conventional' PCR. Journal of Clinical Microbiology. 2008;**46**:1897-1900

[104] Sudarshan M, Weirather JL, Wilson ME, et al. Study of parasite kinetics with antileishmanial drugs using real-time quantitative PCR in Indian visceral leishmaniasis. The Journal of Antimicrobial Chemotherapy. 2011;**66**:1751-1755

[105] Espy MJ, Uhl JR, Sloan LM, et al. Real-time PCR in clinical microbiology : Applications for routine laboratory testing. Clinical Microbiology Reviews. 2006;**19**:165-256

[106] Espinosa D, Boggild AK, Deborggraeve S, et al. Leishmania OligoC-TesT as a simple, rapid, and standardized tool for molecular diagnosis of cutaneous leishmaniasis in Peru. Journal of Clinical Microbiology. 2009;**47**:2560-2563

[107] Palatnik-De-Sousa CB, Dos Santos WR, França-Silva JC, et al. Impact of canine control on the epidemiology of canine and human visceral leishmaniasis in Brazil. The American Journal of Tropical Medicine and Hygiene. 2001;**65**:510-517

[108] Coura-Vital W, Marques MJ, Veloso VM, et al. Prevalence and factors associated with *Leishmania infantum* infection of dogs from an urban area of Brazil as identified by molecular methods. PLoS Neglected Tropical Diseases;**5**. Epub ahead of print 2011. DOI: 10.1371/journal.pntd.0001291

[109] Islam MZ, Itoh M, Mirza R, et al. Direct agglutination test with urine samples for the diagnosis of visceral leishmaniasis. The American Journal of Tropical Medicine and Hygiene. 2004;**70**:78-82

[110] Boelaert M, Verdonck K, Menten J, et al. Rapid tests for the diagnosis of visceral leishmaniasis in patients with suspected disease. Cochrane Database of Systematic Reviews. 2014;**6**:CD009135

[111] Schallig HDFH, Canto-Cavalheiro M, Da Silva ES. Evaluation of the direct agglutination test and the rK39 dipstick test for the sero-diagnosis of visceral leishmaniasis. Memórias do Instituto Oswaldo Cruz. 2002;**97**:1015-1018

[112] Adams ER, Jacquet D, Schoone G, et al. Leishmaniasis direct agglutination test: Using pictorials as training materials to reduce inter-reader variability and improve accuracy. PLoS Neglected Tropical Diseases. 2012;**6**:1-6

[113] Alvar J, Cañavate C, Molina R, et al. Canine leishmaniasis. Advances in Parasitology. 2004;**57**:1-88

[114] Otranto D, Paradies P, Sasanelli M, et al. Rapid immunochromatographic test for serodiagnosis of canine leishmaniasis. Journal of Clinical Microbiology. 2004;**42**:2769-2771

[115] Otranto D, Paradies P, De Caprariis D, et al. Toward diagnosing *Leishmania infantum* infection in asymptomatic dogs in an area where leishmaniasis is endemic. Clinical and Vaccine Immunology. 2009;**16**:337-343

[116] Nolan JP, Mandy F. Multiplexed and microparticle-based analyses? Quantitative tools for the large-scale analysis of biological systems. Cytometry Part A. 2006;**69**:318-325

[117] Silvestre R, Santarém N, Cunha J, et al. Serological evaluation of experimentally infected dogs by LicTXNPx-ELISA and amastigote-flow cytometry. Veterinary Parasitology. 2008;**158**:23-30

[118] Lemos EM, Gomes IT, Carvalho SFG, et al. Detection of anti-Leishmania (Leishmania) chagasi immunoglobulin G by flow cytometry for cure assessment following chemotherapeutic treatment of american visceral leishmaniasis. Clinical and Vaccine Immunology. 2007;**14**:569-576

[119] Cañavate C, Herrero M, Nieto J, et al. Evaluation of two rK39 dipstick tests, direct agglutination test, and indirect fluorescent antibody test for diagnosis of visceral leishmaniasis in a new epidemic site in highland Ethiopia. The American Journal of Tropical Medicine and Hygiene. 2011;**84**:102-106

[120] Biglino A, Bolla C, Concialdi E, et al. Asymptomatic *Leishmania infantum* infection in an area of Northwestern Italy (piedmont region) where such infections are traditionally nonendemic. Journal of Clinical Microbiology. 2010;**48**:131-136

[121] Goto Y, Coler RN, Guderian J, et al. Cloning, characterization, and serodiagnostic evaluation of *Leishmania infantum* tandem repeat proteins. Infection and Immunity. 2006;**74**:3939-3945

[122] Mirsamadi N, Naeini KM, Mamishi S, et al. Application of direct agglutination test (DAT) for the diagnosis and Seroepidemiological studies of visceral leishmaniasis in Iran. Iranian Journal of Parasitology. 2006;**1**:15-25

[123] Miró G, Cardoso L, Pennisi MG, et al. Canine leishmaniosis - new concepts and insights on an expanding zoonosis: Part two. Trends in Parasitology. 2008;**24**:371-377

[124] Quinnell RJ, Carson C, Reithinger R, et al. Evaluation of rK39 rapid diagnostic tests for canine visceral leishmaniasis: Longitudinal study and meta-analysis. PLoS Neglected Tropical Diseases;**7**. Epub ahead of print 2013. DOI: 10.1371/journal.pntd.0001992

[125] Ben-Abid M, Galaï Y, Habboul Z, et al. Diagnosis of Mediterranean visceral leishmaniasis by detection of Leishmania-related antigen in urine and oral fluid samples. Acta Tropica. 2017;**167**:71-72

[126] Sarkari B, Chance M, Hommel M. Antigenuria in visceral leishmaniasis: Detection and partial characterisation of a carbohydrate antigen. Acta Tropica. 2002;**82**:339-348

5

Clinical Application of Coagulation Biomarkers

Makoto Aoki, Shuichi Hagiwara and
Kiyohiro Oshima

Abstract

Coagulopathy is of intense interest in the fields of emergency medicine, with many recent studies of coagulation biomarkers for clinical use. The occurrence of disseminated intravascular coagulation (DIC) also resulted in the activation of studies about the coagulopathy. At present DIC has been admitted in many clinical conditions and many coagulation biomarkers have been studied. Fibrin degradation product (FDP) and D-dimer are one type of coagulation biomarker. A characteristic of FDP and D-dimer is the rapid and dynamic elevation of their levels when fibrinolysis occurs in several acute diseases. In this chapter, we present the clinical application of FDP and D-dimer. In trauma, FDP and -dimer have been used for the evaluation of trauma severity, to predict the likelihood of hemorrhage and to evaluate the need for the transfusion of packed red blood cells. In cardiac pulmonary arrest (CPA), FDP and D-dimer have been useful for predicting the return of spontaneous circulation. Thus, the measurement of coagulation biomarkers is useful in the diagnosis and/or treatment of trauma and CPA.

Keywords: fibrin degradation product, D-dimer, diagnosis, prognosis, emergency medicine

1. Introduction

Fine balance exists between coagulation and fibrinolysis within the coagulation system, with coagulopathy defined as the failure of this balance. Coagulopathy has long been known to occur in several acute diseases such as cardiovascular disease [1], infection [2] and trauma [3]. In response, coagulation biomarkers have been identified and used in clinical practice in recent years to diagnose and treat several diseases of the coagulation system.

There is a variety of coagulation biomarkers used in real clinical situation. Prothrombin time (PT), activated partial thromboplastin time (APTT), fibrinogen has been used to test the coagulation function from long ago in hematologic disorder, liver disease, disseminated intravascular coagulation (DIC) and to monitor the use of anticoagulation drugs. Owing to the recent progress in measuring method, the more minute coagulation biomarkers can be measured and divided into coagulation systems and fibrinolytic systems. Each example is thrombin-antithrombin complex (TAT), soluble fibrin (SF) and soluble fibrin monomer complex (SFMC) in coagulation systems, and Fibrin degradation product (FDP) and D-dimer in fibrinolytic systems. They are relatively new coagulation biomarkers and the characteristics of them are to be rapidly elevated in acute phase. In clinical situation, they are practically used to detect the venous thromboembolism [4–6]. Besides, FDP and D-dimer are more studied, and the clinical applications of these coagulation biomarkers are ranging from diagnosing [7] to the treatment [8].

In this chapter, we present information on the successful use of FDP, D-dimer and fibrinogen in clinical practice. Finally, we demonstrate the prospects of the clinical application of coagulation biomarkers.

2. Disseminated intravascular coagulation (DIC) and clinical use of coagulation biomarkers

The occurrence of DIC has been the definitive trigger for the use of coagulation biomarkers in the diagnosis of this disease. DIC is characterized by the widespread activation of coagulation, which results in the intravascular formation of fibrin and, ultimately, the thrombotic occlusion of small- and mid-sized vessels [9–11]. Intravascular coagulation can also compromise the blood supply to organs and peripheral cells, and, in conjunction with hemodynamic and metabolic derangements, may contribute to the failure of multiple organs [12].

DIC is present in many clinical conditions (**Table 1**) [12].

Of these clinical conditions, coagulation biomarkers have been especially used in the treatment of sepsis. The clinical criteria for the early diagnosis of DIC have incorporated the use of several coagulation biomarkers such as FDP, D-dimer, PT, and fibrinogen [13–16]. In addition, the two endogenous anticoagulants, antithrombin and protein C, are found decreased in patients with DIC, and are useful in predicting the outcome of such patients, as well as those with sepsis [17, 18]. Furthermore, thrombomodulin, tissue factor pathway inhibitor, Von Willebrand factor and Adamts 13 are also useful in clinical situations [19, 20].

Of these coagulation biomarkers, we focused on the use of FDP and D-dimer in several clinical conditions. D-dimer is a specific protein fiber degradation product of cross-linked fibrin in response to hydrolysis by fibrinolytic enzymes [21, 22]. When the thrombus degrades, D-dimer may be released into the circulatory system [23]. In normal blood, the level of D-dimer is low, but once thrombosis occurs, the D-dimer level rises [24]. FDP is the degradation product of fibrous protein. In normal blood, the level of FDP is also low; however, the FDP level also increases when fibrinolysis occurs. FDP is a mitogen for many cell types, promoting the proliferation of endothelial cells, smooth muscle cells, and fibroblasts, as well

Sepsis
Trauma
Serious tissue injury
Head injury
Fat embolism
Cancer
Myeloproliferative diseases
Solid tumors (e.g., pancreatic carcinoma, prostatic carcinoma)
Obstetrical complications
Amniotic-fluid embolism
Abruption placentae
Vascular disorders
Giant hemangioma (Kasabach-Merritt syndrome)
Aortic aneurysm
Severe hepatic failure
Reactions to toxins (e.g., snake venom, drugs and amphetamines)
Immunologic disorders
Severe allergic reaction
Hemolytic transfusion reaction
Transplant rejection

Table 1. Common clinical conditions associated with disseminated intravascular coagulation.

as cholesterol deposition [25]. FDP can also induce the adhesion and accumulation of white blood cells, which results in damage to the blood vessel endothelium [26].

In our facility, FDP and D-dimer are measured by an immunoturbidimetric method using Cs-2000i and Cs-5100 systems (Sysmex Corporation., Hyogo, Japan; **Figure 1**). It takes about 15–20 minutes to measure FDP and D-dimer with this instrument.

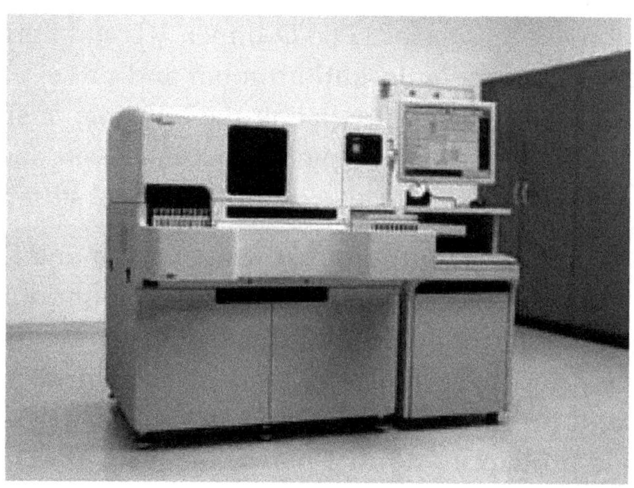

Figure 1. Cs-5100 systems to measure FDP and D-dimer (Sysmex Corporation., Hyogo, Japan).

3. Trauma

DIC has been well known to occur in trauma since the 1960s, especially in relation to head trauma (**Table 1**). Coagulopathy in trauma was believed to originate as a consequence of fluid administration and hypothermia [27]. However, in the 2000s, the concept of acute traumatic coagulopathy (ATC) first appeared [27] with the demonstration that an organ and/or cell injury itself caused the coagulopathy. Using coagulation biomarkers such as PT, APTT and thrombin time (TT), acute traumatic coagulopathy was shown to be associated with mortality and severe trauma.

Initially, the concept of ATC was reported mainly in severe trauma, because PT, APTT and TT were found to have normal values in lightly and mildly traumatized patients. However, using fibrinolytic coagulation biomarkers such as FDP and D-dimer, we also detected ATC in lightly and mildly traumatized patients. This has been described in our first report on the clinical usefulness of coagulation biomarkers [28].

3.1. The relationship between coagulation biomarkers and trauma severity

Our study reported that of all coagulation biomarkers, FDP and D-dimer were associated with the severity of trauma [28]. We have previously demonstrated an association between FDP and D-dimer, and a trauma score such as the Injury Severity Score (ISS) [29]. The ISS has been one of the most common and useful scoring systems to evaluate the severity of trauma and is used widely throughout the world. In clinical practice, the ISS is calculated for each anatomical injury according to the results of physical examinations, surgery and imaging studies; therefore, the ISS cannot be calculated in an initial emergency field. However, we can predict ISS using FDP and D-dimer.

In this study, the area under receiver operating characteristics curves (AUROCs) of FDP and D-dimer for predicting an ISS ≥ 9 were 0.757 and 0.756, and the sensitivity and specificity of FDP and D-dimer based on the Youden's index were 75.9 and 68.4%, and 75.9 and 73.7%, respectively. This demonstrated that we could predict mild to severe injury (ISS ≥ 9) with about 70% sensitivity and specificity; this finding signaled to trauma physicians and surgeons that minor injury was not to be overlooked. Because several minor injuries, such as minute spinal column and rib fractures, are sometimes hard to detect, FDP and D-dimer can be used as supplementary diagnostic tools.

In addition, we have adopted this finding to more severe trauma. In the previous study, we investigated the association between FDP and D-dimer, and an ISS ≥ 9. In a similar setting, we calculated the AUROCs of FDP and D-dimer for predicting ISS ≥ 9, ISS ≥ 16 and ISS ≥ 25 (**Figure 2**).

These figures demonstrated that the predictivity of FDP and D-dimer for ISS was more accurate, especially in severe trauma. In **Table 2**, the AUROC and cut-off points of FDP and D-dimer to predict whether the ISS was over the 25 were the highest at 0.818 and 0.813, respectively. The sensitivities and specificities, based on the Youden's index, of FDP and D-dimer to

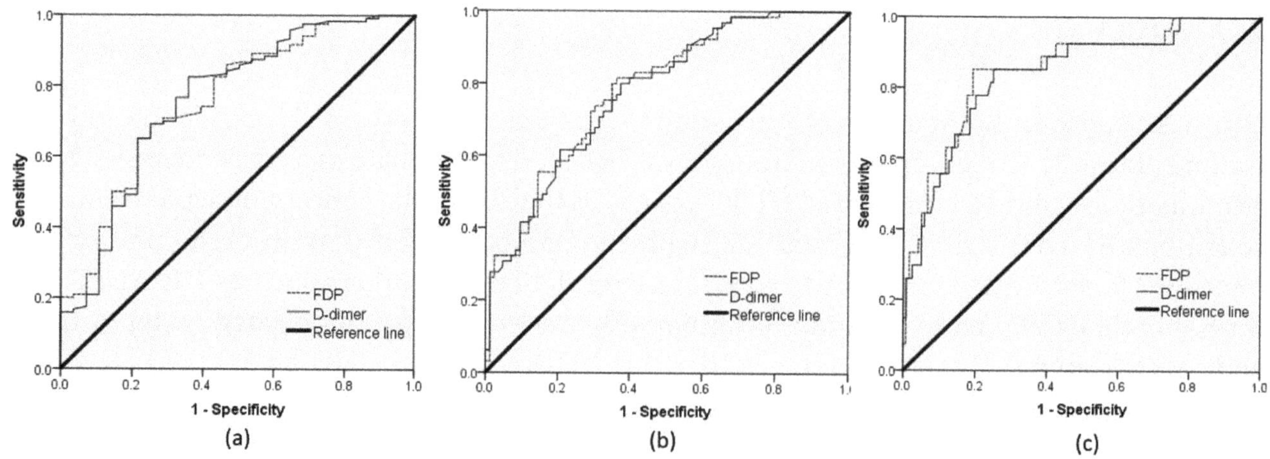

Figure 2. (a) Receiver operating characteristic (ROC) curve of coagulation biomarkers to predict the injury severity score (ISS) of a patient with trauma ≥9 points. FDP, fibrin degradation products. (b) Receiver operating characteristic (ROC) curve of coagulation biomarkers to predict the injury severity score (ISS) of a patient with trauma ≥16 points. FDP, fibrin degradation products. (c) Receiver operating characteristic (ROC) curve of coagulation biomarkers to predict the injury severity score (ISS) of a patient with trauma ≥25 points. FDP, fibrin degradation products.

FDP D-dimer	ISS ≥ 9	ISS ≥ 16	ISS ≥ 25
AUROC (95% CI)	0.743 (0.681–0.806)	0.691 (0.624–0.759)	0.818 (0.735–0.901)
	0.751 (0.689–0.814)	0.694 (0.628–0.761)	0.813 (0.732–0.894)
Cut-off point	32.1 μg/mL	32.1 μg/mL	101.4 μg/mL
	6.5 μg/mL	12.8 μg/mL	28.2 μg/mL
Sensitivity, %	59.4	67.8	73.3
	73.1	65.6	76.7
Specificity, %	79.8	64.9	82.7
	66.7	66.1	78.4

CI, confidence interval; FDP, fibrin degradation product; AUROC, area under the receiver operating characteristic curve; ISS, injury severity score.

Table 2. Area under the receiver operating characteristic curve and cut-off points of FDP and D-dimer to predict whether the ISS is over 9, 16 or 25.

predict an ISS over 25 were 73.3 and 82.7%, and 76.7 and 78.4%, respectively. These findings are novel because they are based on a patient's trauma severity, allowing the development of definitive treatment more rapidly.

3.2. The prediction of extravasation in pelvic fracture using coagulation biomarkers

In the section of the relationship between coagulation biomarkers and trauma severity the ability of FDP and D-dimer to predict trauma severity was demonstrated. Therefore, we also applied this to pelvic fracture [30]. Pelvic fracture is an independent risk factor for death after blunt trauma. It is associated with increased mortality in blunt trauma, with rates up to 30%

[31–33]. In pelvic fracture, retroperitoneal hemorrhage may induce hemodynamic instability, with 5–20% originating from arterial bleeding [34].

In a clinical situation, the standard tool to detect arterial bleeding in a pelvic fracture has been computed tomography (CT) using contrast material; however, several problems exist with CT scanning. One problem is the specificity of CT scanning to detect arterial bleeding in pelvic fracture [35] is decreased. Another problem is that the quality of the CT scanning may be related to the scanning protocol and can be affected by interference caused by vasospasm, consequently affecting the diagnostic ability of physicians [36, 37]. Thus, we evaluated the predictive ability of coagulation biomarkers to detect arterial bleeding and whether these could be used as alternative tools for CT scanning.

Our report highlighted the highly accurate ability of FDP and D-dimer to detect arterial bleeding in a pelvic fracture; the AUROCs of FDP and D-dimer were 0.900 and 0.882, respectively (**Table 3**) [30]. In addition, in this study we calculated the ratios of FDP to fibrinogen, and of D-dimer to fibrinogen. Fibrinogen is said to be an independent risk factor of mortality and severity in blunt trauma patients [38–40], and a predictor of transfusion [41, 42]. We combined the high FDP and D-dimer, and the low fibrinogen, to the ratio of FDP to fibrinogen and the ratio of D-dimer to fibrinogen, this was a novel finding. This ratio was subsequently developed to the next stage [43, 44].

3.3. Prediction of the need for packed red blood cell transfusions using coagulation biomarkers

We applied coagulation biomarkers to the prediction of the need for packed red blood cell transfusions [43]. For a long time, many investigators have discussed how to predict massive transfusion requirements in blunt trauma patients [45–51]. The characteristics of FDP and D-dimer were correlated with the trauma severity: from relatively light to severe trauma [28]. This feature has been utilized to predict not only patients requiring massive transfusions, but also whether patients needed packed red blood cells or not. Coagulation biomarkers,

	FDP	**D-dimer**	**Ratio of FDP to fibrinogen**	**Ratio of D-dimer to fibrinogen**	**Hemoglobin level**	**Lactate level**
AUROC	0.900	0.882	0.918	0.900	0.815	0.765
(95% CI)	(0.765–1.000)	(0.728–1.000)	(0.797–1.000)	(0.773–1.000)	(0.656–0.974)	(0.563–0.967)
Cut-off point	126.8 μg/mL	46.0 μg/mL	0.656	0.215	11.0 g/dL	2.75 mmol/L
Sensitivity, %	94.1	94.1	94.1	94.1	61.1	58.8
Specificity, %	90.0	90.0	90.0	80.0	0.0	85.7

CI, confidence interval; FDP, fibrin degradation product; AUROC, area under the receiver operating characteristic curve.

Table 3. Area under the receiver operating characteristic curves and cut-off points of parameters to predict arterial extravasation in pelvic fracture patients.

	AUROC (95% CI)	Cut-off point	Sensitivity (%)	Specificity (%)
ABC	0.591 (0.420–0.763)	0.5	21.4	96.7
GCS	0.716 (0.547–0.885)	12.5	96.4	42.9
Ht	0.667 (0.503–0.830)	31.3%	97.3	35.7
PT–INR	0.859 (0.760–0.958)	1.065	71.4	90.1
APTT	0.684 (0.501–0.866)	36.45 s	42.9	96.4
Fib	0.877 (0.808–0.947)	245.5 mg/dL	64.3	100
FDP	0.874 (0.784–0.963)	45.65 μg/dL	78.6	80.4
FDP/Fib ratio	0.899 (0.819–0.979)	0.202×10^{-3}	85.7	82.3

AUROC, area under the receiver operating characteristic curve; CI, confidence interval; ABC, assessment of blood consumption score; GCS, Glasgow Coma Scale; Ht, hematocrit; PT-INR, international normalized ratio of prothrombin time; APTT, activated partial thromboplastin time; Fib, fibrinogen; FDP, fibrin degradation product.

Table 4. Results of receiver operating characteristic curves analysis.

especially, the ratio of FDP to fibrinogen, were found to be the most accurate markers for predicting the need for packed red blood cell transfusions (**Table 4**) [43].

4. Cardiac pulmonary arrest

In recent decades, the science of cardiac pulmonary arrest (CPA) has been improving due to the widespread adoption of guidelines by the International Liaison Committee on Resuscitation (ILCOR). The 2015 guidelines by the Japan Resuscitation Council, which is one of the subsidiary organizations of ILCOR, enumerates predictive candidates for outcomes of patients with an out-of-hospital cardiac arrest (OHCA), such as S-100B, neuron specific enolase, imaging findings, brain waves, among others. However, it is presently difficult to predict favorable neurological outcomes or the survival of patients with OHCA [52]. Recently, several reports have suggested that blood coagulation makers reflected the prognosis of patients with CPA. The occurrence of fibrinolysis in patients with CPA has been noticed for a long time [53]; however, coagulation biomarkers has not been clinically applied to CPA until recently, with clinical applications with

	AG	ACAG	FDP	D-dimer
AUROC (95% CI)	0.664 (0.514–0.815)	0.667 (0.516–0.818)	0.714 (0.571–0.858)	0.707 (0.561–0.853)
Cut-off point	27.8 mmol/L	31.7 mmol/L	29.4 μg/mL	10.2 μg/mL
Sensitivity, %	84.4	78.1	87.5	87.5
Specificity, %	45.0	55.0	50.0	55.0

AG, anion gap; ACAG, albumin-corrected anion gap; CI; confidence interval; FDP, fibrin degradation products; AUROC, areas under receiver operating characteristic curves.

Table 5. Areas under receiver operating characteristic curves and cut-off points of parameters that predict whether a patient with cardiopulmonary arrest can achieve a return of spontaneous circulation after effective cardiopulmonary resuscitation.

regard to CPA having appeared since the 2010s. For example, FDP and D-dimer are associated with the return of spontaneous circulation (ROSC) and have been useful for predicting ROSC [54] (**Table 5**) [54]. Other reports have demonstrated that a high D-dimer concentration on admission predicts a poorer outcome [55], and that the FDP level predicts neurological outcomes [56].

5. Conclusion

Coagulation disorders are associated with several diseases and symptoms in emergency medical fields. The occurrence of DIC is a modern topic and has been accelerating the studies about the coagulation biomarkers. We demonstrated that testing for and measuring FDP and/or DD may be advantageous in diagnosing and/or treatment of trauma and CPA.

Acknowledgements

I would like to thank the Department of Clinical Laboratory Medicine, Gunma University Graduate School of Medicine for measuring the coagulation biomarkers.

Conflict of interest

The authors declare that they have no competing interests.

Author details

Makoto Aoki*, Shuichi Hagiwara and Kiyohiro Oshima

*Address all correspondence to: aokimakoto@gunma-u.ac.jp

Department of Emergency Medicine, Gunma University Graduate School of Medicine, Maebashi, Japan

References

[1] Scott J, Humphreys DR. Dissecting aortic aneurysm and disseminated intravascular coagulation. British Medical Journal. 1977;**1**:24

[2] Corrigan Jr JJ, Ray WL, May N. Changes in the blood coagulation system associated with septicemia. The New England Journal of Medicine. 1968;**279**:851-856. DOI: 10.1056/NEJM196810172791603

[3] Salzman EW. Does intravascular coagulation occur in hemorrhagic shock in man? The Journal of Trauma. 1968;**8**:867-871

[4] Lee SY, Niikura T, Iwakura T, Sakai Y, Kuroda T, Kurosaka M. Thrombin-antithrombin III complex tests. Journal of Orthopaedic Surgery (Hong Kong). 2017;**25**:170840616684501

[5] Mitani G, Takagaki T, Hamahashi K, Serigano K, Nakamura Y, Sato M, Mochida J. Associations between venous thromboembolism onset, D-dimer, and soluble fibrin monomer complex after total knee arthroplasty. Journal of Orthopaedic Surgery and Research. 2015;**10**:172

[6] Wells PS, Ihaddadene R, Reilly A, Forgie MA. Diagnosis of venous Thromboembolism: 20 years of progress. Annals of Internal Medicine. 2018;**168**:131-140

[7] Kotani Y, Toyofuku M, Tamura T, Shimada K, Matsuura Y, Tawa H, Uchikawa M, Higashi S, Fujimoto J, Yagita K, Sato F, Atagi Y, Hamasaki T, Tsujimoto T, Chishiro T. Validation of the diagnostic utility of D-dimer measurement in patients with acute aortic syndrome. European Heart Journal. Acute Cardiovascular Care. 2017;**6**:223-231

[8] Suehiro E, Koizumi H, Fujiyama Y, Yoneda H, Suzuki M. Predictors of deterioration indicating a requirement for surgery in mild to moderate traumatic brain injury. Clinical Neurology and Neurosurgery. 2014;**127**:97-100

[9] Marder VJ, Feinstein DI, Francis CW, Colman RW. Consumptive thrombohemorrhagic disorders. In: Colman RW, Hirsh J, Marder VJ, Salzman EW, editors. Hemostasis and Thrombosis: Basic Principles and Clinical Practice. 3rd ed. Philadelphia: J.B. Lippincott; 1994. pp. 1023-1063

[10] Bone RC. Modulators of coagulation. A critical appraisal of their role in sepsis. Archives of Internal Medicine. 1992;**152**:1381-1389. DOI: 10.1001/archinte.1992.00400190023007

[11] Müller-Berghaus G, Ten Cate H, Levi M. Disseminated intravascular coagulation. In: Verstraete M, Fuster V, Topol EJ, editors. Cardiovascular Thrombosis: Thrombocardiology and Thromboneurology. 2nd ed. Philadelphia: Lippincott-Raven; 1998. pp. 781-801

[12] Levi M, Ten Cate H. Disseminated intravascular coagulation. The New England Journal of Medicine. 1999;**341**:586-592. DOI: 10.1056/NEJM199908193410807

[13] Yasunaga K. Diagnostic criteria of disseminated intravascular coagulation (DIC). Nihon Rinsho. 1975;**33**:3380-3388 (article in Japanese)

[14] Kobayashi N, Maekawa T, Takada M, Takada M, Gonmori H. Criteria for diagnosis of DIC based on the analysis of clinical and laboratory findings in 345 DIC patients collected by the research committee on DIC in Japan. Bibliotheca Haematologica. 1983;**49**:265-275

[15] Taylor Jr FB, Toh CH, Hoots WK, Wada H, Levi M, Scientific Subcommittee on Disseminated Intravascular Coagulation (DIC) of the International Society on Thrombosis and Haemostasis (ISTH). Towards definition, clinical and laboratory criteria, and a scoring system for disseminated intravascular coagulation. Thrombosis and Haemostasis. 2001;**86**:1327-1330

[16] Gando S, Iba T, Eguchi Y, Ohtomo Y, Okamoto K, Koseki K, Mayumai T, Murata A, Ikeda T, Ishikura H, Ueyama M, Ogura H, Kushimoto S, Saitoh D, Endo S, Shimazaki S,

Japanese Association for Acute Medicine Disseminated Intravascular Coagulation (JAAM DIC) Study Group. A multicenter, prospective validation of disseminated intravascular coagulation diagnostic criteria for critically ill patients: Comparing current criteria. Critical Care Medicine. 2006;**34**:625-631

[17] Fourrier F, Chopin C, Goudemand J, Hendrycx S, Caron C, Rime A, Marey A, Lestavel P. Septic shock, multiple organ failure, and disseminated intravascular coagulation. Compared patterns of antithrombin III, protein C, and protein S deficiencies. Chest. 1992;**101**:816-823. DOI: 10.1378/chest.101.3.816

[18] Macias WL, Nelson DR. Severe protein C deficiency predicts early death in severe sepsis. Critical Care Medicine. 2004;**32**:S223-S228

[19] Iba T, Ito T, Maruyama l JB, Brenner T, Muller MC, Juffermans NP, Thacil J. Potential diagnostic markers for disseminated intravascular coagulation of sepsis. Blood Reviews. 2016;**30**:149-155. DOI: 10.1016/j.blre.2015.10.002

[20] Wada H, Thachil J, Di Nisio M, Mathew P, Kurosawa S, Gando S, Kim HK, Nielsen JD, Demfle CE, Levi M, Toh CH. The Scientific Standardization Committee on DIC of the International Society on Thrombosis Haemostasis. Guidance for diagnosis and treatment of DIC from harmonization of the recommendations from three guidelines. Journal of Thrombosis and Haemostasis. 2013;**11**:761-767. DOI: 10.1111/jth.12155

[21] Ay C, Vormittag R, Dunkler D, Simanek R, Chiriac AL, Drach J, Quehenberger P, Wagner O, Zielinski C, Pabinger L. D-dimer and prothrombin fragment 1 + 2 predict venous thromboembolism in patients with cancer: Results from the Vienna Cancer and thrombosis study. Journal of Clinical Oncology. 2009;**27**:4124-4129. DOI: 10.1200/JCO/2008.21.7752

[22] Kline JA, Hogg MM, Courtney DM, Miller CD, Jones AE, Smithline HA. D-dimer threshold increase with pretest probability unlikely for pulmonary embolism to decrease unnecessary computerized tomographic pulmonary angiography. Journal of Thrombosis and Haemostasis. 2012;**10**:572-581. DOI: 10.1111/j.1538-7836.2012.04647.x

[23] Suzuki T, Distante A, Zizza A, Trimarchi S, Villani M, Salerno Uriate JA, De Luca Tupputi Schinosa L, Renzulli A, Sabino F, Nowak R, Birkhahn R, Hollander JE, Counselman F, Vijayendran R, Bossone E, Eagle K. IRAD-bio investigators. Diagnosis of acute aortic dissection by D-dimer: The international registry of acute aortic dissection substudy on biomarkers (IRAD-bio) experience. Circulation. 2009;**119**:2702-2707. DOI: 10.1161/CIRCULATIONAHA.108.833004

[24] Raghini M, Van Es J, Den Exter PL, Roy PM, Verschuren F, Ghuysen A, Rutschmann OT, Sanchez O, Jaffrelot M, Trinh-Duc A, Le Gall C, Moustafa F, Principe A, Vanhouten AA, Ten Wolde M, Douma RA, Hazelaar G, Erkens PM, Van Kralingen KW, Grootenboers MJ, Durian MF, Cheung YW, Meyer G, Bounameaux H, Huisman MV, Kamphuisen PW, Le Gal G. Age-adjusted D-dimer cutoff levels to rule out pulmonary embolism: The ADJUST-PE study. Journal of the American Medical Association. 2014;**311**:1117-1124. DOI: 10.1001/jama.2014.2135

[25] Naito M. Effects of fibrinogen, fibrin and their degradation products on the behaviour of vascular smooth muscle cells. Nihon Ronen Igakkai Zasshi. 2000;**37**:458-463 (in Japanese). DOI: 10.3143/geriatrics.37.458

[26] Yakovlev S, Zhang L, Ugarova T, Medved L. Interaction of fibrin(ogen) with leukocyte receptor alpha M beta 2 (Mac-1): Further characterization and identification of a novel binding region within the central domain of the fibrinogen gamma-module. Biochemistry. 2005;**44**:617-626. DOI: 10.1021/bi048266w

[27] Brohi K, Singh J, Heron M, Coats T. Acute traumatic Coagulopathy. The Journal of Trauma. 2003;**54**:1127-1130. DOI: 10.1097/01.TA.0000069184.82147.06

[28] Hagiwara S, Oshima K, Aoki M, Murata M, Ishihara K, Kaneko M, Furukawa K, Ohyama Y, Tamura J. Usefulness of fibrin degradation products and d-dimer levels as biomarkers that reflect the severity of trauma. Journal of Trauma and Acute Care Surgery. 2013;**74**: 1275-1278. DOI: 10.1097/TA.0b013e31828cc967

[29] Baker SP, O'Neill B, Haddon Jr W, Long WB. The injury severity score: A method for describing patients with multiple injuries and evaluating emergency care. Journal of Trauma. 1974;**14**:187-196

[30] Aoki M, Hagiwara S, Tokue H, Shibuya K, Kaneko M, Murata M, Nakajima J, Sawada Y, Isshiki Y, Ichikawa Y, Oshima K. Prediction of extravasation in pelvic fracture using coagulation biomarkers. Injury. 2016;**47**:1702-1706. DOI: 10.1016/j.injury.2016.05.012

[31] Schulman JE, O'Toole RV, Castillo RC, Manson T, Sciadini MF, Whitney A, Pollak AN, Nascone JW. Pelvic ring fractures are an independent risk factor for death after blunt trauma. The Journal of Trauma. 2010;**68**(4):930. DOI: 10.1097/TA.0b013e3181cb49d1

[32] Burgess AR, Eastridge BJ, Young JW, Ellison TS, Ellison Jr PS, Poka A, Bathon GH, Brumback RJ. Pelvic ring disruptions: Effective classification system and treatment protocols. The Journal of Trauma. 1990;**30**:848-856

[33] Dalal SA, Burgess AR, Siegel JH, Young JW, Brumback RJ, Poka A, Dunham CM, Gens D, Bathon H. Pelvic fracture in multiple trauma: Classification by mechanism is key to pattern of organ injury, resuscitative requirements, and outcome. The Journal of Trauma. 1989;**29**:981-1000

[34] Dyer GS, Vrahas MS. Review of the pathophysiology and acute management of haemorrhage in pelvic fracture. Injury. 2006;**37**:602-613. DOI: 10.1016/j.injury.2005.09.007

[35] Kuo LW, Yang SJ, Fu CY, Liao CH, Wang SY, Wu SC. Relative hypotension increases the probability of the need for angioembolisation in pelvic fracture patients without contrast extravasation on computed tomography scan. Injury. 2016;**47**:37-42. DOI: 10.1016/j.injury.2015.07.043

[36] Fu CY, Wang SY, Liao CH, Kang SC, Hsu YP, Lin BC, Yuan KC, Ouyang CH. Computed tomography angiography provides limited benefit in the evaluation of patients with pelvic fractures. The American Journal of Emergency Medicine. 2014;**32**:1220-1224. DOI: 10.1016/j.ajem.2014.07.021

[37] Mongan J, Rathnayake S, Fu Y, Gao DW, Yeh BM. Extravasated contrast material in penetrating abdominopelvic trauma: Dual-contrast dual-energy CT for improved diagnosis – preliminary results in an animal model. Radiology. 2013;**268**:738-742. DOI: 10.1148/radiol.13121267

[38] McQuilten ZK, Wood EM, Bailey M, Cameron PA, Cooper DJ. Fibrinogen is an independent predictor of mortality in major trauma patients: A five-year statewide cohort study. Injury. 2017;**48**:1074-1081. DOI: 10.1016/j.injury.2016.11.021

[39] Hayakawa M, Maekawa K, Kushimoto S, Kato H, Sasaki J, Ogura H, Matauoka T, Uejima T, Morimura N, Ishikura H, Hagiwara A, Takeda M, Kaneko N, Saitoh D, Kudo D, Kanemura T, Shibusawa T, Furugori S, Nakamura Y, Shiraishi A, Murata K, Mayama G, Yaguchi A, Kim S, Takasu O, Nishiyama K. High d-dimer levels predict a poor outcome in patients with severe trauma, even with high fibrinogen levels on arrival: A multicenter retrospective study. Shock. 2016;**45**:308-314. DOI: 10.1097/SHK.0000000000000542

[40] Deras P, Villiet M, Manzanera J, Latry P, Schved JF, Capodevila X, Charbit J. Early coagulopathy at hospital admission predicts initial or delayed fibrinogen deficit in severe trauma patients. Journal of Trauma and Acute Care Surgery. 2014;**77**:433-440. DOI: 10.1097/TA.0000000000000314

[41] Umemura T, Nakamura Y, Nishida T, Hoshino K, Ishikura H. Fibrinogen and base excess levels as predictive markers of the need for massive blood transfusion after blunt trauma. Surgery Today. 2016;**46**:774-779. DOI: 10.1007/s00595-015-1263-7

[42] Yanagawa Y, Ishikawa K, Jitsuiki K, Yoshizawa T, Oode Y, Omori K, Ohsaka H. Fibrinogen degradation product levels on arrival for trauma patients requiring a transfusion even without head injury. World Journal of Emergency Surgery. 2017;**8**:106-109. DOI: 10.5847/wjem.j.1920-8642.2017.02.004

[43] Hagiwara S, Aoki M, Murata M, Kaneko M, Ichikawa Y, Nakajima J, Isshiki Y, Sawada Y, Tamura J, Oshima K. FDP/fibrinogen ratio reflects the requirement of packed red blood cell transfusion in patients with blunt trauma. The American Journal of Emergency Medicine. 2017;**35**:1106-1110. DOI: 10.1016/j.ajem.2017.03.009

[44] Lee DH, Lee BK, Noh SM, Cho YS. High fibrin/fibrinogen degradation product to fibrinogen ratio is associated with 28-day mortality and massive transfusion in severe trauma. European Journal of Trauma and Emergency Surgery. 2018;**44**:291-298. DOI: 10.1007/s00068-017-0844-0. Epub 2017 Sep 18

[45] Nunez TC, Voskresensky IV, Dossett LA, Shinall R, Dutton WD, Cotton BA. Early prediction of massive transfusion in trauma: Simple as ABC (assessment of blood consumption)? The Journal of Trauma. 2009;**66**:346-352. DOI: 10.1097/TA.0b013e3181961c35

[46] Yucel N, Lefering R, Maegele M, Vorweg M, Tjardes T, Ruchholtz S, Neugebauer EA, Wappler F, bouillon B, Rixen D, Polytrauma Study Group of the German Trauma Society. Trauma associated severe hemorrhage (TASH)-score: Probability of mass transfusion as surrogate for life threatening hemorrhage after multiple trauma. The Journal of Trauma. 2006;**60**:1228-1236. DOI: 10.1097/01.ta.0000220386.84102.bf

[47] Schreiber MA, Perkins J, Kiraly L, Underwood S, Wade C, Holcomb JB. Early predictors of massive transfusion in combat casualties. Journal of the American College of Surgeons. 2007;**205**:541-545. DOI: 10.1016/j.jamcollsurg.2007.05.007

[48] Rainer TH, Ho AM, Yeung JH, Cheung NK, Wong RS, Tang N, Ng SK, Wong GK, Lai PB, Graham CA. Early risk stratification of patients with major trauma requiring massive blood transfusion. Resuscitation. 2011;**82**:724-729. DOI: 10.1016/j.resuscitation.2011.02.016

[49] Vandromme MJ, Griffin RL, McGwin Jr G, Weinberg JA, Rue 3rd LW, Kerby JD. Prospective identification of patients at risk for massive transfusion: An imprecise endeavor. The American Surgeon. 2011;**77**:155-161

[50] Ogura T, Nakamura Y, Nakano M, Izawa Y, Nakamura M, Fujizuka K, Suzukawa M, Lefor AT. Predicting the need for massive transfusion in trauma patients: The traumatic bleeding severity score. Journal of Trauma and Acute Care Surgery. 2014;**76**:1243-1250. DOI: 10.1097/TA.0000000000000200

[51] Ohmori T, Kitamura T, Ishihara J, Onishi H, Nojima T, Yamamoto K, Tamura R, Muranishi K, Matsumoto T, Tokioka T. Early predictors for massive transfusion in older adult severe trauma patients. Injury. 2017;**48**:1006-1012. DOI: 10.1016/j.injury.2016.12.028

[52] Japan Resuscitation Council [Internet]. Part 2: Adult basic Life Support and Cardiopulmonary Resuscitation Quality. Japan Resuscitation Council Guideline. Available from: http://www.japanresuscitationcouncil.org/wpcontent/uploads/2016/04/0e5445d84c8c2a31aaa17db0a9c67b76.pdf (in Japanese) [Accessed: November 6, 2017]

[53] Gando S, Kameue T, Nanzaki S, Nakanishi Y. Massive fibrin formation with consecutive impairment of fibrinolysis in patients with out-of-hospital cardiac arrest. Thrombosis and Haemostasis. 1997;**77**:278-282

[54] Hagiwara S, Murata M, Kaneko M, Aoki M, Kanbe M, Ohyama Y, Tamura J, Oshima K. Usefulness of serum fibrin degradation products and d-dimer levels as biomarkers to predict return of spontaneous circulation in patients with cardiopulmonary arrest on arrival: Comparison with acid-base balance. Acute Medicine & Surgery. 2014;**1**:222-227. DOI: 10.1097/TA.0b013e31828cc967

[55] Szymanski FM, Karpinski G, Filipiak KJ, Platek AE, Hrynkiewicz-Szymanska A, Kotkowski M, Opolski G. Usefulness of the D-dimer concentration as a predictor of mortality in patients with out-of-hospital cardiac arrest. The American Journal of Cardiology. 2013;**112**:467-471. DOI: 10.1016/j.amjcard.2013.03.057

[56] Ono Y, Hayakawa M, Maekawa K, Kodate A, Sadamoto Y, Tominaga N, Murakami H, Yoshida T, Katabami K, Wada T, Sageshima H, Sawamura A, Gando S. Fibrin/fibrinogen degradation products (FDP) at hospital admission predict neurological outcomes in out-of-hospital cardiac arrest patients. Resuscitation. 2017;**111**:62-67. DOI: 10.1016/j.resuscitation.2016.08

6

Circulating MicroRNA Profiling in Cancer Biomarker Discovery

Francesca Scionti, Pierosandro Tagliaferri,
Pierfrancesco Tassone and Maria Teresa Di Martino

Abstract

MicroRNAs (miRNAs) are a class of small non-coding RNA molecules of approximately 22 nucleotides that regulate gene expression at the post-transcriptional level. Alterations in miRNA expression patterns correlate with a wide spectrum of pathological conditions, including cancer. miRNA profiling was mostly performed, in solid tissues, obtained by invasive diagnostic procedures. However, miRNAs in biofluids, such as serum and plasma, show high stability resulting from the formation of complexes with specific protein or incorporation within circulating exosomes or other microvesicles. Circulating miRNAs could be reliable biomarkers for early-stage cancer diagnosis, prognosis and response to therapy. In this chapter, we analyze the major pre-analytical and analytical challenges in experimental design for circulating miRNA detection, focusing on exosome fraction and microarray-based approach.

Keywords: miRNAs, exosomes, miRNA profiling, biomarkers discovery

1. Introduction

MicroRNAs (miRNAs) are small evolutionary conserved non-coding RNAs of 19–25 nucleotides that bind to the 3′-untranslated region (3′-UTR) of target mRNAs, resulting in a negative regulation of gene expression by suppressing translation or causing mRNA degradation [1]. The complex miRNA network plays an important role in the regulation of cellular processes such as development, proliferation, differentiation and apoptosis. Significant changes of tissue miRNA "signatures" occur in various diseases, including cancer [2–4]. More than 50% of human miRNAs are mapped to chromosomal region of genomic instability due to extensive repetitive sequences resulting in structural mutations (deletion, duplication and translocation) during tumor development [5]. Regulation of miRNA expression is an important mechanism by which tumor-suppressor proteins and oncogenic proteins exert some of their effects. A decrease or mutation in tumor-suppressor miRNAs can lead to overexpression of oncogenic proteins, in contrast to an overexpression of oncogenic miRNAs which can reduce expression of tumor suppressors. For example, tumor suppressor of the let-7 family targets RAS oncogene, which is involved in cell growth, differentiation and survival; reduced expression of let-7 miRNAs correlates with poor survival in many cancers [6]. In contrast, oncogenic miRNAs in the cluster miR-17-92, comprising six miRNAs (miR-17, miR-18a, miR-19a, miR-20a, miR-19b-1 and miR-92a-1), inhibits PTEN to activate AKT signaling and promote cancer cell survival [7].

miRNAs have been considered promising candidates as diagnostic and prognostic biomarkers for the strong correlation between expression patterns of miRNAs and disease status and for the differences between normal and cancer tissues. This reflects the current evidence that some miRNAs are overexpressed or downregulated exclusively or preferentially in certain cancer types.

Although miRNA profiling of tumors has been reported in solid tissues, obtained by invasive procedures, as an excellent prognostic test [8], routine biopsies from any organ for miRNA profiling are not practical options. Different studies suggest that circulating miRNAs are reliable indicators of pathological change because of their stability and protection against RNase digestion resulting from the formation of complexes with specific protein or incorporation within circulating exosomes or other extracellular vesicles (EV) [9]. In this context, accumulating evidence suggests that tumor cells are able to alter the function of both local and distant normal cells, thereby promoting tumor growth and metastasis, through the transfer of EV cargo [10]. miR-21, which targets the tumor-suppressor gene PTEN and programmed cell death 4 (PDCD4), is one of the first discovered and most investigated circulating miRNAs. Its upregulation seems to be of diagnostic and prognostic value in a variety of solid and hematological malignancies. High serum levels of miR-21 were strongly associated with lymph node metastasis, advanced-stage clinical disease and poor survival [11]. In patients with ovarian cancer, high serum levels of miR-34a were associated with lymph node disease and distant metastases [12].

Also, in patients with prostate cancer, plasma levels of miR-21, miR-141 and miR-221 were significantly higher in patients with metastases as compared to patients with localized or locally advanced-stage disease [13].

Currently, a variety of miRNA detection methods, including northern blotting, in situ hybridization, quantitative reverse transcription PCR (qRT-PCR), microarray and deep sequencing, are commonly used [14]. However, miRNA profiling in biofluid samples is affected by a range of pre-analytical and analytical challenges in experimental design, from sample collection to profiling and data analysis (**Figure 1**). In this chapter, we will propose a workflow for exosomal miRNA detection from sera samples using the Affymetrix GeneChip microarray platform as a powerful molecular approach for biomarker discovery to translate into clinical practice.

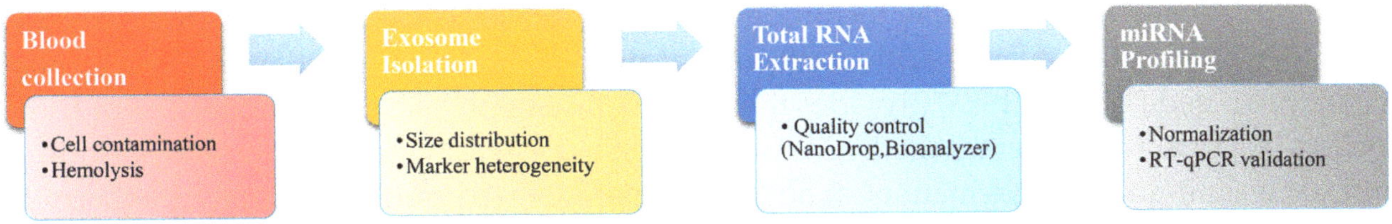

Figure 1. Summary of workflow in designing miRNA profiling from blood serum.

2. Methodological challenges in miRNA profiling design

2.1. Sample collection

Blood sample processing has a substantial impact on the results of miRNA profiling. During blood collection, it is important to avoid cellular contamination and hemolysis that can occur during phlebotomy as miRNAs derived from red and white blood cells risk to mask the intensities of truly circulating miRNA species. Residual platelets and microparticles can also affect the miRNA profile so an additional centrifugation is recommended prior to freezing samples. Moreover, biofluidics contain inhibitors of the reverse transcriptase and polymerase enzymes that can inhibit the enzymatic reactions in RT-qPCR so it is important to minimize the carryover of inhibitors into the RNA.

In our protocol, blood samples were collected and processed according to the national cancer institute (NCI's) Early Detection Research Network (EDRN) standard operating procedures for the collection and preparation of serum [15].

Whole blood samples were collected in red-top vacutainer tubes. Blood samples were incubated at room temperature for 30 min to allow complete coagulation. Coagulated samples were then centrifuged at 1500 × *g* for 20 min at room temperature to separate serum. The serum was transferred to new cryotubes with care so as to not to disturb the red blood layer and then centrifuged for 5 min at 3000 × *g* to remove cells. Aliquots of 1.5 ml of supernatant containing the cell-free serum were stored in cryotubes at −80°C until RNA extraction. Hemolyzed samples were excluded from further analysis.

2.2. Exosome isolation and characterization

The established standard for exosome isolation is ultracentrifugation [16]. However, this method cannot discriminate between exosomes and other microvesicles because different vesicles of similar size as well as protein aggregates can co-sediment at 100,000 × *g*.

Recently, methods claiming fast and simple exosome-purification procedures without ultracentrifugation are commercially available by various firms that use polymer-based precipitation or immune capture by antibody-coated beads.

However, according to the International Society for Extracellular Vesicles (ISEV) the separation of non-vesicular entities, such as protein complexes, from EV is not fully achievable by common EV isolation protocols, including centrifugation protocols or commercial kits. On the other hand, a list of EV-specific markers that distinguish subsets of EVs from each other is not proposed [17]. The ISEV provides minimal requirements to claim the presence of EV in pellets isolated from different methods. They suggested assessing the protein composition in at least a semi-quantitative manner in any EV preparation (Western blots, flow cytometry or mass spectrometry techniques). Size distribution of EVs, such as nanoparticle-tracking analysis (NTA), dynamic light scattering or resistive pulse sensing, needs to be analyzed. However, the values acquired with these techniques should be compared with TEM, AFM or other microscopy techniques, since they do not distinguish membrane vesicles from co-isolated non-membranous particles of similar size.

In our laboratory, serum exosomes underwent isolation by miRCURY™ Exosome Isolation Kit (Exiqon, Vedbaek, Denmark). The process is based on capturing water molecules which otherwise form the hydrate envelope of particles in suspension. The samples (1.5 ml) thawed on ice or at 4°C, were mixed with a precipitation solution in order to reduce the hydration of the particles. This allows precipitation of the subcellular particles below 100 nm with a low-speed centrifugation step after incubation at 4°C for 1 h. The last pellet, containing exosomes, was resuspended using 240 μL of the provided resuspension buffer and used for further RNA extraction or stored at −20°C.

NTA was performed using a NanoSight LM10-HS microscope equipped with NTA software v3.1 (NanoSight Ltd., UK). Background was extracted and the automatic setting for minimum expected particle size, minimum track length and blur settings was employed. Each sample was diluted at 1:10,000 in sterile-filtered PBS (Sigma, USA). A video of typically 60 s duration was made, with a frame rate of 30 frames per second, and particle movement was analyzed by NTA software. Only measurements with >1000 completed tracks were analyzed (**Figure 2**).

We also have used 20 μL of human CD63 coated beads (Thermo Fisher Scientific, Inc) per 50 μL sample in order to isolate CD63 positive sub-populations of exosomes from total exosome isolations derived from serum samples. The isolated exosomes were stained for typical exosome markers, such as CD63, and CD9 was analyzed with the Attune NxT Flow Cytometer (Thermo Fisher Scientific, Inc.) (**Figure 3**).

2.3. RNA purification

RNA extraction method is another important issue in miRNA profiling as the exosomal RNA pattern is highly correlated with the sample source. The principles for isolating miRNA for profiling are, in general, the same for isolation of total RNA, except that miRNA isolation protocols are adapted to retain the small RNA fraction. In different studies describing exosome RNA, a number of alternative RNA extraction methods have been used, including phenol-based techniques, combined phenol and column-based approaches and pure column-based techniques [18–22].

For RNA purification from exosomes, we used the miRCURY™ RNA Isolation Kit (Exiqon, Vedbaek, Denmark) that is based on spin column chromatography using a proprietary resin as the separation matrix. First, membrane particles and cells were lysed using the lysis solution and then proteins were precipitated using the provided protein precipitation solution.

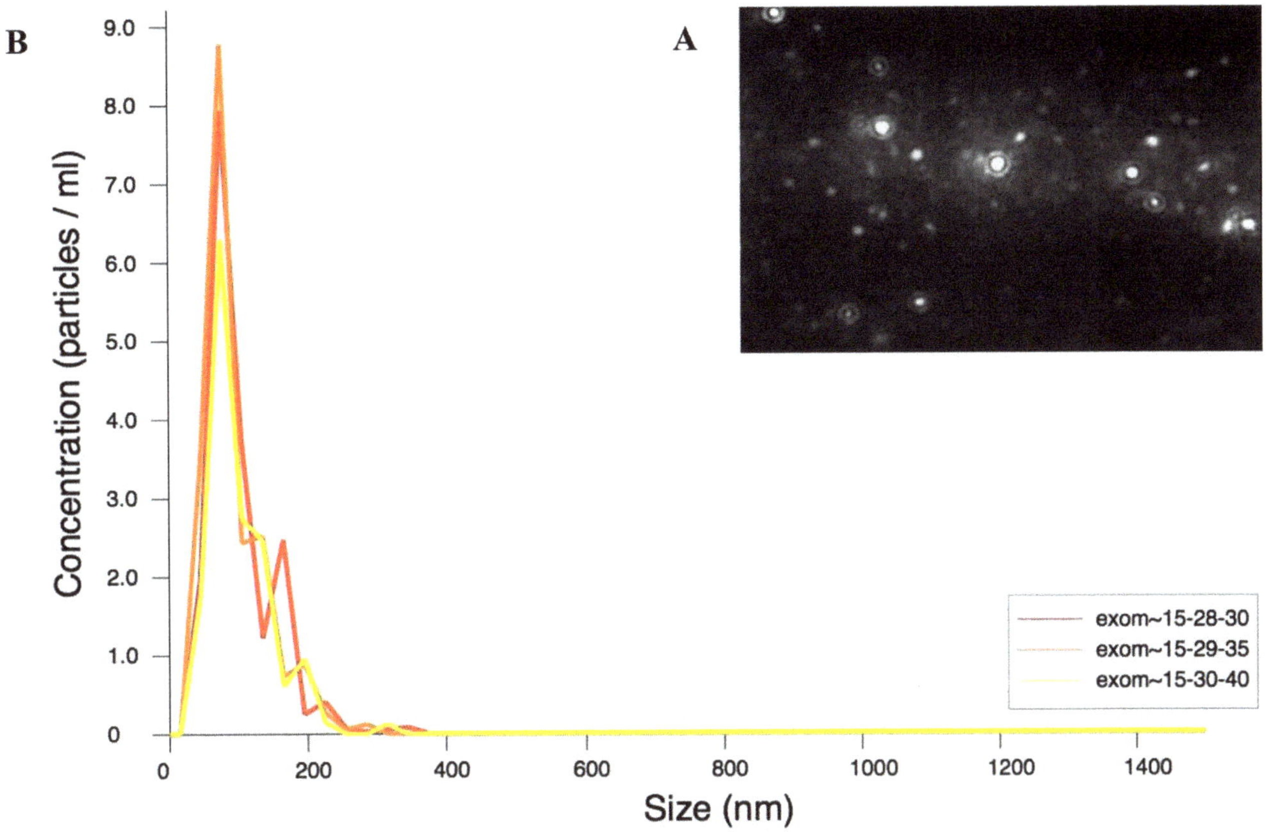

Figure 2. Extracellular vesicle NanoSight data. Example NanoSight NTA video frame (A), NanoSight NTA particle size/concentration for 3 different miRCURY™ Exosome Isolation Kit recovered exosome pellets (B).

Isopropanol was added to the supernatant and the solution was loaded onto a spin column. Thus, only molecules of RNA will bind to the resin, while proteins will be removed in the flow through. The RNA bound to the column was then washed with provided wash solution in order to remove any remaining impurities and then eluted with 100 μL of RNase free water.

We also evaluated miRNA recovery from serum samples by the use of the exogenous synthetic miRNA cel-mir-39 (Applied Biosystems, Inc.) as standard control. For this procedure during RNA isolation, a known amount of cel-mir-39 (25 fmol) was spiked in each serum sample after the denaturation step. Consistent and homogeneous miRNA recovery leads to cel-miR-39 levels that are similar in all samples. A standard curve was generated using five ten-fold dilution of cel-miR-39 (1.4×10^{-4}–1.4×10^{-8} ng) processed in parallel with qRT-PCR of experimental samples. The copy number of spiked cel-miR-39 was estimated, plotting Ct values, versus the copy number of the synthetic miRNA. The recovery of the synthetic miRNA is considered consistent if cel-miR-39 Ct values are within the range of acceptability ($\leq 2 \times$ standard deviation) in replicate isolations.

2.4. RNA quantification and quality control

Exosomal RNA purity was assessed by Nanodrop ND-1000 UV spectrometer (Thermo Scientific, Wilmington, DE) at the absorbance of 230, 260 and 280 nm. RNA samples extracted using the miRCURY™ method produced RNA concentrations above the lower detection limit of 2 ng/µL of the NanoDrop instrument and less than 10 ng/µL. Moreover, the miRCURY™ RNA isolation method showed a high average A260/280 ratio (1.9 ± 0.1) but low average

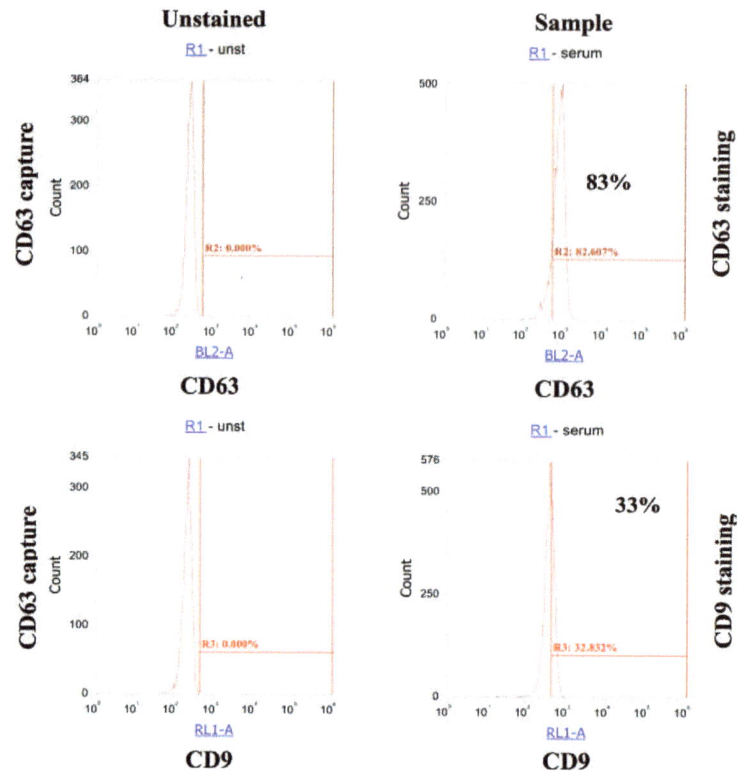

Figure 3. Flow analysis on exosome sub-populations (A). Exosomes isolated with CD63 showed that serum-derived exosome in our samples express high level of CD63 marker (82.6%) and a moderate level of CD9 markers (32.8%) (B).

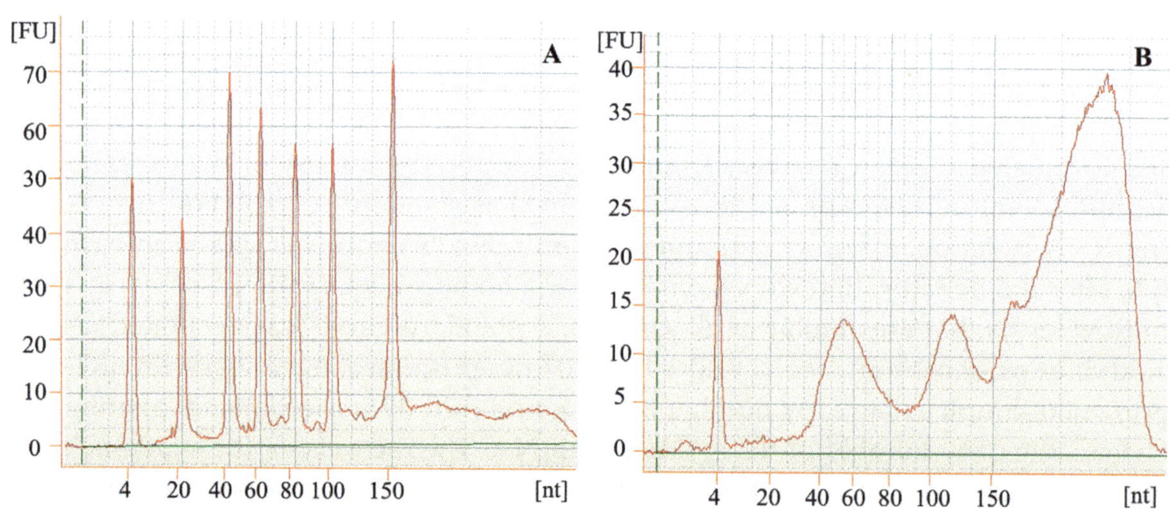

Figure 4. Bioanalyzer analysis of serum exosomal small RNA. Exosome total RNA derived from serum was analyzed using Small RNA Kit in an Agilent 2100 Bioanalyzer. The electropherograms show the size distribution in nucleotides (nt) and fluorescence intensity (FU) of ladder (A) and exosome total RNA (B). The peak at 4 nt is an internal standard. The Small RNA region is visible in the interval of 0–150 nucleotides, including the miRNAs in the sizes between 10 and 40 nucleotides.

A260/230 ratio (<2.0). These values are consistent and acceptable in samples containing very low amounts of RNA, as biofluid samples.

Because of the absence of 18S and 28S rRNA species in serum, the quality of isolated RNA samples might not be assessable by means of RNA integrity number (RIN), as a rule for total RNA samples to use for microarray procedures. On this basis, we used the Agilent Small RNA assays that are able to resolve fragments in the range 0–150 nucleotides (**Figure 4**).

3. MiRNA profiling and data analysis

miRNA expression profiling has allowed the identification of miRNAs that are involved in many biological processes, including organism development and establishment and maintenance of tissue differentiation [23, 24]. Thus, miRNAs are being explored as elements for cell-fate reprogramming in stem-cell applications or as biomarkers for identifying the origin of cancers of unknown primary sites. The expression pattern of miRNAs is widely different being tissue specific and related to developmental stages. Measuring miRNA expression can also be useful for system-level studies of gene regulation, especially when miRNA profiles are integrated with mRNA profiling. Circulating extracellular miRNAs, including exosome miRNA, are quantifiable in a range of specimen types including serum, plasma, urine and formalin-fixed tissue block. Hence, they are important as non-invasive biomarkers for many molecular diagnostic applications, including cancer [25, 26], cardiovascular and autoimmune diseases [27] and forensics [28]. **Table 1** shows new and promising miRNAs as potential biomarkers for diagnosis and prognosis of different cancers.

3.1. General consideration for high-throughput miRNA profiling

The yield of RNA extracted from biofluids is usually very low, in the order of 1–10 ng. If we consider that miRNAs represent only 0.01% of total RNA, the strategies used for their detection and quantification are crucial. Some general consideration must be made in high-throughput miRNA profiling. First, the length of mature miRNA (19–25 nucleotides) is too low to allow annealing to the traditional primers during the reverse transcription step. Second, unlike mRNAs, miRNAs lack poly(A) tail, a region frequently used to anneal complementary and universal primers for RNA enrichment or reverse transcription. Third, miRNAs exist in different isoforms, so-called isomiRs, that are functional and evolutionarily important and, inside the same family (e.g., the let-7 family), can differ by a single base to the reference miRNA sequence. Depending on the goals of an miRNA profiling experiment, measurement of different forms may be required, even if the large majority of miRNAs typically show only modest-length heterogeneity. Another challenge for miRNA high-throughput profiling is variance in miRNA GC content that is reflected in different melting temperatures (Tm) of annealing reactions. To date, three major approaches are used for miRNA profiling: quantitative reverse transcription PCR (qRT-PCR), hybridization-based methods (microarrays) and next-generation sequencing (NGS) (RNA-seq). Microarrays were among the first hybridization-based methods to be used for parallel analysis of large numbers of miRNAs.

Cancer	Samples	miRNAs		Types of biomarkers	Reference
Head and neck	Plasma	miR-21	qRT-PCR	D	[29]
Lung cancer	Serum	miR-182, miR183, miR-210, miR-126	qRT-PCR	D	[30]
	Serum	miR-125b	qRT-PCR	R	[31]
Breast cancer	Serum	miR-1, miR-92a, miR-133a, miR-133b	Microarray	D	[32]
	Serum	miR-125b	qRT-PCR	R	[33]
Ovarian cancer	Serum	miR-34a		P	[12]
Prostate cancer	Plasma	miR-21, miR-141, miR-221	qRT-PCR	D	[13]
Gastric cancer	Serum	miR-1, miR-20a, miR-27a, miR-34, miR-423-5p	qRT-PCR	D	[34]
Renal cancer	Serum	miR-378, miR-451	qRT-PCR	D	[35]
Pancreatic cancer	Serum	miR-16 and miR-196a	qRT-PCR	D	[36]
		miR-21	qRT-PCR	R	[37]
Colorectal cancer	Plasma	miR-409-3p, miR-7, miR-93	qRT-PCR	D	[38]
		miR-126	qRT-PCR	R	[39]
Hepatocellular cancer	Exosome	miR-101, miR-221, miR-221, miR-224	qRT-PCR	D	[40]
Melanoma	Serum	miR-221	qRT-PCR	D, P	[41]
Lymphoma	Serum	miR-221	qRT-PCR	P	[42]
Leukemia	Exosome	miR-29a	qRT-PCR	P	[8]

D = diagnostic; P = prognostic; R = response predictor.

Table 1. Circulating miRNAs as potential biomarkers in different cancers.

3.2. Microarray miRNA profiling

Microarrays provide a high-throughput approach to profile all annotated miRNAs, in different types of samples including biological fluids. This method is relatively less expensive than others, such as qRT-PCR and next-generation sequencing (NGS). Moreover, the integrated analysis of the expression profile of miRNAs and their target genes, together with the analysis of each miRNA gene target pathway, is able to provide information on the function of each miRNA for a given sample. The technique generally begins with the enzymatic or chemical marking of targets followed by their hybridization to oligonucleotides fixed on a solid support. The signal generated by each probe is detected by a scanner and analyzed by specific software able to process the signal intensity. The variables related to the method include the different hybridization efficiencies of each probe, due to their different content in GC, the different melting temperature, due to the reduced size of miRNAs, the bias due to the enzymatic labeling and the relative low dynamic range. Microarray-based methods generally require a larger amount of starting material than qRT-PCR, and it can be challenging to develop probes and hybridization conditions that work well to detect many different miRNAs at once [43, 44]. miRNA profiling by NGS platforms may be the most promising approach, as it largely avoids many miRNA measurement pitfalls [45]. However, NGS remains expensive and labor intensive, both in the sample preparation and data analysis.

3.3. Affymetrix GeneChip microarray platform

To date, oligonucleotide-miRNA microarray analysis is the most common high-throughput technique for assessment of disease-specific expression of hundreds of miRNAs. The Affymetrix GeneChip® miRNA microarrays platform provides the most sensitive, accurate and complete measurement of small non-coding RNA transcripts involved in gene regulation. It represents miRNA sequences from all organisms present in miRBase (http://www.mirbase.org), as well as small nucleolar RNAs (snoRNA) and small Cajal body-specific RNAs (scaRNA) included in snoRNABase (http://www.snorna.biotoul.fr/) and Ensembl (http://www.ensembl.org). This platform has been used in our laboratory with success to profile exosome non-coding RNA from serum samples (unpublished data, manuscript in preparation). The protocols for non-coding RNA profiling include the use of the Affymetrix FlashTag Biotin HSR RNA Labeling Kit (Affymetrix, Santa Clara, CA, USA) and the detection by fluorescent emission. Total RNA samples or total RNA samples enriched for low molecular weight (LMW) RNA were starting materials. The process begins with a poly(A) tailing reaction followed by the ligation of a biotinylated signal molecule to the target RNA samples. The labeled RNA samples are included in the hybridization mix and hybridized overnight to Affymetrix GeneChip miRNA arrays (Affymetrix, Santa Clara, CA, USA), followed by a procedure to wash, stain and scan the array to acquire probe cell intensity data (CEL file). To date, the GeneChip miRNA 4.0 array is the updated array designed to interrogate all mature miRNA sequences contained in miRBase release 20, including 30,424 probe sets, covering 203 organisms and requiring low sample input (130–1000 ng total RNA). CEL files analysis by the Expression Console Software coupled with Transcriptome Analysis Console (TAC) Software (Affymetrix, Santa Clara, CA, USA) leads to a simple, fast and free analysis for Affymetrix GeneChip expression arrays.

3.4. Analysis of raw data

Raw data processing begins with quality control analysis by assessing the performance of internal controls and analyzing replicates to detect biases. For example, microarrays have well-known geographic biases, because some areas of the array perform differently from others. Data normalization, which is the next step after quality assessment, is crucially for obtaining accurate results [46]. The goal of normalization is to adjust the data to remove variation across samples not related to the biological condition and therefore allowing the identification of relevant biological differences. The normalization step is particularly important because some of the discrepancies between miRNA profiling studies are in part due to the application of different normalization approaches. GeneChip array data are normalized by the use of a tool that uses Robust Multichip Analysis (RAM) plus detection above background (DABG) algorithms, as default analysis. RAM is a robust linear normalization model, to minimize the effect of probe-specific affinity differences, and consists of three steps: background adjustment, quantile normalization and summarization. DABG is a detection metric generated by comparing perfect match probes to a distribution of background probes.

miRNA profiling experiments typically involve comparisons between two or more groups, and therefore the next stage of analysis is usually the calculation of differential miRNA expression between groups. The degree of fold difference that constitutes a meaningful difference depends on the experimental context, although it is always useful to assess the statistical significance and false discovery rate that is associated with the differential miRNA expression. This comparison yields a p-value, which is, then, combined into a probe set level p-value using the Fischer equation. Statistical analysis is performed using TAC and a fold change of two is commonly adopted to describe the signal changes between groups.

3.5. Circulating miRNA profiling challenges

Circulating exosome miRNAs are surprisingly stable and show distinct expression profiles among different fluids. Given the instability of most RNA molecules in the extracellular environment, the presence and apparent stability of miRNAs in body fluids such as serum and other body fluids, that are known to contain ribonucleases, suggest that secreted miRNAs are packaged in some manner to protect them against RNase digestion. miRNAs could be shielded from degradation by packaging in lipid vesicles, like exosomes, in complexes with RNA-binding proteins or both [47]. This view supports the idea that extracellular miRNAs are prepared for export in one cell. They can be recognized, taken up and utilized by another cell, working as mediators of cell-cell communication [48–50]. The growing interest in developing circulating miRNAs as blood-based biomarkers requires very careful consideration of the effects of various pre-analytical procedures, such as handling and storage conditions of the sample before processing, which can affect the reliability and reproducibility of circulating miRNA quantification. The main technical difficulty to study miRNA expression profiles is the efficient extraction of miRNAs from biological samples, because of their small size and their attachment to lipids and proteins. The use of commercial extraction kits has become available to optimize the extraction of small RNAs and normalize sample-to-sample variations in isolation procedures. Therefore, it is important to establish standardized protocols for blood collection, sample storage conditions, inclusion of exogenous and endogenous miRNA controls for each clinical sample and standardized calculations for normalization of the results to ensure the reproducible and accurate quantification of circulating miRNA levels so that miRNA analysis can be implemented in the clinical laboratory setting.

3.6. Validation of microarray results by qRT-PCR

miRNA microarrays are less expensive but inclined to have a lower sensitivity and dynamic range and are therefore best used as discovery tools rather than as quantitative assay platforms. Current publication guidelines require that all microarray results are confirmed by an independent gene expression profiling method. Most researchers choose qRT-PCR as the preferred method for the validation of microarray data using both TaqMan and SYBR-green assay.

The TaqMan qRT-PCR method uses a stem-loop RT primer, specifically designed to detect the 3′ end of individual mature miRNAs generating a unique template for RT. In the qPCR step, cDNA is amplified with specific primers and product accumulation is monitored using a fluorogenic probe (TaqMan probe), complementary to the target gene. In SYBR-green-based qRT-PCR, miRNA is typically poly-adenylated at the 3′ end, and oligo-d(T) is used as an RT primer while a double-strand DNA binding dye (SYBR-green) allows for the detection of PCR products during qPCR.

We routinely use TaqMan® microRNA assays (Applied Biosystems, Inc.) to validate microarray data on the same clinical samples as described [51] and perform qPCR in triplicate reactions and the $2^{-\Delta\Delta Ct}$ method to estimate the relative quantity of each miRNA [52]. An important issue is the choice of normalizer. Typically, "housekeeping" genes selected as endogenous controls allow normalization of qPCR data as they are affected by the same experimental variability as the target genes. In a cellular context, stable small RNA controls, such as RNU44, RNU48 and RNU6, are usually used. However, for circulating miRNAs, there is growing evidence that the abovementioned small RNAs are highly variable or not stably detectable [53]. This lack of consensus has resulted in the generation of various normalization strategies. An approach widely used and employed in our group is the selection, from each microarray study, of several genes as a normalizer based on their stable expression.

4. Conclusion

Circulating miRNAs are attractive as clinical biomarkers for diagnostic purposes, as well as for monitoring disease progression and response to treatment. However, the nature of circulating miRNAs places several challenges. The success of the circulating miRNA profiling requires rigorous control of pre-analytic and analytic variables, specifically when investigating potential circulating miRNA markers. Here, we provided a consistent and reproducible method for circulating miRNA detection, profiling and analysis. We discussed the main issues associated with miRNA measurement that is crucial for miRNA profiling, especially for exosomal circulating miRNA. In addition, it needs to take into account that it is difficult to measure specific miRNA levels because they are short and conserved sequences, paralogs or distinguish between precursor and mature forms. In our work experience, the use of standard protocols for sample preparation, and of exogenous synthetic miRNA as the standard control, helps to solve a part of these problems. Microarray data processing such as normalization procedures among different samples is challenging especially for extracellular miRNA. In our work experience, it can be concluded that the use of robust algorithms and software may avoid errors and false positive discovery. However, the validation of array results by the use of an alternative methodology, especially when using different protocols and platforms for profiling purposes, is mandatory.

Objective assessment of these technical metrics is an important step toward understanding the appropriate use of microarray technology application in general and more specifically for circulating miRNA to be used as clinical markers as well as in regulatory settings.

Acknowledgements

This chapter has been supported by the Italian Association for Cancer Research (AIRC), PI: PT. "Special Program Molecular Clinical Oncology - 5 per mille" n. 9980, 2010/15.

Conflict of interest

The authors declare no conflicts of interest.

Author details

Francesca Scionti, Pierosandro Tagliaferri, Pierfrancesco Tassone and Maria Teresa Di Martino*

*Address all correspondence to: teresadm@unicz.it

Department of Experimental and Clinical Medicine, Medical Oncology, Magna Graecia University of Catanzaro, Italy

References

[1] Bartel DP. MicroRNAs: Genomics, biogenesis, mechanism, and function. Cell. 2004;**116**: 281-297. DOI: 10.1016/S0092-8674(04)00045-5

[2] Xiao C, Rajewsky K. MicroRNA control in the immune system: Basic principles. Cell. 2009;**136**:26-36. DOI: 10.1016/j.cell.2008.12.027

[3] Slack FJ, Weidhaas JB. MicroRNA in cancer prognosis. The New England Journal of Medicine. 2008;**359**:2720-2722. DOI: 10.1056/NEJMe0808667

[4] Romaine SP, Tomaszewski M, Condorelli G, Samani NJ. MicroRNAs in cardiovascular disease: An introduction for clinicians. Heart. 2015;**101**:921-928. DOI: 10.1136/heartjnl-2013-305402

[5] Esquela-Kerscher A, Slack FJ. Oncomirs—microRNAs with a role in cancer. Nature Reviews. Cancer. 2006;**6**:259-269. DOI: 10.1038/nrc184

[6] Hayashita Y, Osada H, Tatematsu Y, Yamada H, Yanagisawa K, Tomida S, Yatabe Y, Kawahara K, Sekido Y, Takahashi T. A polycistronic microRNA cluster, miR-17-92, is

overexpressed in human lung cancers and enhances cell proliferation. Cancer Research. 2005;**65**:9628-9632. DOI: 10.1158/0008-5472.CAN-05-2352

[7] Mogilyansky E, Rigoutsos I. The miR-17/92 cluster: A comprehensive update on its genomics, genetics, functions and increasingly important and numerous roles in health and disease. Cell Death and Differentiation. 2013;**20**:1603-1614. DOI: 10.1038/cdd.2013.125

[8] Yeh YY, Ozer HG, Lehman AM, Maddocks K, Yu L, Johnson AJ, Byrd JC. Characterization of CLL exosomes reveals a distinct microRNA signature and enhanced secretion by activation of BCR signaling. Blood. 2015;**125**:3297-3305. DOI: 10.1182/blood-2014-12-618470

[9] Mitchell PS, Parkin RK, Kroh EM, Fritz BR, Wyman SK, Pogosova-Agadjanyan EL, Peterson A, Noteboom J, O'Briant KC, Allen A, Lin DW, Urban N, Drescher CW, Knudsen BS, Stirewalt DL, Gentleman R, Vessella RL, Vessella RL, Nelson PS, Martin DB, Tewari M. Circulating microRNA as stable blood-based markers for cancer detection. PNAS. 2008;**105**:105013-105018. DOI: 10.1073/pnas.0804549105

[10] Valadi H, Ekstrom K, Bossios A, Sjostrand M, Lee JJ, Lotvall JO. Exosome-mediated transfer of mRNAs and microRNAs is a novel mechanism of genetic exchange between cells. Nature Cell Biology. 2007;**9**:654-659. DOI: 10.1038/ncb1596

[11] Huang Y, Yang YB, Zhang XH, Yu XL, Wang ZB, Cheng XC. MicroRNA-21 gene and cancer. Medical Oncology. 2013;**30**:376. DOI: 10.1007/s12032-012-0376-8

[12] Roth C, Rack B, Muller V, Janni W, Pantel K, Schwarzenbach H. Circulating microRNAs as blood-based markers for patients with primary and metastatic breast cancer. Breast Cancer Research. 2010;**12**:R90. DOI: 10.1186/bcr2766

[13] Yaman Agaoglu F, Kovancilar M, Dizdar Y, Darendeliler E, Holdenrieder S, Dalay N, Gezer U. Investigation of miR-21, miR-141, and miR-221 in blood circulation of patients with prostate cancer. Tumour Biology. 2011;**32**:583-588. DOI: 10.1007/s13277-011-0154-9

[14] Pritchard CC, Cheng HH, Tewari M. MicroRNA profiling: Approaches and considerations. Nature Reviews. Genetics. 2012;**13**:358-369. DOI: 10.1038/nrg3198

[15] Tuck MK, Chan DW, Chia D, Godwin AK, Grizzle WE, Krueger KE, Rom W, Sanda M, Sorbara L, Stass S, Wang W, Brenner DE. Standard operating procedures for serum and plasma collection: Early detection research network consensus statement standard operating procedure integration working group. Journal of Proteome Research. 2009;**8**:113-117. DOI: 10.1021/pr800545q

[16] Thery C, Amigorena S, Raposo G, Clayton A. Isolation and characterization of exosomes from cell culture supernatants and biological fluids. Current Protocols in Cell Biology. 2006;**3**:3.22.1-3.22.29. DOI: 10.1002/0471143030.cb0322s30

[17] Lotvall J, Hill AF, Hochberg F, Buzas EI, Di Vizio D, Gardiner C, Gho YS, Kurochkin IV, Mathivanan S, Quesenberry P, Sahoo S, Tahara H, Wauben MH, Witwer KW, Thery C. Minimal experimental requirements for definition of extracellular vesicles and their functions: A position statement from the International Society for Extracellular Vesicles. Journal of Extracellular Vesicles. 2014;**3**:26913. DOI: 10.3402/jev.v3.26913

[18] Skog J, Wurdinger T, van Rijn S, Meijer DH, Gainche L, Sena-Esteves M, Curry WT Jr, Carter BS, Krichevsky AM, Breakefield XO. Glioblastoma microvesicles transport RNA and proteins that promote tumour growth and provide diagnostic biomarkers. Nature Cell Biology. 2008;**10**:1470-1476. DOI: 10.1038/ncb1800

[19] Taylor DD, Gercel-Taylor C. MicroRNA signatures of tumor-derived exosomes as diagnostic biomarkers of ovarian cancer. Gynecologic Oncology. 2008;**110**:13-21. DOI: 10.1096/fj.08-119131

[20] Kesimer M, Scull M, Brighton B, DeMaria G, Burns K, O'Neal W, Pickles RJ, Sheehan JK. Characterization of exosome-like vesicles released from human tracheobronchial ciliated epithelium: A possible role in innate defense. The FASEB Journal. 2009;**23**:1858-1868. DOI: 10.1096/fj.08-119131

[21] Michael A, Bajracharya SD, Yuen PS, Zhou H, Star RA, Illei GG, Alevizos I. Exosomes from human saliva as a source of microRNA biomarkers. Oral Diseases. 2010;**16**:34-38. DOI: 10.1111/j.1601-0825.2009.01604.x

[22] Ohshima K, Inoue K, Fujiwara A, Hatakeyama K, Kanto K, Watanabe Y, Muramatsu K, Fukuda Y, Ogura S, Yamaguchi K, Mochizuki T. Let-7 microRNA family is selectively secreted into the extracellular environment via exosomes in a metastatic gastric cancer cell line. PLoS One. 2010;**5**:e13247. DOI: 10.1371/journal.pone.0013247

[23] Wienholds E, Kloosterman WP, Miska E, Alvarez-Saavedra E, Berezikov E, de Bruijn E, Horvitz HR, Kauppinen S, Plasterk RH. MicroRNA expression in zebrafish embryonic development. Science. 2005;**309**:310-311. DOI: 10.1126/science.1114519

[24] Alvarez-Garcia I, Miska EA. MicroRNA functions in animal development and human disease. Development. 2005;**132**:4653-4662. DOI: 10.1242/dev.02073

[25] Lu J, Getz G, Miska EA, Alvarez-Saavedra E, Lamb J, Peck D, Sweet-Cordero A, Ebert BL, Mak RH, Ferrando AA, Downing JR, Jacks T, Horvitz HR, Golub TR. MicroRNA expression profiles classify human cancers. Nature. 2005;**435**:834-838. DOI: 10.1038/nature03702

[26] Rosenfeld N, Aharonov R, Meiri E, Rosenwald S, Spector Y, Zepeniuk M, Benjamin H, Shabes N, Tabak S, Levy A, Lebanony D, Goren Y, Silberschein E, Targan N, Ben-Ari A, Gilad S, et al. MicroRNAs accurately identify cancer tissue origin. Nature Biotechnology. 2008;**26**:462-469. DOI: 10.1038/nbt1392

[27] Tili E, Michaille JJ, Costinean S, Croce CM. MicroRNAs, the immune system and rheumatic disease. Nature Clinical Practice. Rheumatology. 2008;**4**:534-541. DOI: 10.1038/ncprheum0885

[28] Courts C, Madea B. Specific micro-RNA signatures for the detection of saliva and blood in forensic body-fluid identification. Journal of Forensic Sciences. 2011;**56**:1464-1470. DOI: 10.1111/j.1556-4029.2011.01894.x

[29] Hsu CM, Lin PM, Wang YM, Chen ZJ, Lin SF, Yang MY. Circulating miRNA is a novel marker for head and neck squamous cell carcinoma. Tumour Biology. 2012;**33**:1933-1942. DOI: 10.1007/s13277-012-0454-8

[30] Zhu W, Zhou K, Zha Y, Chen D, He J, Ma H, Liu X, Le H, Zhang Y. Diagnostic value of serum miR-182, miR-183, miR-210, and miR-126 levels in patients with early-stage non-small cell lung cancer. PLoS One. 2016;**11**:e0153046. DOI: 10.1371/journal

[31] Cui E, Li H, Hua F, Wang B, Mao W, Feng X, Li J, Wang X. Serum microRNA 125b as a diagnostic or prognostic biomarker for advanced NSCLC patients receiving cisplatin-based chemotherapy. Acta Pharmacologica Sinica. 2016;**34**:309-313. DOI: 10.1038/aps.2012.125

[32] Chan M, Liaw CS, Ji SM, Tan HH, Wong CY, Thike AA, Tan PH, Ho GH, Lee AS. Identification of circulating microRNA signatures for breast cancer detection. Clinical Cancer Research. 2013;**19**:4477-4487. DOI: 10.1158/1078-0432.CCR-12-3401

[33] Wang H, Tan G, Dong L, Cheng L, Li K, Wang Z, Luo H. Circulating MiR-125b as a marker predicting chemoresistance in breast cancer. PLoS One. 2012;**7**:e34210. DOI: 10.1371/journal.pone.0034210

[34] Liu R, Zhang C, Hu Z, Li G, Wang C, Yang C, Huang D, Chen X, Zhang H, Zhuang R, Deng T, Liu H, Yin J, Wang S, Zen K, Ba Y, Zhang CY. A five-microRNA signature identified from genome-wide serum microRNA expression profiling serves as a fingerprint for gastric cancer diagnosis. European Journal of Cancer. 2011;**47**:784-791. DOI: 10.1016/j.ejca.2010.10.025

[35] Redova M, Poprach A, Nekvindova J, Iliev R, Radova L, Lakomy R, Svoboda M, Vyzula R, Slaby O. Circulating miR-378 and miR-451 in serum are potential biomarkers for renal cell carcinoma. Journal of Translational Medicine. 2012;**10**:55. DOI: 10.1186/1479-5876-10-55

[36] Liu J, Gao J, Du Y, Li Z, Ren Y, Gu J, Wang X, Gong Y, Wang W, Kong X. Combination of plasma microRNAs with serum CA19-19 for early detection of pancreatic cancer. International Journal of Cancer. 2012;**131**:683-691. DOI: 10.1002/ijc.26422

[37] Wang P et al. The serum miR-21 level serves as a predictor for the chemosensitivity of advanced pancreatic cancer, and miR-21 expression confers chemoresistance by targeting FasL. Molecular Oncology. 2013;**7**:334-345

[38] Wang S, Xiang J, Li Z, Lu S, Hu J, Gao X, Yu L, Wang L, Wang J, Wu Y, Chen Z, Zhu H. A plasma microRNA panel for early detection of colorectal cancer. International Journal of Cancer. 2015;**136**:152-161. DOI: 10.1002/ijc.28136

[39] Hansen TF, Carlsen AL, Heegaanrd NH, Sorensen FB, Jakobsen A. Changes in circulating microRNA-126 during treatment with chemotherapy and bevcizumab predicts treatment response in patients with metastatic colorectal cancer. British Journal of Cancer. 2015;**112**:624-629. DOI: 10.1038/bjc.2014.652

[40] Sohn W, Kim J, Kang SH, Yang SR, Cho JY, Cho HC, Shim SG, Paik YP. Serum exosomal microRNAs as novel biomarkers for hepatocellular carcinoma. Experimental & Molecular Medicine. 2015;**47**:e184. DOI: 10.1038/emm.2015.68

[41] Kanemaru H, Fukushima S, Yamashita J, Honda N, Oyama R, Kakimoto A, Masuguchi S, Ishihara T, Inoue Y, Jinnin M, Ihn H. The circulating microRNA-221 level in patients

with malignant melanoma as a new tumor marker. Journal of Dermatological Science. 2011;**61**:187-193. DOI: 10.1016/j.jdermsci.2010.12.010

[42] Guo HQ, Huang GL, Guo CC, Pu XX, Lin TY. Diagnostic and prognostic value of circulating miR-221 for extranodal natural killer/T-cell lymphoma. Disease Markers. 2010; **29**:251-258. DOI: 10.3233/DMA-2010-0755

[43] Sato F, Tsuchiya S, Terasawa K, Tsujimoto G. Intra-platform repeatability and inter-platform comparability of microRNA microarray technology. PLoS One. 2009;**4**:e5540. DOI: 10.1371/journal.pone.0005540

[44] Chen Y, Gelfond JA, McManus LM, Shireman PK. Reproducibility of quantitative RT-PCR array in miRNA expression profiling and comparison with microarray analysis. BMC Genomics. 2009;**10**:407. DOI: 10.1186/1471-2164-10-407

[45] Thomas MF, Ansel KM. Construction of small RNA cDNA libraries for deep sequencing. Methods in Molecular Biology. 2010;**667**:93-111. DOI: 10.1007/978-1-60761-811-9_7

[46] Meyer SU, Pfaffl MW, Ulbrich SE. Normalization strategies for microRNA profiling experiments: A 'normal' way to a hidden layer of complexity? Biotechnology Letters. 2010;**32**:1777-1788. DOI: 10.1007/s10529-010-0380-z

[47] Gibbings DJ, Ciaudo C, Erhardt M, Voinnet O. Multivesicular bodies associate with components of miRNA effector complexes and modulate miRNA activity. Nature Cell Biology. 2009;**11**:1143-1149. DOI: 10.1038/ncb1929

[48] Iguchi H, Kosaka N, Ochiya T. Secretory microRNAs as a versatile communication tool. Communicative & Integrative Biology. 2010;**3**:478-481. DOI: 10.4161/cib.3.5.12693

[49] Camussi G, Deregibus MC, Bruno S, Cantaluppi V, Biancone L. Exosomes/microvesicles as a mechanism of cell-to-cell communication. Kidney International. 2010;**78**:838-848. DOI: 10.1038/ki.2010.278

[50] Muralidharan-Chari V, Clancy JW, Sedgwick A, D'Souza-Schorey C. Microvesicles: Mediators of extracellular communication during cancer progression. Journal of Cell Science. 2010;**123**:1603-1611. DOI: 10.1242/jcs.064386

[51] Kroh EM, Parkin RK, Mitchell PS, Tewari M. Analysis of circulating microRNA biomarkers in plasma and serum using quantitative reverse transcription-PCR (qRT-PCR). Methods. 2010;**50**:298-301. DOI: 10.1016/j.ymeth.2010.01.032

[52] Schmittgen TD, Livak KJ. Analyzing real-time PCR data by the comparative C(T) method. Nature Protocols. 2008;**3**:1101-1108. DOI: 10.1038/nprot.2008.73

[53] Turchinovich A, Weiz L, Langheinz A, Burwinkel B. Characterization of extracellular circulating microRNA. Nucleic Acids Research. 2011;**39**:7223-7233. DOI: 10.1093/nar/gkr254

7

Neutrophil/Lymphocyte Ratio, Platelet/ Lymphocyte Ratio, and Mean Platelet Volume for Detection of Resectable Pancreas Cancer

Kemal Turker Ulutas, Inanc Samil Sarici and Ozgul Duzgun

Abstract

Several biomarkers have been preferred for the early diagnosis of pancreatic adenocancer (PAC), but most are not ready to be included as part of the routine diagnostic algorithm because they still lack sensitivity, specificity or reproducibility. CA19-9 is the most widely used serum-based marker for the diagnosis and follow-up of pancreatic cancer. However, CA19-9 lacks sensitivity for early or small-diameter pancreatic cancers. For more than 3 decades, information on neutrophil/lymphocyte ratio (NLR), platelet/lymphocyte ratio (PLR), mean platelet volume (MPV) has been widely available to health care practitioners, as part of the data provided in the full blood count. However, these biomarkers have more than used in the routine. The present chapter shares the prognostic significance of the hematological parameters in the light of our own findings and recent studies in the literature.

Keywords: NLR, PLR, MPV, resectable pancreas cancer, biomarker

1. Introduction

Pancreatic adenocarcinoma is a devastating disease with an extremely poor prognosis and prompt diagnostic evaluation is vital when PAC is suspected. CA19-9 is the most widely used serum-based marker for the diagnosis and follow-up of pancreatic cancer [1]. The diagnostic role of CA19-9 as a test for the detection of pancreatic malignancy remains poorly defined, because, as in other diagnostic modalities, the utility of CA19-9 has several confounding limitations. The sensitivity and specificity of CA19-9 vary, ranging from 70 to 90% and 68 to 91%, respectively. However, CA19-9 lacks sensitivity for early or small-diameter pancreatic cancers. Poorly differentiated pancreatic cancers also appear to produce less CA19-9 than either moderately or well-differentiated cancers. Another limitation is that CA19-9 can also be elevated in benign inflammatory and cholestatic diseases of the pancreaticobiliary tract [2, 3].

After inflammatory processes have emerged as key mediators of pancreatic cancer development and progression, many inflammatory pathways have been identified in recent years. Neutrophil/lymphocyte ratio (NLR), platelet/lymphocyte ratio (PLR), and mean platelet volume (MPV) are the most used in the literature [4–6]. Elevated NLR has reportedly been associated with poor survival following resection or chemotherapy in a variety of cancer. In colorectal cancer, an increasing number of studies have reported an association between elevated NLR and poor prognosis [7]. The first study done by us, including a total of 41 resectable PAC patients and 43 age-matched and sex-matched healthy participants [8]. NLR, PLR, and MPV were significantly higher in preoperative stage 1 and stage 2 PAC patients compared with age-matched and sex matched healthy participants (5.51 vs. 2.5, P = 0.002; 180 vs. 134, P = 0.017; 9.2 vs. 2.5 fl, P = 0.004) (**Table 1**). Our results suggested that NLR, PLR and MPV might be used as easily available additional biomarkers for PAC in screening general population (**Figure 1**).

The role of new tumor marker PLR has been defined recently in the prognosis of PAC [9]. Miglani et al. reported that PLR has been at least as good as CA 19-9 as diagnostic marker to differentiate between malignant and inflammatory head mass of pancreas. This is based on the fact that PAC causes thrombosis and lymphocytopenia. Platelet activation is a link in the pathophysiology of diseases prone to thrombosis and inflammation. Lymphocytopenia occurs due to systemic inflammation caused by cancers that release a number of inhibitory immunologic mediators [10]. The diagnostic value of platelet size has recently been shown to be elevated in neoplastic disorders particularly in gastric cancer. Moreover, it has been determined that platelet size has a predictive value for bone marrow metastasis in patients with solid tumors [11]. Numerous platelet markers, including MPV, have been investigated in connection with both thrombosis and inflammation.

	PAC	Control	P value
Neutrophil	6092 ± 4212	3944 ± 1219	*0.002*
PLT	230 ± 84	244 ± 64	0.39
MPV	9.21 ± 1.2	8.5 ± 0.82	*0.004*
NLR	5.51 ± 7.3	2.5 ± 1.1	*0.002*
PLR	180 ± 103	135 ± 65	0.017

Abbreviations: PLT: platelet; MPV: mean platelet volume; NLR: neutrophil/lymphocyte ratio; PLR: platelet/lymphocyte ratio; PAC: pancreatic cancer

Table 1. Hematological results of the patients and controls.

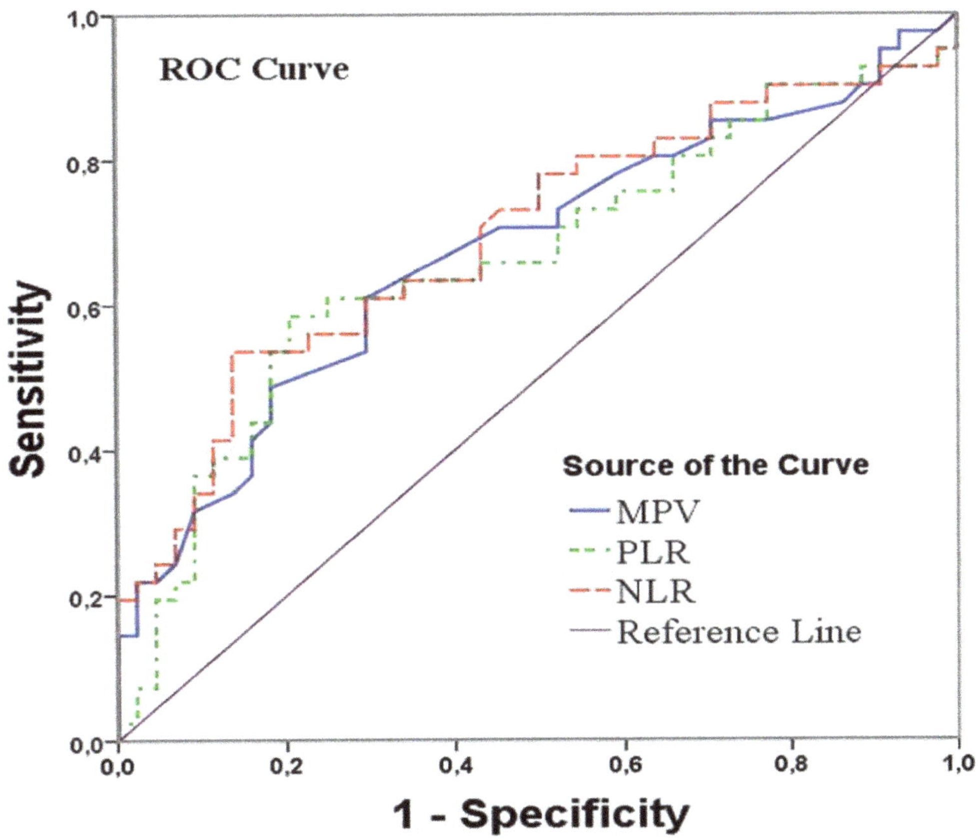

Figure 1. Receiver operating characteristic curves NLR, PLR and MPV for predicting stage 1 and stage 2 pancreatic cancer. Abbreviations: MPV: mean platelet volume; NLR: neutrophil/lymphocyte ratio; PLR: platelet/lymphocyte ratio.

2. Inflammation and PAC

In the development and progression of cancer, inflammation is a crucial and essential process [12]. Persistence of the inflammatory process within the tumor leads to an increase in the proliferation of tumor cells, angiogenesis, and the inhibition of apoptosis [13, 14]. Several reports have suggested that markers of systemic inflammation including cytokines, C-reactive protein, NLR, and PLR may provide useful information on the prognosis of colorectal gastrointestinal cancer [15, 16]. Thus, pathogenesis of PAC appears to be an inflammation-driven malignancy, as well as colorectal gastrointestinal cancer. Usually, cancer cells are a source of inflammatory cytokines and growth factors. Interleukin-6 (IL-6) is an inflammatory cytokine that can cause carcinogenesis through several signal pathways involved in carcinogenesis, as well as metastasis of a variety of malignancies, including PAC [17].

It has been shown that PAC patients have higher levels of IL-6 compared with a healthy control group [18]. We acknowledged that IL-6 is released from leukocytes and is also able to activate the production of IL-6 by tumor cells through the IL-6 receptor. Besides their role in homeostasis, platelets and leucocytes take part in the pathophysiology of tumor angiogenesis [19]. Platelets are known to be the major transporter of vascular endothelial growth factor, which is the target for antiangiogenic therapies. Vascular endothelial growth factor accelerates the formation of blood vessels in the tumor and facilitates infiltration and spread to adjacent tissues, which in turn promotes the formation of metastases [20]. Solid tumors such as renal, gastric, and colon malignancies produce IL-6, which induces the proliferation and differentiation of megakaryocyte progenitors through specific receptors. This process causes platelet activation and aggregation. Platelet size has been shown to reflect changes in the level of platelet stimulation and the rate of platelet production.

According to the literature, lymphocytes play a key role in cytotoxic cell death and the production of cytokines that inhibit proliferation and metastatic spread of tumor cells. In contrast, neutrophils have a protumor effect by being the primary source of circulating angiogenesis-regulating chemokines, growth factors, and proteases [4]. Elevated neutrophil levels may result in an increase in angiogenesis, which promotes development and progression of the neoplasm [6]. Therefore, NLR can be considered as the balance between protumor inflammatory status and antitumor immune status. At present, there is little information on the relevance of these prognostic markers to both diagnosis and monitoring of PAC. Similarly as being in our experience, newly diagnosed PAC patients have high NLR and PLR values than healthy human.

3. Diagnostic weakness and missing points

Even with decades passed, measurement of this parameter is still not standardized, as it can easily be obtained with electronic meters. This is a major flaw because many pre-analytical and analytical variables can affect platelet size. The pre-analytical variables include vascular occlusion method, the correctness of the filling of the vial and the mixing of the sample, the type of anticoagulant, the storage temperature and the duration of the analysis. Any inflammatory or malignant process can lead to an increase in these parameters [21].

In practice, these markers, if used alone, may have a low positive predictive value in screening an asymptomatic population. Getting in touch with EDTA, *ethylene diamine tetra acetic acid*, the most common anticoagulant used in laboratory practice, effects the platelet morphology and leads to swelling and an increase in volumes. The differences in the methodology of platelet counting with different automated analytics are most like to be major analytical variable for the measurement [22].

The poor standardization of the number of physiological variables affecting platelet size and the poor standardization of this parameter makes it very unlikely that small differences in this parameter, defined by clinical trials in various clinical conditions, could be used for clinical purposes. In the future, better methodological standardization and more personalized reference intervals may make them as a reliable parameter for differential diagnosis and prognostic identification in daily clinical practice, but there is a need for well-designed clinical trials to confirm this hypothesis [23].

4. Diagnostic efficiency and strengths

Certainly, the most important advantage is their cost-efficiency. In routine analyzes of PAC, several parameters have been being used at high cost. These parameters have so low cost which cannot be easily overlooked. Additionally, we speculate that increased MPV in a patient group newly diagnosed with PAC may be a reflection of ongoing inflammation, and it can be related to increased levels of cytokines, particularly IL-6. Thus, we suggest that MPV could be used for detection of PAC instead of CA19-9. Increased MPV value, an indicator of platelet volume, points the presence of a subpopulation of young, metabolically and enzymatically more active platelets taking part in the process of homeostasis. NLR and PLR are two representative indices of systemic inflammation [24]. It has been shown that a preoperative NLR of greater than 4 or 5 is associated with a poor outcome in gastric cancer, non-small-cell lung cancer, and ovarian cancer. Neutrophils and leukocytes play a crucial role in the host systemic inflammatory response. A nonspecific systemic inflammatory response due to a tumor leads to an increase in the levels of circulating neutrophils and an elevated NLR, all of which are also clearly demonstrated in our study.

5. Conclusion

As in our results and the literature, the patients with PAC have higher levels of these biomarkers than healthy people. Thus, patients with high NLR, PLR, and MPV with suspicious symptoms and/or signs of PAC are candidates for early evaluation, which can prevent delay in the diagnosis of PAC. Therefore, prospective studies with inflammatory marker screening as IL-6, TNF on a larger number of asymptomatic patients are needed to compare the performance of NLR, PLR, and MPV with that of other diagnostic and monitoring tests to confirm their diagnostic utility.

Author details

Kemal Turker Ulutas[1], Inanc Samil Sarici[2*] and Ozgul Duzgun[3]

*Address all correspondence to: issarici2015@gmail.com

1 Department of Clinical Biochemistry, Antakya State Hospital, Hatay, Turkey

2 Department of General Surgery, Kanuni Sultan Suleyman Training and Research Hospital, Istanbul, Turkey

3 Department of Surgical Oncology, Umraniye Training and Research Hospital, Istanbul, Turkey

References

[1] Zhang GM, Bai SM, Zhang GM, Ma XB. Reference intervals of carbohydrate antigen 19-9 in the apparently healthy adult population. Journal of Clinical Laboratory Analysis. 2018;e22380. https://doi.org/10.1002/jcla.22380

[2] Bedi MMS, Gandhi MD, Jacob G, Lekha V, Venugopal A, Ramesh H. CA 19-9 to differentiate benign and malignant masses in chronic pancreatitis: Is there any benefit? Indian Journal of Gastroenterology. 2009;**28**(1):24-27

[3] Goonetilleke KS, Siriwardena AK. Systematic review of carbohydrate antigen (CA 19-9) as a biochemical marker in the diagnosis of pancreatic cancer. European Journal of Surgical Oncology (EJSO). 2007;**33**(3):266-270

[4] Gaitanidis A, Patel D, Nilubol N, Tirosh A, Sadowski S, Kebebew E. Markers of systemic inflammatory response are prognostic factors in patients with pancreatic neuroendocrine tumors (PNETs): A prospective analysis. Annals of Surgical Oncology. 2018; **25**(1):122-130

[5] Mannaerts D, Heyvaert S, De Cordt C, Macken C, Loos C, Jacquemyn Y. Are neutrophil/lymphocyte ratio (NLR), platelet/lymphocyte ratio (PLR), and/or mean platelet volume (MPV) clinically useful as predictive parameters for preeclampsia? The Journal of Maternal-Fetal & Neonatal Medicine: the Official Journal of the European Association of Perinatal Medicine, the Federation of Asia and Oceania Perinatal Societies, the International Society of Perinatal Obstet. 2017:1-8. DOI: 10.1080/14767058.2017.1410701

[6] Rejec A, Butinar J, Gawor J, Petelin M. Evaluation of complete blood count indices (NLR, PLR, MPV/PLT, and PLCRi) in healthy dogs, dogs with periodontitis, and dogs with oropharyngeal tumors as potential biomarkers of systemic inflammatory response. Journal of Veterinary Dentistry. 2017;**34**(4):231-240

[7] Zhou WW, Chu YP, An GY. Significant difference of neutrophil-lymphocyte ratio between colorectal cancer, adenomatous polyp and healthy people. European Review for Medical and Pharmacological Sciences. 2017;**21**(23):5386-5391

[8] Ulutas KT, Sarici IS. Could neutrophil/lymphocyte ratio, platelet/lymphocyte ratio, and mean platelet volume serve as potential biomarkers for detection of resectable pancreas ca? International Journal of Clinical and Experimental Medicine. 2016;**9**(6):11865-11870

[9] Miglani RK, Bhateja N, Bhat RS, Kumar KV. Diagnostic role of platelet lymphocyte ratio(PLR) in pancreatic head masses. The Indian Journal of Surgery. 2013;**75**(1):4-9

[10] Kishiki T, Masaki T, Mastuoka H, Abe N, Mori T, Sugiyama M. New prognostic scoring system for incurable stage IV colorectal cancer. Asian Pacific Journal of Cancer Prevention: APJCP. 2016;**17**(2):597-601

[11] Buergy D, Wenz F, Groden C, Brockmann M. Tumor-platelet interaction in solid tumors. International Journal Cancer. 2012;**130**(12):2747-2760. DOI: 10.1002/ijc.27441

[12] Hait NC, Maiti A. The role of sphingosine-1-phosphate and ceramide-1-phosphate in inflammation and cancer. Mediators of Inflammation. 2017;**2017**:4806541

[13] Ikwegbue PC, Masamba P, Oyinloye BE, Kappo AP. Roles of Heat Shock Proteins in Apoptosis, Oxidative Stress, Human Inflammatory Diseases, and Cancer. Pharmaceuticals. 2018;**11**(1):2. DOI: 10.3390/ph11010002

[14] Lujan DA, Ochoa JL, Hartley RS. Cold-inducible RNA binding protein in cancer and inflammation. Wiley Interdisciplinary Reviews RNA. 2018;**9**(2). DOI: 10.1002/wrna.1462

[15] Kakkat S, Rajan R, Sindhu RS, Natesh B, Raviram S. Comparison of platelet-lymphocyte ratio and CA 19-9 in differentiating benign from malignant head masses in patients with chronic pancreatitis. Indian Journal of Gastroenterology: Official Journal of the Indian Society of Gastroenterology. 2017;**36**(4):263-267

[16] Rammohan A, Cherukuri SD, Palaniappan R, Perumal SK, Sathyanesan J, Govindan M. Preoperative platelet-lymphocyte ratio augments CA 19-9 as a predictor of malignancy in chronic calcific pancreatitis. World Journal of Surgery. 2015;**39**(9):2323-2328

[17] Joshi RK, Lee SA. Obesity related adipokines and colorectal cancer: A review and meta-analysis. Asian Pacific Journal of Cancer Prevention: APJCP. 2014;**15**(1):397-405

[18] Knüpfer H, Preiss R. Serum interleukin-6 levels in colorectal cancer patients—A summary of published results. International Journal of Colorectal Disease. 2009;**25**(2):135-140

[19] Belluco C, Nitti D, Frantz M, Toppan P, Basso D, Plebani M, et al. Interleukin-6 blood level is associated with circulating carcinoembryonic antigen and prognosis in patients with colorectal Cancer. Annals of Surgical Oncology. 2000;**7**(2):133-138

[20] Ashizawa T, Okada R, Suzuki Y, Takagi M, Yamazaki T, Sumi T, et al. Clinical significance of interleukin-6 (IL-6) in the spread of gastric cancer: Role of IL-6 as a prognostic factor. Gastric Cancer. 2005;**8**(2):124-131

[21] Buttarello M, Mezzapelle G, Plebani M. Effect of preanalytical and analytical variables on the clinical utility of mean platelet volume. Clinical Chemistry and Laboratory Medicine. 2018;**56**(5):718-725. DOI: 10.1515/cclm-2017-0730

[22] Ulutas KT, Celik M. Preanalytical error occurrence rate in Central Clinic Laboratory of a Public Hospital in Turkey. Journal of Pharmacy and Pharmacology. 2016;**4**(1):318-321

[23] Raleigh JS, Jandrey KE, Burges J, Kent MS. Factors affecting platelet concentration in platelet concentrates from canine blood donors. Journal of Veterinary Internal Medicine. 2017;**31**(3):759-763

[24] Ulutas KT, Dokuyucu R, Sefil F, Yengil E, Sumbul AT, Rizaoglu H, et al. Evaluation of mean platelet volume in patients with type 2 diabetes mellitus and blood glucose regulation: A marker for atherosclerosis? International Journal of Clinical and Experimental Medicine. 2014;**7**(4):955-961

8

Biomarkers Utility for Sepsis Patients Management

Agustin Iskandar, Hani Susianti,
Muhammad Anshory and Salvatore Di Somma

Abstract

Sepsis is a global problem in either developing or developed countries and it is expected that the number of patients with sepsis and septic shock will tremendously increase in next decades also because of the antibiotic resistance growing issue worldwide. Criteria for sepsis diagnosis and prognosis have been recently established, but still a further understanding of the role of biomarkers in this setting is needed. Better utilization of biomarkers such as white blood cell count, CRP, lactate, procalcitonin, presepsin and bioadrenomedullin in sepsis patients, a state of the art on how to use them is needed. This review will focus on the actual recognized role of sepsis biomarkers not only for diagnosis purpose but also to improve patients treatment results in order to reduce mortality, hospital length of stay and cost related.

Keywords: biomarkers, sepsis, patient management

1. Introduction

For about a century, sepsis has been defined as a systemic inflammatory response of the host to an infection. The lack of precise definitions and diagnostic criteria had also made difficult or even impossible to compare different studies and research. It was necessary to find a precise and standardized definition of sepsis, a common nomenclature to correctly diagnose the disease, allowing the creation of a targeted therapy for the patient [1]. The SIRS criteria were considered too sensitive and unspecific to be used in the identification of sepsis in most clinical practice [1, 2]. This scheme is based on four specific characteristics defined by the acronym PIRO:

- Predisposition, indicates pre-existing conditions potentially able to reduce septic patient survival;

- Insult or infection, reflects the pathogenicity of the microorganism;
- Response of the organism to the infectious event, including the manifestation of the SIRS;
- Organ dysfunction, which includes both organ failure and the failure of the coagulation system.

Sepsis

Documented or suspected infection.

Pathological process caused by the invasion of tissues, fluids or cavities of the host normally sterile by pathogenic or potentially pathogenic microorganisms, associated with some of the following signs and symptoms:

Variables:

1. Temperature > 38.3°C or < 36°C.
2. Heart rate > 90 min^{-1} or > 2 SD above the normal value for age.
3. Tachypnea.
4. Alteration of the state of consciousness.
5. Important edema or positive fluid balance (>20 mL/kg in 24 h).
6. Hyperglycaemia (>120 mg/dL) in the absence of diabetes.

- Inflammatory variables:

1. White blood cells >12,000 mL^{-1} or < 4000 mL^{-1}.
2. White blood cells in the standard but >10% of immature forms.
3. C-reactive protein>2 SD normal values.
4. Procalcitonin>2SD normal values.

- Hemodinamic variables:

1. Arterial hypotension (SBP <90 mmHg, MAP <70 mmHg, or a reduction in SBP > 40 mmHg in adults or < 2 SD below normal for age).
2. SvO2 > 70%.
3. Cardiac Index>3.5 L min^{-1} m^2.

- Organ defunction variables:

1. Hypoxemia (PaO2/FiO2 < 300).
2. Acute oliguria (<0.5 mL/kg/h).
3. Increase of creatinine>0.5 mg/dL.
4. Abnormality of coagulation (INR > 1.5 or APTT>60 s).
5. Ileus (absence of peristalsis).
6. Platelet decrease (<100,000 mL^{-1}).
7. Hyperbilirubinemia (> 4 mg/dL).

- Tissue perfusion variables:

1. Hyperlactacidemia (> 1 mmol/L).

Severe sepsis

Sepsis associated with organ dysfunction (hypotension, hypoxemia, oliguria, metabolic acidosis and thrombocytopenia).

Septic shock

Severe sepsis with hypotension despite adequate fluid rehydration, along with the presence of organ perfusion abnormalities.

Table 1. SCCM/ESICM/ACCP/ATS/SIS – 2001 [3].

The use of this scheme is useful for defining, diagnosing and treating patients with sepsis but above all for obtaining better results in situations of severe sepsis and septic shock. The PIRO model is not yet fully defined and it has been debated [2]. **Table 1** summarizes the different definitions obtained after the two Consensus Conferences [3]:

Therefore, given the need to reexamine the current definitions, the "European Society of Intensive Care Medicine" and the "Society of Critical Care Medicine" have organized a task force of 19 specialists among infectiologists, surgeons, pulmonologists and anesthesiologists in order to review the data in the literature so far available.

Although SIRS criteria may be useful in the general diagnosis of an infection, they representative of an appropriate adaptive response of the organism, while sepsis involves an organ dysfunction that underlies a much more complex pathology; in this context the pro- and anti-inflammatory endogenous factors play a fundamental role and they are responsible for the inter-individual differences between patients [4–6].

The task force therefore suggests to use new values to decide to further investigate the search for organ dysfunction damage, to initiate or modify a therapy that is more appropriate and to consider patient's hospitalization in an Intensive Care [7]. **Table 2** reflects the conclusions reached by the task force and the implications in everyday practice, with the exemplification of the new diagnostic criteria and the new classification recognized by the International Classification of Diseases (ICD) [7].

Current guidelines and terminology	Sepsis	Septic shock
1991 and 2001 consensus terminology	Severe sepsis Sepsis-induced hypoperfusion	Septic shock
2015 definition	Sepsis is life-threatening organ dysfunction caused by a dysregulated host response to infection	Septic shock is a subset of sepsis in which underlying circulatory and cellular/metabolic abnormalities are profound enough to substantially increase mortality
2015 clinical criteria	Suspected or documented infection and an acute increase of ≥2 SOFA points (a proxy for organ dysfunction)	Sepsis and vasopressor therapy needed to elevate MAP ≥65 mmHg and lactate >2 mmol/L (18 mg/dL) despite adequate fluid resuscitation
Recommended primary ICD codes		
ICD-9	995.92	785.52
ICD-10	R65.20	R65.21
Framework for implementation for coding and research	Identify suspected infection by using concomitant orders for blood cultures and antibiotic (oral or parenteral) in a specified period Within specified period around suspected infection: 1. Identify sepsis by using a clinical criterion for life-threatening organ dysfunction 2. Assess for shock criteria, using administration of vasopressors, MAP <65 mmHg and lactate >2 mmol/L (18 mg/dL)	

Table 2. Terminology and International Classification of Disease coding [7].

2. Sepsis in emergency department

Sepsis is a complex clinical syndrome that still represents a major challenge for today's medicine. In fact, despite the current possibilities of treatment, sepsis remains burdened by a high prevalence in the population and above all by a severe prognosis, representing one of the pathologies with the highest rate of morbidity and mortality. It is responsible for about one-third of all hospital admissions, and about 50% of ICU admissions. Mortality would reach 40%, of which 25% of deaths would occur within 48 h of entry into ICU [8].

In this complex scenario, the emergency doctor plays a key role. In fact, it depends on early diagnosis and treatment, the two factors that are recognized today as fundamental in the correct management of the septic patient as it is able to improve the prognosis. The enigmatic and often heterogeneous nature of sepsis, the absence of specific clinical and laboratory elements causes the lack of valid diagnostic tools, strongly influencing early intervention [9].

The recent literature has therefore placed great attention in the search for all clinical and laboratory factors, which can help in the rapid identification of sepsis and in the stratification of the risk of such patients, in order to make the treatment as aggressive as possible in terms of timeliness and effectiveness. More than two decades ago, sepsis was defined by the combination of an SIRS and an infection. This criterion, therefore useful for the correct diagnosis of sepsis, is also endowed with prognostic capacity, proving to be effective for the gravity stratification of patients with suspected infection due to the linking of these criteria with the presence of organ damage. However, the role of SIRS has been recently revised because although it has high prognostic power, it has little specificity being involved in a wide variety of pathologies regardless the presence of infection, in which the differential diagnosis often becomes difficult. Furthermore, it has been calculated that a certain number of patients with sepsis may not present SIRS criteria (about 1 in 8) [10]. The "Third International Consensus Definitions for Sepsis and Septic Shock" (Sepsis-3) [7] has therefore decided to go beyond the concept of SIRS, emphasizing rather the role of the organism's response to infection and organ damage (identified by a SOFA value ≥2) in the pathogenesis of sepsis.

3. Diagnosis

Sepsis diagnosis is established on the basis of patient's symptoms and clinical signs combined with radiological examinations and laboratory tests such as the search for biomarkers and identification of the microorganism responsible for the infection. In cases of sepsis, delay in diagnosis and antibiotic therapy affects the mortality of critically ill patients. Establishing diagnosis and therapy is very important but to hinder their definition it is difficult in differentiating sepsis from non-infectious stimuli in SIRS situations, symptoms and clinical signs, radiological and laboratory tests used for the diagnosis of sepsis are those reported in the previously reported tables, used in the definition of sepsis itself. The use of clinical scores, blood cultures and biomarkers for the diagnosis of sepsis will be discussed later.

4. Clinical scores

Since 2004, worldwide, the "Surviving Sepsis Campaign", consisting of a multidisciplinary team of specialists, periodically deals with the preparation and updating of documents on the general management of the septic patient and some specific aspects, such as timing and the optimal choice of antibiotic therapy, blood pressure support, glycemic control and oxygenation. In particular, at the last revision, the bundle of measures are implemented within the first hours after admission of the patient to reduce mortality was well defined [11].

At the same time, over the years, the need arose, especially in an intensivist environment, to identify those factors capable of predicting clinical severity and, in particular, the risk of death; for this purpose, many patient severity scores have been proposed and validated, useful from the moment of diagnosis to stratify the patient's clinical severity and, indirectly, to assess the risk of mortality [12].

The ideal prognostic score should have high sensitivity and high predictive value, be able to predict early mortality or clinical evolution, be rapidly usable, available everywhere, economic, objective and non-observer-dependent. Currently, no clinical score has all these characteristics. In particular, the two basic requirements of a prognostic system are the power of discrimination and calibration [13].

There are several works that have evaluated in the emergency medicine settings, the applicability of different gravity scores. In particular, simpler models to be calculated than those commonly used in Intensive Care Unit (ICU) have been proposed [11]. In 2003, Shapiro et al. have proposed the adoption of a new prognostic model, called Mortality in Emergency Department Sepsis (MEDS), as a method for stratifying patients afferent in emergency medicine with suspected sepsis [14]. Sankoff et al. resumed the MEDS score and carried out a multi-center prospective study to verify its reproducibility and validity [15]. The MEDS is the only score designed to be used in the septic patient in settings different from ICU. Numerous prognostic models born to be used in ICU were subsequently applied in different care settings, primarily in emergency medicine.

In one of the best known studies, Jones et al. have proposed the adoption of the Sequential Organ Failure Assessment (SOFA) score as a tool to predict the outcome of patients with severe sepsis with signs of hypoperfusion or septic shock. The authors considered all patients over the age of 18 with sepsis and evidence of hypoperfusion (systolic BP <90 mmHg or lactate levels>4 mmol/L); calculated the SOFA score at time zero and after 72 h (delta SOFA). The outcome of the study was to evaluate in-hospital mortality, the possible correlation between the difference in SOFA between admission and after 72 h, and finally mortality. The authors have shown a good correlation between the SOFA score at the entrance and the delta SOFA with the risk of in-hospital mortality. The limit of the work, similar to the studies on the MEDS score, is that it is an experience conducted only in a single center, which should be validated and extended to several centers to obtain a useful risk assessment tool [16, 17]. Alan E Jones et al. also demonstrated the usefulness of SOFA as a predictive prognosis score in patients with sepsis, and in particular in patients with severe sepsis with signs of hypoperfusion already on arrival in the emergency room [16].

The SOFA score (**Table 3**) is therefore a prognostic score, used for the prediction of mortality, based on the degree of dysfunction of six different systems and apparatuses, involved in the pathophysiology of the sepsis response. In particular, the respiratory, cardiovascular, renal, neurological, coagulative and hepatic systems are examined. The alteration of each of them indicates a condition of particular gravity, and the progression of the number of systems involved represents a negative prognostic variable. Thus, values < 9 predict mortality <33%, values between 9 and 11 a mortality of 40–50% and values>11 of 95%. Only one work assessed the accuracy of different prognostic models in septic patient assessment in a care setting of this kind [18]. The study, conducted in a single center, evaluated five different prognostic models MEDS, APACHE II, SAPS II, SOFA score (at time 0 and 24 h) and the Charlson index. The outcome examined was 28-day mortality, the number of patients examined was 140. The most accurate result was the 24-hour SOFA; however, also the SOFA at time 0, the maximum SOFA and increasing values of SOFA were related to mortality. It is useful to underline that the patients enrolled in the study already had a diagnosis of sepsis-septic shock with a mortality equal to 29%, much higher than the previously reported jobs (close to that of the IT departments). It is therefore reasonable to think that for a population of this kind, the use of a score

System	Score				
	0	**1**	**2**	**3**	**4**
Respiration					
PaO_2/FiO_2, mmHg (kPa)	≥400 (53.3)	<400 (53.3)	<300 (40)	<200 (26.7) with respiratory support	<100 (13.3) with respiratory support
Coagulation					
Platelets, ×10³/uL	≥150	<150	<100	<50	<20
Liver					
Bilirubin, mg/dL (umol/L)	<1.2 (20)	1.2–1.9 (20–32)	2.0–5.9 (33–101)	6.0–11.9 (102–204)	>12 (204)
Cardiovascular	MAP ≥70 mmHg	MAP <70 mmHg	Dopamine <5 or dobutamine (any dose)[b]	Dopamine 5.1–15 or epinephrine ≤0.1 or norepinephrine ≤0.1[b]	Dopamine >15 or epinephrine >0.1 or norepinephrine >0.1[b]
Central nervous system					
Glasgow Coma Scale score[b]	15	13–14	10–12	6–9	<6
Renal					
Creatinine, mg/dL (umol/L)	<1.2 (110)	1.2–1.9 (110–170)	2.0–3.4 (171–299)	3.5–4.9 (300–440)	>5.0 (440)
Urine output, mL/d				<500	<200

Abbreviations: FiO_2: fraction of inspired oxygen; MAP: mean arterial pressure; PaO_2: partial pressure of oxygen.
[a]Catecholamine doses are given as ug/kg/min for at least 1 h.
[b]Glasgow Coma Scale scores range from 3 to 15; higher score indicates better neurological function.

Table 3. Sequential (sepsis-related) organ failure assessment score [7].

validated in ICU (such as SOFA) may be more reliable than models validated in emergency medicine (such as MEDS) .

The shorter version of SOFA score, the qSOFA, evaluates only three clinical variables that are easily obtainable "bedside" which are systolic arterial pressure ≤ 100 mmHg, respiratory rate ≥ 22 times/min and alteration of the mental state (GCS ≤ 13 or other alteration). A ≥ 2 qSOFA would allow rapid detection of the septic patient and would be associated with 10% mortality. However, recent scientific studies have questioned the role of qSOFA, comparing it with the previous SIRS diagnostic criteria. In particular, a qSOFA ≥2 would seem to have high specificity but low sensitivity compared to a SIRS ≥2 value in the recognition of organ damage, and this could limit its use as a screening method [9].

5. Blood cultures

Blood culture is the "gold standard" exam to diagnose sepsis because it allows the etiological agent to be determined and provides the clinician with useful information for targeted therapy [11].

Several factors can influence the effectiveness and clinical significance of blood culture. In the pre-analytical phase, the withdrawal methods and the number of samples are very important. The sampling must be done when the first suspicions of infection arise and above all before the administration of any antibiotic, otherwise the therapy should be discontinued for a few hours or taken before the next administration of the antibiotic. In most episodes of bacteremia, it is necessary to collect two or three blood culture sets within 24 h to identify the pathogen, in case a single sample set is taken the probability of not identifying a patient with sepsis is about 35–40% [19].

An important factor for the accuracy of the diagnosis is the volume of blood present in the blood culture flask, in fact it is necessary to inoculate at least three colony forming units (CFU) per milliliter to get 100% positive; however, it is considered that in adult patients, in sepsis, the concentration per milliliter of blood is normally 0.1–1 CFU/mL, while in pediatric age the bacterial load is equal to 10–100 CFU/mL [20, 21].

Therefore, in the adult, the ideal amount of blood will therefore be 5–10 mL per vial and for pediatric patients of 1–5 mL. The ratio between the volume of the sample and that of the culture broth must allow the growth of many microorganisms, this ratio is 1:5–1:10 even if with the addition of substances that disable the inhibitory factors the optimal ratio is 1:5 [22–24]. Another important factor for a successful blood culture is incubation time.

The Clinical and Laboratory Standards Institute (CLSI) established that 5 days of incubation are sufficient to detect 95% growth of clinically significant bacteria (CLSI, 2007). Several studies have shown that in 97.5% of blood cultures containing a pathogen are positive after 3 days using automated systems [25, 26].

In the case of suspected endocarditis supported by demanding bacteria, or yeast septicemia or in pediatric patients, the incubation times are prolonged. Moreover, a possible administration of a therapy prior to sampling or the presence of a pathogen with particular nutritional needs lowers the ability of the investigation to identify the microorganism, in fact it has been shown that the levels of analytical sensitivity vary between 8 and 88% [27].

A limitation of blood culture is the lack of sensitivity in the search for particular bacteria that are often responsible for community-acquired pneumonia, such as *Mycoplasma pneumoniae*, *Legionella pneumophila* and *Chlamydia pneumoniae* and other germs that are difficult to grow or even non-cultivable such as *Coxiella burnetii*, *Francisella tularensis*, *Bartonella* spp., *Rickettsia* spp. and *Nocardia* spp. [28, 29].

The value of blood culture as a diagnostic test for bacteraemia and sepsis is limited, in fact, it emerges that in 50% of cases, the blood culture is negative even if the diagnosis of sepsis is certain and also the first results are provided after 48 h to conclude analysis with the identification and sensitivity to the pathogen's antibiotics after 5 days or more [1, 30, 31].

6. Sepsis biomarkers

6.1. Introduction

The current gold standard for the diagnosis of infections of the circulatory stream is blood culture, unfortunately its important limitation is the time necessary to complete the survey that goes from 1 to 5 or more days in the case of suspected sepsis caused by yeasts. The ideal situation would be to analyze the patient's on-site blood and provide all the necessary information to immediately target a targeted antibiotic therapy, and then the test should provide data for therapy evaluation by measuring the clearance of pathogenic nucleic acids in the blood in a certain period of time.

The ideal molecular test does not exist but these characteristics will have to be set as a long-term objective in the design of new molecular techniques for the diagnosis of sepsis.

A short-term objective is to analyze blood in parallel to culture methods and identify pathogens responsible for infection including non-cultivable organisms, and also to detect some of the determinants of drug resistance [30]. The molecular techniques currently available on the market can be distinguished in those based on the principle of amplification of the bacterial and/or fungal genome and those that exploit the principle of hybridization. Blood culture coupled with molecular investigations involves some disadvantages inherent to the traditional method such as delay in response with its possible alteration due to an unsuitable collection and the inability to provide the nutrients necessary for the development of demanding microorganisms. In the market, there are several kits in molecular biology that identify the pathogen from positive blood culture samples.

In the medical field, a circulating biochemical marker is defined as a demonstrable, therefore measurable, substance in the blood whose variation in concentration constitutes the signal of the presence of a pathology [32].

Regarding the role of biomarkers in the management of sepsis, over time various molecules were analyzed that, taken singly or combined in a panel, could be able to allow rapid diagnosis and prognosis, and that in the near future could also be able to guide the therapy itself to improve the clinical response and management of these patients [33]. Among the various biomarkers, some are used daily in clinical practice. Among these great importance has always been attributed to the role of lactates. They are considered useful by the guidelines because they have a prognostic value, being related to disease severity especially for values

≥ 2 mmol/L. However, according to other authors, the additive prognostic role of lactates to qSOFA would not be significant [34].

CRP and PCT are routinely used in patients with suspected first aid infection. CRP, released as an acute phase protein in inflammatory states, has a high specificity but low sensitivity and is therefore used for its negative predictive value. PCT, on the other hand, has been shown to have diagnostic and prognostic value in the management of sepsis. It is released in the course of bacterial infections, being therefore aids in the differential diagnosis, and is also included within the guidelines as a valid aid in guiding antibiotic therapy, representing a "mirror" of the therapeutic response to infection, and for its high prognostic power.

More recently, however, we have focused on the role of adrenomedullin (ADM). It is a peptide that several studies have shown to increase in septic patients [35]. The secretion mechanism depends to a large extent on stimulation by the lipopolysaccharide of bacteria, and its plasma levels derive mainly from secretion by endothelial cells [36]. ADM plays a fundamental role in hyperdynamic response during the early stages of sepsis and its main function is vasodilator [37]. After demonstrating the prognostic role of its precursor MR-proADM [38], thanks to a novel instrument based on a chemiluminescent sandwich detection (in which specific monoclonal antibodies are used against the C-terminal part of the peptide), today, it is possible directly measure the biologically active molecule (Bio-ADM or ADM). Thus, in a study published in 2014, our group showed that ADM values are significantly higher in patients with severe sepsis and septic shock than those with sepsis [39]; in particular, ADM, considered one of the most potent endogenous vasodilators, was found to be closely related to low mean arterial pressure (PAM) values and to the need to use vasopressors, thus detecting septic shock markers. Furthermore, higher values have been correlated with greater probability of death; and finally, the detection of multi-stroke ADM has proved to be fundamental in identifying patients with a worse prognosis [39].

From what has emerged, considering that sepsis determines endothelial dysregulation, excessive vasodilatation and consecutively collapse of arterial pressure and micro-vascular homeostasis and that ADM has as its main function vasodilator and therefore regulator of vascular tone, new studies currently in progress and still in the experimental phase, are directed to the development of a murine anti-ADM monoclonal antibody (HAM1101) that can become a therapy in septic shock, according to the hypothesis that it can improve the hemodynamics and perfusion of the organs and, consequently, also reduce the incidence of acute renal failure. To date, a humanized antibody has been selected, the HAM8101, which will be the subject of phase III experimental studies in the near future [39, 40].

Establishing diagnosis and therapy is very important but to hinder their definition is the difficulty in differentiating sepsis from non-infectious stimuli in SIRS situations, especially in those critically ill patients who may have developed SIRS for other causes such as pancreatitis, trauma, burns, etc. Therefore, the detection of an accurate biomarker in sepsis is decisive in critical situations with the ability to exclude or confirm an acute bacterial infection, to evaluate the systemic inflammatory response to infection and the host response to the established therapy [41].

An ideal biological marker must have different characteristics:

- useful in early diagnosis, provide information for a definitive diagnosis or help to identify a probable diagnosis;

- provide information regarding the prognosis including the patient in subpopulations whose outcome is better/worse than the population in question;
- provide, in the clinical course, useful information on how the patient responds to therapy and eventually help in modulating the therapeutic strategy;
- high specificity and sensitivity;
- have a clinically useful half-life time;
- be easily determinable and reproducible and difficult to influence by disturbing factors;
- have low costs and be easily used to quantify intervention actions, costs and benefits;
- in the case of sepsis, allow differential diagnosis between infectious and non-infectious etiology.

The use of biomarkers must always be integrated with the information deriving from a careful medical history collection, from a complete clinical objective examination, from the results of laboratory analyzes and diagnostic methods required in different cases. In fact, only the set of all these elements make it possible to reduce the number of evaluation errors deriving from a hasty decision, often dictated by superficiality or by incorrect knowledge. At present, there is no biomarker that ensures 100% correlation with a single pathology. In fact, we speak of "highly significant values" for a given pathological condition. Other potential uses of biomarkers include their prognostic role and, consequently, the ability to drive antibiotic therapy and to evaluate the response to the therapy itself, identifying those patients who most likely will face complications and organ dysfunction [32].

In the literature, there are many biomarkers already evaluated, such biomarkers for chemokine, cellular, receptor, hemostasis and vascular and others [42].

The available markers for the diagnosis of sepsis are numerous. There are leukocyte count, C-reactive protein (CRP), procalcitonin (PCT), endotoxin, cytokine, IL-1 receptor, complement factors, endothelin-1, ICAM-1 and VCAM-1, fosofolipase A2, PGE2, lactoferrin, neopterin, elastase, different interleukins (ILS), adrenomedullin (ADM) and proADM, atrial natriuretic peptide (ANP) and proANP, pro-vasopressin (copeptin), interferon-γ (IFN-γ), triggering receptor expressed on myeloid cells 1 (TREM-1) and resistin [41–44]. In several recently published studies, the most relevant biomarkers used, as they have a high diagnostic and prognostic capacity are CRP [45], PCT [46], ADM [47], copeptin [48], natriuretic peptide (MR-proANP) [49], presepsin (or CD 14 ligand) [50] and suPAR [51].

Unfortunately, in the sepsis, an ideal marker has not yet been identified and those normally used (fever, leukocytosis, CRP, PCT, etc.) often have little sensitivity and specificity, consequently they have limited use in patient management. Their dosage should be used and evaluated in the context of the clinical situation in which the patient is located and therefore it is essential to determine the appropriateness of the individual markers' request in collaboration with the clinician to exploit their potential to the full diagnostics, therapeutic monitoring and prognosis.

This section will discuss about white blood cell count (WBC), serum lactate, C-reactive protein (CRP), procalcitonin (PCT), presepsin and bioadrenomedullin as biomarker of sepsis.

6.2. White blood cell count (WBC)

White blood cell is a part of innate immune response by localizing infection. Otherwise in systemic sepsis process, there is profound leucocyte activation. Systemic sepsis also leading to organ damage and organ dysfunction attenuated by inhibition of leukocyte-endothelial interactions, systemic leukocyte activation and disseminated leukocyte adhesion [52].

The WBC results were considered abnormal if both the total number of neutrophils and the immature/total neutrophil ratio were abnormal simultaneously [53]. The sensitivity and specificity WBC for sepsis diagnosis in the literature vary widely, since there are significant differences in definitions used to count total neutrophils and sub-fractions; with sensitivity varying from 17 to 100% and specificity from 31 to 100%. A study by Caldas et al., reported that combination of WBC and CRP had sensitivity better than WBC alone [54].

In 2001, Zahorec introduced the use of neutrophil and lymphocyte count ratio (NLCR) as one of infection marker [55]. There is also correlation between NLCR and disease severity, also predictor for bacteremia [56].

The sepsis criteria recently changed from Sepsis-2 to Sepsis-3 highlighting on life-threatening organ damage caused by dysregulated host response to infection. This also affecting the use of biomarker in the diagnosis of sepsis, based on Ljungstrom et al., the AUC of NLCR to predict positive culture was 0.71, similar to previous study by Loonen showed AUC of 0.73 and 0.77 [56–58].

6.3. Serum lactate

Lactate is an important source of energy, particularly during starvation. Lactate also contributes to acidic environment by converting to lactic acid. Lactate value of 1400–1500 mmol/L per day resulted from anaerobic glycolysis activity as the reduction of pyruvate, moreover in tissue hypoxia [59]. Excretion of lactate mostly occurs in liver (60%) followed by kidney (30%) and other organs [60]. Shock status, such as cardiogenic or septic shock, is an important source of lactate production. The mortality rate was 46.1% for patients with both hypotension and lactate ≥4 mmol/L, 36.7% for septic patients with hypotension alone and 30% for patients with lactate ≥4 mmol/L alone [61, 62].

According to the new definition, septic shock can be diagnosed under two circumstances. The first one is persistent hypotension and the second one is increase of lactate serum level for more than 2 mmol/L, with additional note that lactate cut off were changed from 4 to 2 mmol/L. Therefore, increase of lactate serum level for more than 2 mmol/L can be recognized as a sign of septic shock. This condition greatly affects by hypotension and the use of vasopressor which caused further tissue hypoxia [62].

Ljungstrom et al. showed lactate correlate well with Sepsis-2 criteria in diagnosis of sepsis and septic shock, with specificity, accuracy and DOR were 97, 92 and 56.3%, respectively, by using cutoff 3.5 mmol/L. The downside of lactate is that even lactate level alone is widely used for diagnosis in early sepsis, the elevated level is not considered specific for sepsis diagnosis, hence it is proven to be more valuable in predicting mortality. The suggestion is to use combination of several biomarkers including lactate in diagnosing septic and septic shock [56].

6.4. C-reactive protein (CRP)

C-reactive protein (CRP) is synthesized by the liver after the action of various inflammation mediators such as IL-1, IL-6 and IL-8. This biomarker is produced 4–6 h after the phlogistic stimulus, and doubles its concentration in the circulation within 8 h and reaches its peak in 36–50 h [2, 63, 64].

CRP has both pro-inflammatory and anti-inflammatory characteristics, its half-life is 19 h and its levels in the blood stream remain elevated for a few days after the infection has disappeared [63]. Elevated plasma CRP levels indicate the presence of an infection and/or organ damage while protein synthesis will be significantly reduced in the case of hepatic failure [65]. The normal value of plasma CRP is <1 mg/dL, while it may increase up to 50 mg/dL in case of acute severe infection. The increase in CRP does not appear to be related to the severity of inflammation and also increases in cases of non-infectious diseases such as autoimmune diseases, acute coronary syndromes, rheumatic disorders, malignant tumors and after traumas or surgical interventions [66].

In conclusion, the values of CRP do not allow to distinguish between sepsis and SIRS of a non-infectious nature. This marker appears to be more sensitive than parameters such as the leukocyte count and the temperature but less specific than others such as PCT. However, CRP is a commonly used low cost and widely available marker.

6.5. Procalcitonin (PCT)

"Procalcitonin" (PCT) is a protein consisting of 116 amino acids, with a molecular weight of approximately 13 kDalton. The amino acid sequence of PCT is identical to that of calcitonin prohormone; it comprises the sequence of calcitonin from position 60 to 91 (32 amino acids). Through specific proteolysis, PCT (116 amino acids) and, in healthy intracellular individuals, calcitonin (32 amino acids) are released from this protein. Currently, four genes corresponding to calcitonin with homologies in the nucleotide sequence are known. These genes are all called "genetic family of calcitonin", although not all of them produce the calcitonin peptide hormone. The "CALC-I" gene, a candidate responsible for the production of procalcitonin induced by the inflammatory state, is one of the first examples of a process called "alternative splicing". The primary transcript can give rise to different mRNAs for inclusion or exclusion of the different exons present. Calcitonin encoding mRNA is the main product of CALC-I transcription in thyroid C cells, whereas CGRP-I mRNA (CGRP = calcitonin gene-related peptide) is produced in the nervous tissue of the central and peripheral nervous system (115). The plasma concentrations of procalcitonin in healthy individuals are very low, on the order of picograms, and in any case below the limits of determination of the test used for the immunoluminometric assay (<0.1 ng/mL, LUMItest PCT, BRAHMS Diagnostica, Berlin). PCT is a very stable protein in vivo and in vitro. In plasma it does not degrade to active calcitonin hormone; its in vivo half-life time is approximately 25–30 h [67] [115]. PCT production was stimulated in healthy volunteers through the intravenous injection of small amounts of bacterial endotoxin (lipopolysaccharide). PCT can be observed in the plasma 2 h after endotoxin injection; between 6 and 8 h after the concentration of PCT increases rapidly up to a plateau about 12 h after injection. Over the next 2–3 days, the PCT values decrease until they reach their normal value [67, 68].

PCT concentrations above 0.5 ng/mL always indicate an acute infection or inflammation, with particularly high values in patients with severe bacterial infections in the acute phase and with septic inflammation. Plasma PCT concentration in the presence of serious infections and sepsis; however, can vary from 1 to 1000 ng/mL and PCT, in these cases, is probably not produced by C cells of the thyroid, but is inclined to believe that origin from neuroendocrine cells of the lung or intestine [67].

The release of PCT is determined only by the systemic reaction of the organism toward the infection, therefore local bacterial colonizations, encapsulated abscesses and localized and limited infections do not cause PCT release. In addition to bacterial infections, plasma PCT concentration has been shown to increase in acute forms of malaria and fungal infections. PCT, on the other hand, does not appear or appear to be not very significant, in the presence of viral infections, autoimmune diseases, neoplasia or traumatic surgery [69]. It could thus become one of the first-choice tests to be performed in patients with fever of unknown origin in the emergency room, to unmask an underlying bacterial infection [46, 70].

Bacterial endotoxins play the most important role in the mechanism of PCT release. At the end of the acute inflammatory reaction, the PCT concentration decreases according to the plasma half-life time. From these considerations it is clear that PCT, besides being a diagnostic marker of systemic bacterial infections, also has an important prognostic value. The medical literature, in fact, has shown the correlation between the severity of the clinical picture, the risk of development of multi-organ failure (MOF), long-term outcomes and one-year mortality, with plasma PCT values; in particular it was established that:

- high values of PCT protracted over time indicate an inflammation in progress;
- constantly increasing PCT levels are an unequivocal sign of poor prognosis;
- decreased PCT levels indicate favorable prognosis, improvement of inflammation or adequate therapeutic treatment of infection.

PCT thus becomes essential for the identification of patients at greatest risk, for guiding their therapy and for monitoring them over time [69, 71].

The areas in which the PCT could be used are numerous. In addition to patients who come to the emergency room with fever or suspected sepsis, PCT has been evaluated as both diagnostic [72, 73] and prognostic [74, 75] markers in pneumonia of bacterial origin. Even in this case, if associated with the clinical picture, the radiographic imaging and the values of the inflammatory indexes (CRP and white blood cells in particular), the PCT has shown to have a high predictive value as a biomarker. For the same reasons listed above, PCT should be measured in patients with significant dyspnea affected by COPD. The bacterial origin of exacerbations is often responsible for hospitalizations and mortality, and early intervention could reduce both of these two harmful consequences [76, 77].

Finally, an increase in PCT has also been shown in bacterial endocarditis [78] and in acute coronary syndromes [79, 80], while its prognostic use as a marker of infection has been exploited in the monitoring of patients undergoing major surgery [81].

Despite the wide space that scientific research has devoted to PCT, its exact mechanism of action still remains partially unknown. The rapid induction of PCT after administration of bacterial endotoxins and its relationship to cytokines, such as TNF-α, suggest the existence of a close correlation between PCT and pro-inflammatory cytokines, which earned him the name "ormokina" [82]. In the clinic, it was observed that there is a correlation between the timing of PCT, IL-6 and TNF-α. In acute inflammation, PCT values increase a few hours after the increase of IL-6 and TNF-α; at the end of the inflammation, the PCT begins to decrease after the decrease of the IL-6 and in any case before the CRP values start to decrease. This would demonstrate a pathophysiological function of PCT in the immune response. It would be responsible for increasing nitric oxide synthesis and monocyte migration to the site of infection [83].

6.6. Presepsin

Presepsin is another name for the sCD14 subtype (sCD14-ST), is a new biomarker associated with sepsis. Soluble CD14 subtype is one fragment of CD14 soluble that is a molecular fragment produced by plasma protease activity during the inflammatory process [84]. Presepsin is present in the cell membranes of macrophages, monocytes and granulocyte cells and said to play a role for the intracellular transduction of endotoxin signals [85]. Presepsin has close relation with infection and is found to increase significantly in sepsis.

Behnes et al. showed that presepsin was moderately significant to determine between sepsis and non sepsis patient, with slightly overlapping value of 817.9 ± 572.7 and 294.2 ± 121.4 pg/mL for sepsis and non sepsis patient, respectively [50]. The level of presepsin in serum usually raised within 2 h after infection and reach maximum level within 3 h, therefore it is useful in diagnosis of sepsis patient during early stages [86, 87].

Wu et al. reported a meta-analysis about diagnostic value of presepsin of some studies. The result showed that the sensitivity of presepsin ranged from 0.67 to 1.0, while the specificity of presepsin ranged from 0.33 to 0.98. The pooled sensitivity and specificity obtained by the HSROC method were 0.84 (95% CI 0.80–0.87) and 0.76 (95% CI 0.67–0.84), respectively. While ROC for presepsin showed the AUC was 0.88 (95% CI 0.85–0.90 [88].

When compared to PCT, presepsin showed similar diagnostic accuracy for sepsis with sensitivity 0.78 [95% CI: 0.76–0.80] and 0.77 [95% CI: 0.72–0.81], specificity 0.83 [95% CI: 0.80–0.85] and 0.79 [95% CI: 0.74–0.84], AUCs 0.89 [95% CI: 0.84–0.94] and 0.85 [95% CI: 0.81–0.88], for presepsin and procalcitonin, respectively, to diagnose patient with sepsis and SIRS without infection [89].

However, there are some superiority of presepsin over PCT. Presepsin raised earlier in the event of infection therefore can be used in earlier and faster in sepsis. The PATHFAST analysis system also allow presepsin assay on takes 17 min to be done, therefore can be used accordingly with the guidelines of diagnosis and treatment of sepsis.

6.7. Bioadrenomedullin

Adrenomedullin (ADM) is a peptide with 52 amino acids initially isolated from the adrenal gland. It is produced in many organs and tissues including the vasculature. ADM has numerous actions, including vasodilation, natriuresis, antiapoptosis and stimulation of NO production. ADM is released from the vascular wall and acts as an autocrine or a paracrine hormone to regulate vascular tone and blood pressure. It may also be involved in the different stages of the cardiovascular continuum as well as in the hemodynamic changes in septic shock [90, 91].

A study by Crain et al. showed that in critically ill patients on admission, there was a stepwise increase in MR-proADM levels from patients without infection (e.g. SIRS) to patients with sepsis, severe sepsis and septic shock. Median proADM levels was 1.1 nmol/L (0.3–3.7 nmol/L) in patients with SIRS, 1.8 nmol/L (0.4–5.8 nmol/L) in patients with sepsis, 2.3 nmol/L (1.0–17.6 nmol/L) in patients with severe sepsis and in patients with septic shock it was 4.5 nmol/L (0.9–21 nmol/L). There are two primary mechanisms that might be responsible for the marked increase in circulating MR-proADM and mature ADM levels in sepsis. The first mechanism, as a member of the CALC gene family, ADM is widely expressed and extensively synthesized during sepsis, just like other calcitonin peptides including PCT, that upregulated by bacterial endotoxins and pro-inflammatory cytokines [92]. The second potential mechanism is the decreased clearance of MR-proADM by the kidneys in sepsis that may be responsible for its increased level. This hypothesis is also supported by a significant correlation between MR-proADM and creatinine levels ($r = 0.76$; $P < 0.001$). The study showed increase of plasma ADM five times higher that normal individuals, that did not changed after hemodialysis. An ideal sepsis marker should permit early diagnosis, should inform about the course of disease, and should help one to differentiate bacterial from non-infectious and viral causes of systemic inflammation [90].

Recently, the combined use of two biomarkers, procalcitonin (PCT) and mid-regional pro-adrenomedullin (MR-proADM) has been reported in sepsis diagnosis and prognosis. In the last years, many articles have been published on the role of PCT and MR-proADM in the diagnosis and prognosis of bacterial infections in different settings. Angeletti et al. showed that MR-proADM differentiates sepsis from non-infectious systemic inflammatory response syndrome with high specificity and that the simultaneous measurement of MR-proADM and PCT in septic patients increases the post-test diagnostic probability compared to the independent determination of individual markers. A score derived from the combination of PCT and MR-proADM has been recently proposed as a useful clinical tool to provide rapid diagnosis as well as to suggest prognosis of bacterial infections. The combined score, calculated on the basis of defined score assigned for each PCT and MR-proADM value, can predict bacterial infections and differentiate localized infections from systemic infections, as suggested by receiver operating characteristic curve analysis. On the basis of the score values, localized infections could be differentiated from systemic infections and the severity of the infectious disease can be predicted. The importance of the use of this multi-marker approach in the diagnosis and prognosis of sepsis is more evident since the publication of the new definition of sepsis that has been updated assigned an important role to the organ dysfunction [93].

6.8. Comparison between biomarker of sepsis

Lactate should be evaluated at least within 24 h after emergency admission, the decrease of lactate after 24 h related to poor prognosis of the patients [94]. CRP can increase within 24–48 h duration to 1000 folds during the acute phase and decrease to low normal value after the acute phase [95]. Procalcitonin start to rise 3–6 h after infection occur and reach its peak on 6–8 h, then remained in the blood until 12–48 h [96]. Meanwhile presepsin increase faster within 2–3 h after sepsis developed and rapidly decreased after symptoms resolved [97] so it can be used to determine whether the treatment is successful in patient with sepsis.

Several conditions can increase lactate in any person, such condition as inadequate oxygen delivery oxygen demands mismatch and inadequate oxygen utilization [94]. CRP increase in bacterial infection as part of innate immune response [95, 98]. It can also increase in condition of inflammation even can predict the cardiovascular event such as the sign of atherogenesis and pathogenesis of myocardial injury and used as predictor in healthy individuals [99, 100]. It also can be a predictor of mortality in hemodialysis patient [101, 102]. Procalcitonin will rise in the event of sepsis, systemic infection and severe inflammation. Procalcitonin will not rise in the event of viral infection, autoimmune and neoplasma, but it can rise in some people with some neuroendocrine tumor such as medullare carcinoma of thyroid, small cell lung carcinoma and renal failure [96, 103]. Procalcitonin is also known to rise in person with trauma [97]. Some inflammation can trigger the rise of procalcitonin are pancreatitis [104], appendicitis [105], burns [106], heat stroke [107], multitrauma [108] and extensive surgery [109]. Presepsin do not increase in patient with trauma without associated infection, thus make it specific in patient with sepsis [97]. Presepsin also reliable in patient with sepsis and both acute kidney injury and those who do not, but it has caveats in patient with advanced kidney injury and end stage renal disease [110].

Head to head study by cochrane comparing procalcitonin, presepsin and CRP is still ongoing [111]. Several data about sensitivity and specificity of these parameters are already covered by some journal. The study about diagnostic value of lactate in cancer patient with sepsis showed for the cutoff value of lactate more than 1 mmol/L could predict sepsis with sensitivity of 86.36% and specificity of 28.12%, with additional data that the value were not different in patient with and without cancer [112]. Another study showed 34.0% sensitivity and 82.0% specificity at the cutoff point of 2.0 mmol/L that emphasized the low sensitivity but high specificity in diagnosing sepsis [113]. While other study measures prognostic value of lactate showed that lactate value over 4.0 mmol/L have increased mortality with sensitivity and specificity of 36 and 92%, respectively [114]. CRP found to be useful as part of screening in sepsis patient with sensitivity and specificity 98.5 and 75%, respectively, for cutoff value 5 mg/dL or more [115]. Another study use CRP as parameter for successful treatment in ICU patient showed that decreasing level of CRP by 25% or more are good indicator with sensitivity of 97% and specificity of 95% [116]. A study showed that sensitivity and specificity of procalcitonin were 75 and 79%, respectively [117]. While another study in patient with renal impairment proposed different cutoff to determine if patient is in septic condition, due to the caveats of procalcitonin in renal failure patient [118]. Another study comparing CRP, procalcitonin and presepsin showed advantage of presepsin, with AUC of presepsin was 0.845, compared to PCT (0.652), and CRP (0.815). With sensitivity and specificity of presepsin with cutoff value 600 pg./mL was 87.8 and 81.4%, respectively [84].

Availability and cost of these examination will be favored more on white blood cell count because it is part of routine practice everywhere, while for lactate, the difference between patient examined for lactate around $39.53/patient whereas the usual care cost $33.20/patient but the effectiveness in term of patient outcome and survival are better in those with lactate examination [119]. On the other hand, the use of CRP in England shows the use of CRP can also increase quality of treatment and decrease cost for patient which leads to fewer antibiotic prescriptions [120]. One study about procalcitonin use as part of management of patient with pneumonia find that procalcitonin although promising not significantly reduce cost of care, due to lack of data, since non adherence of the physician. This condition might be due to lack of experience of using procalcitonin and need for more guided protocol of procalcitonin use in patient [121].

Author details

Agustin Iskandar[1], Hani Susianti[1], Muhammad Anshory[2] and Salvatore Di Somma[3]*

*Address all correspondence to: salvatore.disomma@uniroma1.it

1 Clinical Pathology Department, Faculty of Medicine, Universitas Brawijaya, Malang, Indonesia

2 Internal Medicine Department, Faculty of Medicine, Universitas Brawijaya, Malang, Indonesia

3 Department of Medical-Surgery Sciences and Translational Medicine, Sapienza University of Rome, Italy

References

[1] Russell JA. Management of sepsis. New England Journal of Medicine. 2006;**355**(16): 1699-1713

[2] Ventetuolo CE, Levy MM. Biomarkers: Diagnosis and risk assessment in sepsis. Clinics in Chest Medicine. 2008;**29**(4):591-603

[3] Levy MM, Fink MP, Marshall JC, Abraham E, Angus D, Cook D, et al. 2001 SCCM/ ESICM/ACCP/ATS/SIS international sepsis definitions conference. Critical Care Medicine. 2003;**31**(4):1250-1256

[4] Angus DC, Van der Poll T. Severe sepsis and septic shock. The New England Journal of Medicine. 2013;**369**(9):840-851

[5] Wiersinga WJ, Leopold SJ, Cranendonk DR, van der Poll T. Host innate immune responses to sepsis. Virulence. 2014;**5**(1):36-44

[6] Hotchkiss RS, Monneret G, Payen D. Sepsis-induced immunosuppression: From cellular dysfunctions to immunotherapy. Nature Reviews. Immunology. 2013;**13**(12):862

[7] Singer M, Deutschman CS, Seymour CW, Shankar-Hari M, Annane D, Bauer M, et al. The third international consensus definitions for sepsis and septic shock (sepsis-3). Journal of the American Medical Association. 2016;**315**(8):801-810

[8] Howell MD, Davis AM. Management of sepsis and septic shock. Journal of the American Medical Association. 2017;**317**(8):847-848

[9] Williams JM, Greenslade JH, McKenzie JV, Chu K, Brown AF, Lipman J. Systemic inflammatory response syndrome, quick sequential organ function assessment, and organ dysfunction: Insights from a prospective database of ED patients with infection. CHEST Journal. 2017;**151**(3):586-596

[10] Finkelsztein EJ, Jones DS, Ma KC, Pabón MA, Delgado T, Nakahira K, et al. Comparison of qSOFA and SIRS for predicting adverse outcomes of patients with suspicion of sepsis outside the intensive care unit. Critical Care. 2017;**21**(1):73

[11] Dellinger RP, Levy MM, Rhodes A, Annane D, Gerlach H, Opal SM, et al. Surviving sepsis campaign: International guidelines for management of severe sepsis and septic shock, 2012. Intensive Care Medicine. 2013;**39**(2):165-228

[12] Moemen ME. Prognostic categorization of intensive care septic patients. World Journal of Critical Care Medicine. 2012;**1**(3):67

[13] Bouch DC, Thompson JP. Severity scoring systems in the critically ill. Continuing Education in Anaesthesia, Critical Care & Pain. 2008;**8**(5):181-185

[14] Shapiro NI, Wolfe RE, Moore RB, Smith E, Burdick E, Bates DW. Mortality in emergency department sepsis (MEDS) score: A prospectively derived and validated clinical prediction rule. Critical Care Medicine. 2003;**31**(3):670-675

[15] Sankoff JD, Goyal M, Gaieski DF, Deitch K, Davis CB, Sabel AL, et al. Validation of the mortality in emergency department sepsis (MEDS) score in patients with the systemic inflammatory response syndrome (SIRS). Critical Care Medicine. 2008;**36**(2):421-426

[16] Jones AE, Trzeciak S, Kline JA. The sequential organ failure assessment score for predicting outcome in patients with severe sepsis and evidence of hypoperfusion at the time of emergency department presentation. Critical Care Medicine. 2009;**37**(5):1649

[17] Calle P, Cerro L, Valencia J, Jaimes F. Usefulness of severity scores in patients with suspected infection in the emergency department: A systematic review. The Journal of Emergency Medicine. 2012;**42**(4):379-391

[18] Innocenti F, Bianchi S, Guerrini E, Vicidomini S, Conti A, Zanobetti M, et al. Prognostic scores for early stratification of septic patients admitted to an emergency department-high dependency unit. European Journal of Emergency Medicine. 2014;**21**(4):254-259

[19] Cockerill F III, Wilson J, Vetter E, Goodman K, Torgerson C, Harmsen W, et al. Optimal testing parameters for blood cultures. Clinical Infectious Diseases. 2004;**38**(12):1724-1730

[20] Kreger BE, Craven DE, McCabe WR. Gram-negative bacteremia: IV. Re-evaluation of clinical features and treatment in 612 patients. The American Journal of Medicine. 1980;**68**(3):344-355

[21] Reimer LG, Carroll KC. Role of the microbiology laboratory in the diagnosis of lower respiratory tract infections. Clinical Infectious Diseases. 1998;**26**(3):742-748

[22] Auckenthaler R, Ilstrup D, Washington J. Comparison of recovery of organisms from blood cultures diluted 10%(volume/volume) and 20%(volume/volume). Journal of Clinical Microbiology. 1982;**15**(5):860-864

[23] Herzke CA, Chen LF, Anderson DJ, Choi Y, Sexton DJ, Kaye KS. Empirical antimicrobial therapy for bloodstream infection due to methicillin-resistant Staphylococcus aureus: No better than a coin toss. Infection Control and Hospital Epidemiology. 2009;**30**(11): 1057-1061

[24] Riedel S, Carroll KC. Blood cultures: Key elements for best practices and future directions. Journal of Infection and Chemotherapy. 2010;**16**(5):301-316

[25] Bourbeau PP, Foltzer M. Routine incubation of BacT/ALERT FA and FN blood culture bottles for more than 3 days may not be necessary. Journal of Clinical Microbiology. 2005;**43**(5):2506-2509

[26] Baron EJ, Scott JD, Tompkins LS. Prolonged incubation and extensive subculturing do not increase recovery of clinically significant microorganisms from standard automated blood cultures. Clinical Infectious Diseases. 2005;**41**(11):1677-1680

[27] Carrigan SD, Scott G, Tabrizian M. Toward resolving the challenges of sepsis diagnosis. Clinical Chemistry. 2004;**50**(8):1301-1314

[28] Peters RP, van Agtmael MA, Danner SA, Savelkoul PH, Vandenbroucke-Grauls CM. New developments in the diagnosis of bloodstream infections. The Lancet Infectious Diseases. 2004;**4**(12):751-760

[29] Fenollar F, Raoult D. Molecular diagnosis of bloodstream infections caused by non-cultivable bacteria. International Journal of Antimicrobial Agents. 2007;**30**:7-15

[30] Ecker DJ, Sampath R, Li H, Massire C, Matthews HE, Toleno D, et al. New technology for rapid molecular diagnosis of bloodstream infections. Expert Review of Molecular Diagnostics. 2010;**10**(4):399-415

[31] Tsalik EL, Jones D, Nicholson B, Waring L, Liesenfeld O, Park LP, et al. Multiplex PCR to diagnose bloodstream infections in patients admitted from the emergency department with sepsis. Journal of Clinical Microbiology. 2010;**48**(1):26-33

[32] Visconti GLI. Marcatori Biochimici. Dipartimento di Laboratorio Gove e Carle Cuneo. Cuneo: Sezione immunometria,laboratorio analisi chimico cliniche e microbiologia; 2007

[33] Di Somma S, Magrini L, Travaglino F, Lalle I, Fiotti N, Cervellin G, et al. Opinion paper on innovative approach of biomarkers for infectious diseases and sepsis management in the emergency department. Clinical Chemistry and Laboratory Medicine. 2013;**51**(6):1167-1175

[34] Freund Y, Lemachatti N, Krastinova E, Van Laer M, Claessens Y-E, Avondo A, et al. Prognostic accuracy of sepsis-3 criteria for in-hospital mortality among patients with suspected infection presenting to the emergency department. Journal of the American Medical Association. 2017;**317**(3):301-308

[35] Be3towski J, Jamroz A. Adrenomedullin–what do we know 10 years since its discovery? Polish Journal of Pharmacology. 2004;**56**:5-27

[36] Wong LY, Cheung BM, Li Y-Y, Tang F. Adrenomedullin is both proinflammatory and antiinflammatory: Its effects on gene expression and secretion of cytokines and macrophage migration inhibitory factor in NR8383 macrophage cell line. Endocrinology. 2005; **146**(3):1321-1327

[37] Hirata Y, Mitaka C, Sato K, Nagura T, Tsunoda Y, Amaha K, et al. Increased circulating adrenomedullin, a novel vasodilatory peptide, in sepsis. The Journal of Clinical Endocrinology & Metabolism. 1996;**81**(4):1449-1453

[38] Travaglino F, De Berardinis B, Magrini L, Bongiovanni C, Candelli M, Silveri NG, et al. Utility of Procalcitonin (PCT) and mid regional pro-Adrenomedullin (MR-proADM) in risk stratification of critically ill febrile patients in emergency department (ED). A comparison with APACHE II score. BMC Infectious Diseases. 2012;**12**(1):184

[39] Marino R, Struck J, Maisel AS, Magrini L, Bergmann A, Di Somma S. Plasma adrenomedullin is associated with short-term mortality and vasopressor requirement in patients admitted with sepsis. Critical Care. 2014;**18**(1):R34

[40] Guignant C, Voirin N, Venet F, Poitevin F, Malcus C, Bohé J, et al. Assessment of pro-vasopressin and pro-adrenomedullin as predictors of 28-day mortality in septic shock patients. Intensive Care Medicine. 2009;**35**(11):1859

[41] Kibe S, Adams K, Barlow G. Diagnostic and prognostic biomarkers of sepsis in critical care. The Journal of Antimicrobial Chemotherapy. 2011;**66**(suppl_2):ii33-ii40

[42] Marshall JC, Reinhart K. Biomarkers of sepsis. Critical Care Medicine. 2009;**37**(7):2290-2298

[43] Pierrakos C, Vincent J-L. Sepsis biomarkers: A review. Critical Care. 2010;**14**(1):R15

[44] Figueras-Aloy J, Gómez-López L, Rodríguez-Miguélez J-M, Salvia-Roiges MD, Jordán-García I, Ferrer-Codina I, et al. Serum soluble ICAM-1, VCAM-1, L-selectin, and P-selectin levels as markers of infection and their relation to clinical severity in neonatal sepsis. American Journal of Perinatology. 2007;**24**(06):331-338

[45] Lobo SM, Lobo FR, Bota DP, Lopes-Ferreira F, Soliman HM, Melot C, et al. C-reactive protein levels correlate with mortality and organ failure in critically ill patients. CHEST Journal. 2003;**123**(6):2043-2049

[46] de Kruif MD, Limper M, Gerritsen H, Spek CA, Brandjes DP, ten Cate H, et al. Additional value of procalcitonin for diagnosis of infection in patients with fever at the emergency department. Critical Care Medicine. 2010;**38**(2):457-463

[47] Wang R-l, F-x K. Prediction about severity and outcome of sepsis by pro-atrial natriuretic peptide and pro-adrenomedullin. Chinese Journal of Traumatology (English Edition). 2010;**13**(3):152-157

[48] Christ-Crain M. The stress hormone copeptin: A new prognostic biomarker in acute illness. Swiss Medical Weekly. 2010;**140**:w13101

[49] Morgenthaler NG, Struck J, Christ-Crain M, Bergmann A, Müller B. Pro-atrial natriuretic peptide is a prognostic marker in sepsis, similar to the APACHE II score: An observational study. Critical Care. 2004;**9**(1):R37

[50] Behnes M, Bertsch T, Lepiorz D, Lang S, Trinkmann F, Brueckmann M, et al. Diagnostic and prognostic utility of soluble CD 14 subtype (presepsin) for severe sepsis and septic shock during the first week of intensive care treatment. Critical Care. 2014;**18**(5):507

[51] Donadello K, Scolletta S, Covajes C, Vincent J-L. suPAR as a prognostic biomarker in sepsis. BMC Medicine. 2012;**10**(1):2

[52] Ploppa A, Schmidt V, Hientz A, Reutershan J, Haeberle HA, Nohé B. Mechanisms of leukocyte distribution during sepsis: An experimental study on the interdependence of cell activation, shear stress and endothelial injury. Critical Care. 2010;**14**(6):R201

[53] Manroe BL, Weinberg AG, Rosenfeld CR, Browne R. The neonatal blood count in health and disease. I. Reference values for neutrophilic cells. The Journal of Pediatrics. 1979;**95**(1): 89-98

[54] Caldas JP, Marba S, Blotta MH, Calil R, Morais SS, Oliveira RT. Accuracy of white blood cell count, C-reactive protein, interleukin-6 and tumor necrosis factor alpha for diagnosing late neonatal sepsis. Jornal de Pediatria. 2008;**84**(6):536-542

[55] Zahorec R. Ratio of neutrophil to lymphocyte counts-rapid and simple parameter of systemic inflammation and stress in critically ill. Bratislavské Lekárske Listy. 2001;**102**(1):5-14

[56] Ljungström L, Pernestig A-K, Jacobsson G, Andersson R, Usener B, Tilevik D. Diagnostic accuracy of procalcitonin, neutrophil-lymphocyte count ratio, C-reactive protein, and lactate in patients with suspected bacterial sepsis. PLoS One. 2017;**12**(7):e0181704

[57] Loonen AJ, de Jager CP, Tosserams J, Kusters R, Hilbink M, Wever PC, et al. Biomarkers and molecular analysis to improve bloodstream infection diagnostics in an emergency care unit. PLoS One. 2014;**9**(1):e87315

[58] Passantino A, Monitillo F, Iacoviello M, Scrutinio D. Predicting mortality in patients with acute heart failure: Role of risk scores. World Journal of Cardiology. 2015;**7**(12):902

[59] Jeppesen JB, Mortensen C, Bendtsen F, Møller S. Lactate metabolism in chronic liver disease. Scandinavian Journal of Clinical and Laboratory Investigation. 2013;**73**(4):293-299

[60] Park WM, Gloviczki P, Cherry KJ, Hallett JW, Bower TC, Panneton JM, et al. Contemporary management of acute mesenteric ischemia: Factors associated with survival. Journal of Vascular Surgery. 2002;**35**(3):445-452

[61] Levy MM, Dellinger RP, Townsend SR, Linde-Zwirble WT, Marshall JC, Bion J, et al. The surviving sepsis campaign: Results of an international guideline-based performance improvement program targeting severe sepsis. Intensive Care Medicine. 2010;**36**(2): 222-231

[62] Lee SM, An WS. New clinical criteria for septic shock: Serum lactate level as new emerging vital sign. Journal of Thoracic Disease. 2016;**8**(7):1388

[63] Ansar W, Ghosh S. Inflammation and Inflammatory Diseases, Markers, and Mediators: Role of CRP in some Inflammatory Diseases. Biology of C Reactive Protein in Health and Disease. New Delhi: Springer; 2016. pp. 67-107

[64] Meisner M, Adina H, Schmidt J. Correlation of procalcitonin and C-reactive protein to inflammation, complications, and outcome during the intensive care unit course of multiple-trauma patients. Critical Care. 2005;**10**(1):R1

[65] Pepys MB, Hirschfield GM. C-reactive protein: a critical update. The Journal of Clinical Investigation. 2003;**111**(12):1805

[66] Bozza FA, Bozza PT, Castro Faria Neto HC. Beyond sepsis pathophysiology with cytokines: What is their value as biomarkers for disease severity? Memórias do Instituto Oswaldo Cruz. 2005;**100**:217-221

[67] Christ-Crain M, Müller B. Biomarkers in respiratory tract infections: Diagnostic guides to antibiotic prescription, prognostic markers and mediators. The European Respiratory Journal. 2007;**30**(3):556-573

[68] Meisner M. Procalcitonina: un nuovo, innovativo parametro di infezione. Caleidosc Italiano. 1997;**15**:5-20

[69] Caterino JM, Scheatzle MD, Forbes ML, D'Antonio JA. Bacteremic elder emergency department patients: Procalcitonin and white count. Academic Emergency Medicine. 2004;**11**(4): 393-396

[70] Ruiz-Alvarez MJ, Garcia-Valdecasas S, De Pablo R, Sanchez García M, Coca C, Groeneveld T, et al. Diagnostic efficacy and prognostic value of serum procalcitonin concentration in patients with suspected sepsis. Journal of Intensive Care Medicine. 2009;**24**(1):63-71

[71] Hausfater P, Juillien G, Madonna-Py B, Haroche J, Bernard M, Riou B. Serum procalcitonin measurement as diagnostic and prognostic marker in febrile adult patients presenting to the emergency department. Critical Care. 2007;**11**(3):R60

[72] Stolza D, Christ-Craind M, Gencaya MM, Bingisserb R, Huberc PR, Müllerd B, et al. Diagnostic value of signs, symptoms and laboratory values in lower respiratory tract infection. Coronary Artery Disease. 2006;**59**:24

[73] Müller F, Christ-Crain M, Bregenzer T, Krause M, Zimmerli W, Mueller B, et al. Procalcitonin levels predict bacteremia in patients with community-acquired pneumonia: A prospective cohort trial. CHEST Journal. 2010;**138**(1):121-129

[74] Schuetz P, Suter-Widmer I, Chaudri A, Christ-Crain M, Zimmerli W, Mueller B. Prognostic value of procalcitonin in community-acquired pneumonia. The European Respiratory Journal. 2011;**37**(2):384-392

[75] Krüger S, Ewig S, Marre R, Papassotiriou J, Richter K, von Baum H, et al. Procalcitonin predicts patients at low risk of death from community-acquired pneumonia across all CRB-65 classes. The European Respiratory Journal. 2008;**31**(2):349-355

[76] Daubin C, Parienti J-J, Fradin S, Vabret A, Ramakers M, Terzi N, et al. Procalcitonin levels and bacterial aetiology among COPD patients admitted to the ICU with severe pneumonia: A prospective cohort study. BMC Infectious Diseases. 2009;**9**(1):157

[77] Blasi F, Stolz D, Piffer F. Biomarkers in lower respiratory tract infections. Pulmonary Pharmacology & Therapeutics. 2010;**23**(6):501-507

[78] Crain CMMC, Müller B. What cardiologists do need to know about procalcitonin. Clinical Laboratory. 2005;**51**:1-4

[79] Biasucci LM, Biasillo G, Stefanelli A. Procalcitonin and acute coronary syndromes: A new biomarker for an old disease. Internal and Emergency Medicine. 2009;**4**(5):363-365

[80] Picariello C, Lazzeri C, Chiostri M, Gensini G, Valente S. Procalcitonin in patients with acute coronary syndromes and cardiogenic shock submitted to percutaneous coronary intervention. Internal and Emergency Medicine. 2009;**4**(5):403-408

[81] Castelli GP, Pognani C, Cita M, Paladini R. Procalcitonin as a prognostic and diagnostic tool for septic complications after major trauma. Critical Care Medicine. 2009;**37**(6): 1845-1849

[82] Boussekey N, Leroy O, Alfandari S, Devos P, Georges H, Guery B. Procalcitonin kinetics in the prognosis of severe community-acquired pneumonia. Intensive Care Medicine. 2006;**32**(3):469-472

[83] Meisner M, Tschaikowsky K, Spiessl C, Schüttler J. Procalcitonin—A marker or modulator of the acute immune response? Intensive Care Medicine. 1996;**22**:S14-S

[84] Zou Q, Wen W, Zhang X. Presepsin as a novel sepsis biomarker. World Journal of Emergency Medicine. 2014;**5**(1):16-19

[85] Agilli M, Sener I, Yesildal F, Honca T, Aydin I, Akgul EO, et al. A new marker for the diagnosıs of sepsis: Presepsin. Journal of Investigational Biochemistry. 2012;**1**(1):55-57

[86] Vodnik T, Kaljevic G, Tadic T, Majkic-Singh N. Presepsin (sCD14-ST) in preoperative diagnosis of abdominal sepsis. Clinical Chemistry and Laboratory Medicine. 2013;**51**(10): 2053-2062

[87] Ulla M, Pizzolato E, Lucchiari M, Loiacono M, Soardo F, Forno D, et al. Diagnostic and prognostic value of presepsin in the management of sepsis in the emergency department: A multicenter prospective study. Critical Care. 2013;**17**(4):R168

[88] Wu C-C, Lan H-M, Han S-T, Chaou C-H, Yeh C-F, Liu S-H, et al. Comparison of diagnostic accuracy in sepsis between presepsin, procalcitonin, and C-reactive protein: A systematic review and meta-analysis. Annals of Intensive Care. 2017;**7**(1):91

[89] Wu J, Hu L, Zhang G, Wu F, He T. Accuracy of presepsin in sepsis diagnosis: A systematic review and meta-analysis. PLoS One. 2015;**10**(7):e0133057

[90] Christ-Crain M, Morgenthaler NG, Struck J, Harbarth S, Bergmann A, Müller B. Mid-regional pro-adrenomedullin as a prognostic marker in sepsis: An observational study. Critical Care. 2005;**9**(6):R816

[91] Wong HK, Cheung TT, Cheung BM. Adrenomedullin and cardiovascular diseases. JRSM Cardiovascular Disease. 2012;**1**(5):1-7

[92] Becker K, Nylen E, White J, Muller B, Snider R Jr. Procalcitonin and the calcitonin gene family of peptides in inflammation, infection, and sepsis: A journey from calcitonin back to its precursors. The Journal of Clinical Endocrinology & Metabolism. 2004;**89**(4): 1512-1525

[93] Angeletti S, Battistoni F, Fioravanti M, Bernardini S, Dicuonzo G. Procalcitonin and mid-regional pro-adrenomedullin test combination in sepsis diagnosis. Clinical Chemistry and Laboratory Medicine. 2013;**51**(5):1059-1067

[94] Blomkalns A. LACTATE – A marker for sepsis and trauma; 2017

[95] Volanakis JE. Human C-reactive protein: Expression, structure, and function. Molecular Immunology. 2001;**38**(2):189-197

[96] Maruna P, Nedelnikova K, Gurlich R. Physiology and genetics of procalcitonin. Physiological Research. 2000;**49**(Suppl 1):S57-S61

[97] Endo S, Takahashi G, Shozushima T, Matsumoto N, Kojika M, Suzuki Y, et al. Usefulness of Presepsin (soluble CD14 subtype) as a diagnostic marker for sepsis. **日本救急医学会雑誌**. 2012;**23**(2):27-38

[98] Du Clos TW. Function of C-reactive protein. Annals of Medicine. 2000;**32**(4):274-278

[99] Ridker PM, Buring JE, Cook NR, Rifai N. C-reactive protein, the metabolic syndrome, and risk of incident cardiovascular events. Circulation. 2003;**107**(3):391-397

[100] Ridker PM, Rifai N, Rose L, Buring JE, Cook NR. Comparison of C-reactive protein and low-density lipoprotein cholesterol levels in the prediction of first cardiovascular events. The New England Journal of Medicine. 2002;**347**(20):1557-1565

[101] Helal I, Zerelli L, Krid M, ElYounsi F, Maiz HB, Zouari B, et al. Comparison of C-reactive protein and high-sensitivity C-reactive protein levels in patients on hemodialysis. Saudi Journal of Kidney Diseases and Transplantation. 2012;**23**(3):477

[102] Takahashi R, Ito Y, Takahashi H, Ishii H, Kasuga H, Mizuno M, et al. Combined values of serum albumin, C-reactive protein and body mass index at dialysis initiation accurately predicts long-term mortality. American Journal of Nephrology. 2012;**36**(2):136-143

[103] Becker KL, Snider R, Nylen ES. Procalcitonin in sepsis and systemic inflammation: A harmful biomarker and a therapeutic target. British Journal of Pharmacology. 2010;**159**(2):253-264

[104] Ammori B, Becker K, Kite P, Snider R, Nylen E, White J, et al. Calcitonin precursors in the prediction of severity of acute pancreatitis on the day of admission. The British Journal of Surgery. 2003;**90**(2):197-204

[105] Kafetzis D, Velissariou I, Nikolaides P, Sklavos M, Maktabi M, Spyridis G, et al. Procalcitonin as a predictor of severe appendicitis in children. European Journal of Clinical Microbiology & Infectious Diseases. 2005;**24**(7):484-487

[106] Von Heimburg D, Stieghorst W, Khorram-Sefat R, Pallua N. Procalcitonin—A sepsis parameter in severe burn injuries. Burns. 1998;**24**(8):745-750

[107] Nylen ES, Al Arifi A, Becker KL, Snider RH, Alzeer A. Effect of classic heatstroke on serum procalcitonin. Critical Care Medicine. 1997;**25**(8):1362-1365

[108] Maier M, Wutzler S, Lehnert M, Szermutzky M, Wyen H, Bingold T, et al. Serum procalcitonin levels in patients with multiple injuries including visceral trauma. Journal of Trauma and Acute Care Surgery. 2009;**66**(1):243-249

[109] Meisner M, Tschaikowsky K, Hutzler A, Schick C, Schmidt J. Postoperative plasma concentrations of procalcitonin after different types of surgery. In. Critical Care: BioMed Central; 1998:P040

[110] Nakamura Y, Ishikura H, Nishida T, Kawano Y, Yuge R, Ichiki R, et al. Usefulness of presepsin in the diagnosis of sepsis in patients with or without acute kidney injury. BMC Anesthesiology. 2014;**14**:88

[111] Onyenekwu CP, Okwundu CI, Ochodo EA. Procalcitonin, C-reactive protein, and presepsin for the diagnosis of sepsis in adults and children. The Cochrane Library. 2017

[112] Keçe E, Yaka E, Yılmaz S, Doğan NÖ, Alyeşil C, Pekdemir M. Comparison of diagnostic and prognostic utility of lactate and procalcitonin for sepsis in adult cancer patients presenting to emergency department with systemic inflammatory response syndrome. Turkish Journal of Emergency Medicine. 2016;**16**(1):1-7

[113] Singer AJ, Taylor M, Domingo A, Ghazipura S, Khorasonchi A, Thode HC, et al. Diagnostic characteristics of a clinical screening tool in combination with measuring bedside lactate level in emergency department patients with suspected sepsis. Academic Emergency Medicine. 2014;**21**(8):853-857

[114] Shapiro NI, Howell MD, Talmor D, Nathanson LA, Lisbon A, Wolfe RE, et al. Serum lactate as a predictor of mortality in emergency department patients with infection. Annals of Emergency Medicine. 2005;**45**(5):524-528

[115] Povoa P, Almeida E, Moreira P, Fernandes A, Mealha R, Aragao A, et al. C-reactive protein as an indicator of sepsis. Intensive Care Medicine. 1998;**24**(10):1052-1056

[116] Yentis S, Soni N, Sheldon J. C-reactive protein as an indicator of resolution of sepsis in the intensive care unit. Intensive Care Medicine. 1995;**21**(7):602-605

[117] Riedel S, Melendez JH, An AT, Rosenbaum JE, Zenilman JM. Procalcitonin as a marker for the detection of bacteremia and sepsis in the emergency department. American Journal of Clinical Pathology. 2011;**135**(2):182-189

[118] El-sayed D, Grotts J, Golgert WA, Sugar AM. Sensitivity and Specificity of Procalcitonin in Predicting Bacterial Infections in Patients With Renal Impairment. Open Forum Infectious Diseases. 2014;1:ofu068-ofu

[119] Ward MJ, Self WH, Singer A, Lazar D, Pines JM. Cost-effectiveness analysis of early point-of-care lactate testing in the emergency department. Journal of Critical Care. 2016;**36**:69-75

[120] Hunter R. Cost-effectiveness of point-of-care C-reactive protein tests for respiratory tract infection in primary care in England. Advances in Therapy. 2015;**32**(1):69-85

[121] Smith KJ, Wateska A, Nowalk MP, Raymund M, Lee BY, Zimmerman RK, et al. Cost-effectiveness of procalcitonin-guided antibiotic use in community acquired pneumonia. Journal of General Internal Medicine. 2013;**28**(9):1157-1164

9

Topological Biomarker of Alzheimer's Disease

Sanja Josef Golubic

Abstract

For years, it has been assumed that the cerebral accumulation of pathologic protein forms is the main trigger of Alzheimer's disease (AD) pathology; however, recent studies revealed strong evidences that the alternations in synaptic activity precede and affect the homeostasis of amyloid-beta and tau, both of which aggregate during AD. Given that the neuropathological changes, characteristic for AD, start decades before the onset of the first symptoms, when alternations become irreversible, it is crucial to find a biomarker that can detect the preclinical signs of disease, presumably synaptic dysfunction of specific cerebral areas. Here is presented a novel, a high potential neuroimaging biomarker that can detect the postsynaptic dysfunction of specific neural substrate located in medial prefrontal cortex (mPFC) during sensory gating processing of a simple auditory stimulus. The magnetoencephalography-based localization of mPFC gating activation has the potential not only to detect symptomatic AD but also to become a predictor of cognitive decline related to the pathophysiological processes of AD, both at the individual level. The strengths of proposed biomarker lie in the simplicity of using a binary value, i.e., activated or not activated a neural generator along with its potential to follow the evolution of the pathophysiological process of disease from preclinical phase. The novel biomarker does not require estimation of uniform cutoff levels and standardization processes, the main problems of so far proposed biomarkers. Ability to individually detect AD pathology during putative preclinical and clinical stages, absolute noninvasiveness, and large effect size give this biomarker a high translation capacity and clinical potential.

Keywords: Alzheimer's disease, preclinical Alzheimer's disease, Alzheimer's disease biomarker, neuroimaging biomarker, auditory sensory gating, prefrontal cortex, magnetoencephalography

1. Introduction

Alzheimer's disease (AD), a long-lasting progressive neurodegeneration, characterized by synaptic dysfunction, an increase in extracellular amyloid plaques, intracellular tauopathy, extensive neuronal loss in several cerebral areas, and enhanced neuroinflammation. Highly disrupted cholinergic transmission is proving to be a featured biochemical sign of disease. Clinical manifestations include progressive loss of ability to encode new memories, impairment of both declarative and non-declarative memory, and finally the invincible decline of overall intellectual capacity. Today, worldwide spreading of Alzheimer's type dementia is one of the major public health challenges confronting this generation.

Extensive AD research, especially in the last 40 years, brought a significant progress in the development of diagnostic approaches and understanding the etiology. However, despite accumulated knowledge, the cause of the disease has not been found, a postmortem histopathological evaluation is still required to confirm the clinical diagnosis, and finally, effective treatment that would at least slow progression of the disease has not yet been found. As a result, if Augusta Deter, the first patient who had been described with the hallmarks of the disease, was alive today, her prognosis would be the same as in 1906.

1.1. Amyloid hypothesis

Since the first documentation by Alois Alzheimer, spread of abnormal protein filaments (plaque) throughout the brain, the main histopathological sign of Alzheimer's dementia, had a prominent role in a broad spectrum of proposed mechanisms related to disease pathogenesis. Amyloidogenic fragments were described structurally in extracellular plaques, and tau protein was documented as the main component of intracellular neurofibrillary tangles [1, 2].

According to amyloid hypothesis, the neurotoxic forms of amyloid-beta polypeptides, derived from amyloid precursor protein (APP), induce synaptic injuries followed by substantial intracellular damage in form of tauopathy and subsequently produce the pathological presentations of neurodegeneration leading to dementia [3]. There are reliable evidences, provided by the systematic work of Braak and Braak [4, 5], that the pathological progression of extracellular and intracellular deposits of pathological protein forms starts decades before the onset of clinical symptoms.

The genetic mutations identified on chromosome 21 are conferred to trigger AD through abnormal processing of APP, causing the elevated cerebral concentrations of amyloid-beta or increased production of its specific forms [6]. Also, three other different autosomal dominant mutations that might cause AD have been identified on chromosomes 14 and 1, leading to mutations of presenilin 1 and presenilin 2 proteins, respectively, along with late-onset apolipoprotein genotype ἐ4 [7–9].

The discoveries of mutations in amyloid-beta-related proteins have had significant influence in promoting the amyloid theory. However, while these mutations account for the majority of early-onset AD (<65 years; familial AD), the risk genes linked with late-onset AD (> 65 years; 95% of all AD cases) are subtle, with no direct genetic relation to the APP gene or its enzymes [10]. In addition, recent neuroimaging results strongly indicate that some non-demented individuals can have amyloid-beta aggregates equivalent in concentration to those found in demented patients [11], and also symptoms of AD can emerge regardless of amyloid deposition [12].

The evidences, provided by the animal studies, that amyloid clearance produces decreased symptoms of disease in mouse models of AD [13, 14] had turned the drug development in the direction of targeting beta-amyloid in human brains. The deployment of drugs comprised active and passive immunization directly against amyloid-beta accumulation and inhibition of beta- and gamma-secretase APP cleaving enzyme. Regrettably, none of testing drugs have resulted in recovery of functional abilities or alleviating symptoms of the disease in humans. The treatments did not slow down the course of the disease; on the contrary, some drugs even accelerate the progression of the symptoms. The recently emerged evidences confirmed the low correlation of the cerebral distribution of beta-amyloid plaques with neuropathology, decrease of neural function, or cognitive deficits [3]. A possibility that insoluble plaque is not the primary cause of progressive AD pathology is a strong argument for failure of anti-amyloid vaccination trials to improve patient outcome, even when cerebral amyloid plaque was removed [15]. Consequently, failure of amyloid-based AD treatments shifts research hypothesis to the soluble amyloid beta oligomers rather than plaques to be the main cause of neuronal degeneration [16]. However, there is still not reliable evidence in human studies that soluble amyloid oligomers are toxic in vivo. Notably, the cause of pathological cascade, resulting in redundant amyloid forms production and ejection, is still poorly understood along with the issue concerning the role of different amyloid beta forms in AD pathogenesis [17].

1.2. Synaptic function failure hypothesis

Synapse loss generates a loss of dendritic mass [18] and promotes neuron loss [19], a hallmark of AD pathology. It is interesting that amyloid plaque can show up without synapse loss [20]; moreover, synapse loss can occur without associated amyloid deposition [21]. High quantitative correlations of postmortem cytopathology to premortem cognitive impairments suggest that the decrease in density of synapses and decrease in the number of synapses per neuron are more linked to AD symptoms than are the concentration of amyloid plaques, the number of intracellular tau-tangles, or cortical gliosis [22]. These results appoint synapses as the key feature of AD, strongly indicating that the disease pathogenesis could be the outcome of synaptic failure [23].

It has been shown that the early AD symptoms significantly correlate with a specific dysfunction of cholinergic synapses [24]. Interestingly, acetylcholine receptor agonists affect several of AD hallmarks, including cholinergic deficits, cognitive dysfunction, but also tau and amyloid-beta pathological burdens [25]. The electrophysiological measurements of basal synaptic transmission and long-term potentiation in transgenic mouse with mutations analog of human mutations causing AD suggest that change in synaptic function precedes amyloid plaque production. Increased synaptic activity increases amyloid secretion, while decreasing activity inhibits it [26, 27]. In turn, beta-amyloid burden inhibits synapses and alerts synaptic plasticity [28], implying the existence of a feedback loop between synaptic dynamics and associated amyloid production that might serve as a mechanism to prevent synaptic hyperactivation and excitotoxicity [26]. In addition, recent studies demonstrate an important physiological role of cortical amyloid secretion, showing that low concentrations of beta-amyloid peptides increase long-term potentiation, needed for successful memory formation [29, 30]. There are also evidences that synaptic dysfunction occurs before changes in synaptic morphology or the number of synapses per neuron [31, 32]. These breakthroughs in the field provide strong evidences that amyloid homeostasis is controlled by the synaptic functions and emphasize prominent amyloid involvement in healthy memory coding.

Cerebral dysfunction found in non-demented elderly individuals with amyloid plaques before any memory disturbances [33] points at impairment in neural function as a very early pathophysiological sign of AD. Interestingly, functional changes may be driven in both directions, increased [34, 35] or decreased [36, 37] neuronal excitability, usually depending on the disease stage and a specific brain area and its function. The increased synaptic activity, found in early stages of symptomatic AD, might be an adaptive response driving neuroprotection [38]. On the other hand, the decreased neural network excitability could be induced by activation of gamma-aminobutyric acid (GABA) receptors, which decrease glutamate excitatory transmission, implying that in vivo glutamate-mediated neuronal excitability is controlled by interactions between inhibitory systems [39]. The co-transmission of acetylcholine and GABA, first found within the cholinergic system only, recently was demonstrated as a common feature of nearly all cholinergic forebrain neurons [40, 41]. These results appoint GABA as a fast neurotransmitter utilized throughout the forebrain cholinergic system and emphasized acetylcholine-GABA co-release as a major modulation factor of cortical functions transmitted by cholinergic neurons. Moreover, there is evidence that GABA receptor agonists defend neurons in culture from the toxicity of beta amyloids and of different glutamate receptor agonists [42]. In conclusion, given their major role in both sensory processing and cognition, and high susceptibility to AD pathology, the ability of the cholinergic neurons to co-release GABA could explain the failure of specific synaptic inhibitory processes found in AD that may trigger the cascade of events resulting in characteristic neuropathology.

1.3. Dynamic model of AD pathogenesis

The presence of cerebral amyloid aggregation in cognitively normal individuals, the lack of systematic correlation between amyloid plaque deposition and cognition, insufficiently explained influence of soluble amyloid oligomeric *in vivo*, the bias of preclinical disease models toward the amyloid hypothesis, and finally failures of clinical trials with anti-amyloid drugs are the strong arguments for urgent need to revise present model of AD to include alternative possibilities that could account for all the research results associated to AD.

Failures of clinical trials of anti-amyloid drugs in symptomatic AD patients (mild cognitive impairment (MCI) and moderate Alzheimer's disease patients) in addition to reliable evidence that the hallmarks of disease could be found in the brain decades before symptom onset set up a view that the onset of clinical symptoms is a sign of irreversible neural damage. Consequently, the concept of AD pathogenesis is evolving toward a view of the disease as a long-term continuum, which differs only by symptom appearance; that is, a non-symptomatic (preclinical) AD phase and an irreversible symptomatic AD phase [43, 44]. This dynamic concept of the disease emphasizes the neurobiological advantage of early intervention before of widespread neurodegeneration, during the preclinical stage of disease, when neural injuries may still be reversible. Consequently, it is crucial to detect very early, possibly reversible, pathological changes related to AD in cognitively intact individuals, before the occurrence of the first symptoms, i.e., to reveal the reliable preclinical biomarker of the disease.

1.4. Conclusion

A wealth of evidence suggests that the amyloid hypothesis of AD etiology is insufficient to explain all pathological changes associated with AD and their temporal evolution. Considering the wide spectra of data in AD research, it cannot be overlooked their common link: synaptic dysfunction and degradation as a very early characteristic of the disease. Unlike neuron death, changes in synaptic functions are very likely still reversible. These subtle neurofunctional alternations are likely detectable by functional neuroimaging techniques. The neuroimaging has the capability to provide an assessment of the altered neurophysiology, before anatomical abnormalities and divergent neuropathology of the later disease stages. Focusing the synaptic level, at the phase when the neuron cell potentially is still healthy, provides an excellent opportunity to intervene at a reversible stage of the disease when neural networks are vulnerable, but not lost. With regard to focal neural activation during the early phases of processing external inputs, studying the early sensory responses enable unique insight into the synchronized synaptic activity of functionally related neural substrates, which are on the larger scale recognized as sensory networks. The first manifestations of declining synaptic function could involve desynchronization of synaptic transmission, which may cause the "virtual" absence of activation when it is measured extracranially. These alterations in topology of sensory networks could be even associated with specific patterns of attention, memory, or behavioral disorder that could indicate the preclinical stage of disease.

2. Biomarkers of AD

A biomarker in medicine is conceptualized as a measurable detector of a physiological, anatomic, or biochemical alternation that can distinct normal biologic processes from pathological. Biomarker should be able to provide reliable diagnosis, follow the development of disease, and measure responses to a therapeutic intervention. The development of a new biomarker for any clinical condition is based on the ability to accurately detect specific pathophysiology against the gold or reference standard. This creates problem specifically to AD because there is no in vivo gold standard. Currently, the final diagnosis of AD requires both the presence of amnestic symptoms and postmortem histopathological confirmation. Premortem diagnosis of AD is only "probable" or "possible" based on symptoms characteristic of Alzheimer's type of dementia and neuroimaging findings.

The growing body of evidences evolves AD research field toward the concept of disease pathogenesis as a continuum of long-term phases in which clinical symptomatology and underlying pathophysiological process have different temporal development rates [45]. The existing findings indicate that the onset of the first symptoms marked the already irreversible stage of the disease [44]. Therefore, only detection of preclinical phase, before the occurrence of the first symptoms, but with present neuropathological changes characteristic of AD, would provide a major opportunity for therapeutic intervention in possible still reversible stage of disease. The main problem of AD research lies in the fact that is not yet found a solid link between the specific biomarker occurrence in presymptomatic individuals and the subsequent appearance of clinical symptoms [44, 45]. Although major advances in brain imaging, neurochemistry, and genetic research that highly accelerated the field, there still remains a need for the establishment of accurate biomarkers of preclinical AD, which will differentiate subjects without the risk of progression to dementia from those at risk for developing symptomatic AD. Today, five state-of-the-art diagnostic measures of AD are proposed for diagnostic criteria [46, 47]. Three of these are neuroimaging measures, and the other two are the laboratory indicators related to cerebrospinal fluid (CSF) proteins. Laboratory measures of AD include a reduced level of amyloid-beta 42 or an increase in p-tau concentration in the CSF. Imaging measures include tracers that allow detection of fibrillary amyloid-beta deposits in the cortex by positron emission tomography (PET) and detectors, also known as injury or topographical biomarkers, of a medial temporal lobe atrophy and reduced glucose metabolism in temporoparietal regions, as determined by magnetic resonance imaging (MRI) and fluorodeoxyglucose (FDG) PET, respectively. However, proposed biomarkers have limited efficiency in detecting preclinical changes associated with the disease [45–50] and are invasive for subjects because there are risks associated with lumbar puncture (CSF), exposure to radiation (PET/CT), or claustrophobic time-consuming scanning (MRI). Moreover, the classification results of proposed biomarkers are based on the difference between group means of measured variables that generally cannot provide a clear boundary between normal and pathological responses. The underlying reason for the limited discriminatory accuracy of proposed biomarkers lies in the high individual heterogeneity and variability of neural responses, cerebral anatomy, and metabolism [51], especially in the elderly population. Consequently, there is an urgent need for additional, noninvasive, more accurate tool that can be used to differentiate presymptomatic and symptomatic AD from normal aging.

2.1. Topological biomarker of AD

Besides high sensitivity and specificity, ideal AD biomarker should be individual, robust, and must be able to follow the evolution of the pathophysiological process of AD from early preclinical changes to symptomatic aggravation of the disease. A promising, but so far underutilized line of biomarker research is the alternation of basic neural network topography as a consequence of AD pathology [52]. An efficient way to start topographic search for AD biomarker is studying the most fundamental, still focal neural mechanisms that occur very early in the processing stream of simple sensory inputs. Dominantly cholinergic modulation of a sensory gating processing [53, 54] indicates that sensory gating network would likely be alerted in AD pathophysiology because the leading neurochemical feature of AD is a deterioration of the cholinergic signal transmission by selective impact on the plasticity of nicotinic (nAChr) and muscarinic (mAChr) synaptic receptors [55]. On a large scale, this synaptic dysfunction is likely to cause subtle alterations in sensory gating processing years before meeting criteria for symptomatic AD [56, 57].

2.2. Sensory gating

Sensory gating is a fundamental process of sensory processing, arising within the first 50 ms of exposure to a stimulus, much earlier than conscious perception. It is a phenomenon by which the neural system rapidly adjusts its response to subsequent stimuli, a neural feature with an essential impact in everyday life [58, 60]. This fast inhibition or enhancement of the neural response provoked by the external stimuli refers to different gating mechanisms: by gating-out neural system selectively suppresses its responses to irrelevant or redundant stimuli and by gating-in reinforcing responses on task-relevant or novel stimuli [59, 60]. Gating-out has been proposed as a mechanism of habituating to redundant stimuli that protect working memory overload by preventing irrelevant information from recurrent sensory processing, while at the same time, gating-in processing enables recognition of relevant environment inputs that are essential for survival [59–61].

2.2.1. *Clinical correlates of sensory gating*

Sensory gating deficits have been associated with several clinical conditions. Patients with schizophrenia [62–64], Alzheimer's disease [60, 64, 65], bipolar disorder [66], post-traumatic stress disorder [67], Parkinson's disease [68], or Huntington's disease [69] show alerted sensory gating dynamics compared to controls. Abnormality in extracranially measured auditory gating responses is recognized as one of the best established marks for schizophrenia [70, 71]. In addition, alerted sensory gating has been associated with impaired performance on tasks measuring sustained attention [72], inhibition of distractors [73], or performance on neurocognitive tasks [64].

2.2.2. *Neurochemistry of sensory gating*

Multiple neurotransmitters are found to be involved in sensory gating processing, including the cholinergic, dopaminergic, GABAergic, glutamatergic, noradrenergic, and serotonergic systems [74]. Pharmacological studies have emphasized the particular importance of the cholinergic system in regulating the decreased response to repeated stimuli (gating-out) through stimulation of the α-7 nicotinic receptor [75] and the muscarinic M1 receptor [76]. More recently, a marker of the gene for the α-7 nicotinic receptor has been strongly linked to sensory gating abnormalities [75]. Notably, α7-containing receptors are also known for fast desensitization in the presence of agonist and high Ca^{2+} permeability [77].

2.2.3. *Assessment of sensory gating*

Sensory gating is typically assessed using a paired stimulus or oddball paradigm during an electrophysiological recording. In a paired-click paradigm, the event-related potential (ERP) component P50 or its magnetic counterpart M50, elicited about 50 ms after stimulus presentation, is measured during the presentation of two identical stimuli (S1 and S2) with an interstimulus interval (ISI) of 500 ms [72, 78]. The habituation of the response to the redundant second stimulus, expressed as the ratio between responses amplitudes (S2/S1), indicates the strength of gating-out inhibition [79]. Auditory oddball paradigm is characterized by the varying occurrence probability of a deviant (novel) stimulus between a series of repeated standard stimuli and therefore evokes both gating mechanisms, habituation of redundant information (standard stimuli) and pre-attentive memory-based comparison processes (deviant stimuli) [60, 64].

2.2.4. Neuroimaging of sensory gating

Notably, there is a problem in noninvasively studying the gating function in vivo. Only functional neuroimaging technique with millisecond temporal resolution can capture the sensory gating dynamics, which occurs within the first 100 ms after stimulus input. Positron emission tomography (PET), functional magnetic resonance imaging (fMRI), single-photon emission computed tomography (SPECT), and near-infrared spectroscopy (NIRS) are neuroimaging techniques that provide indirect look at the brain at work. These techniques provide measures of metabolic and vascular signals that are associated with neuronal activity, which are assumed to be linearly correlated, although reliable functional relations are not yet established. The temporal resolution of these functional techniques is rather low, on a minute scale, compared to underlying neural activity, which extends from 1 to 3 ms of action potential firing to a few tens of milliseconds of synchronous synaptic activity of thousands of postsynaptic neurons.

Unlike other functional neuroimaging techniques, electroencephalography (EEG) and magnetoencephalography (MEG) provide a critical opportunity to directly and noninvasively study the brain activity [80, 81]. Neurons in the human cortex generally process their information by means of electromagnetic signals and thus enable the direct recording of their activity. EEG and MEG are electrophysiological techniques that are both sensitive to the electrochemical currents within and between the brain cells. With sub-millisecond temporal resolution, these techniques can easily capture the dynamics of spontaneous and evoked neural responses. MEG and EEG provide a complimentary information about the underlying electromagnetic brain activity. MEG measures the magnetic field generated by the primary intracellular ionic currents through postsynaptic dendrites, while EEG measures the voltage scalp distribution generated by the secondary extracellular ionic flow, both produced by the normal brain activity [80, 81].

Though EEG can capture both radial and tangential components of a produced extracellular electrical field [80, 81], there was a widely accepted assumption that MEG detects only sources that are tangential to the scalp surface. However, recently, it was shown that source orientation is not a significant factor in limiting MEG sensitivity. Using both numerical simulation and empirical measurements, it has been demonstrated that source depth and spatial extent of activated assembly on convoluted cortical surface are the main factors that compromise the sensitivity of MEG to neural activity in the human cortex [82]. Although both techniques have high temporal resolution, MEG outperforms EEG in spatiotemporal localization of neural substrate underlying extracranially captured electromagnetic activity. Using modern signal analysis methods the centimeter spatial resolution of EEG approach that of conventional fMRI [83]. On the other hand, MEG technique has an excellent, millimeter spatial accuracy [82, 84]. Moreover, MEG can detect low-amplitude dipole current source in the deep tissue of dislocate cortex, which is simultaneously active with several times higher-magnitude dipole sources in the superficial regions of primary sensory areas [60], demonstrating a high spatial resolution of synchronously active sources within a neural network. Therefore, MEG can be used in two basic ways. The first, similar to the ordinary EEG recordings, utilizes studies of rhythmic brain activity, evoked neural processing, and clinical diagnostics to detect the presence or signs of abnormality in spontaneous or evoked brain activity. The second and more ambitious use of MEG is in the estimation of the location, strength, and time courses of neuronal current sources of spontaneous and evoked magnetic signals recorded outside the head. In conclusion, MEG is a unique method that enables the noninvasive spatiotemporal mapping of elementary sensory gating processing that rises within first 100 ms after stimulus presentation. Moreover, the sources of MEG signals, primarily cortical intracellular postsynaptic currents, make MEG the first choice technique for the noninvasive study of synaptic function in real time. Consequently, MEG has an advantage in the neuroimaging search for early neurodegenerative biomarkers associated with synaptic alterations.

2.2.5. Cortical network underlying sensory gating

In line with the hierarchical model of neural processing [85], sensory gating responses have been long conceptualized to originate in the primary sensory areas [86, 87], due to the very early appearance in a sensory process stream. However, a report of the gating response presence after bilateral damage of the primary auditory areas [88] suggested a contribution from at least one source related to arousal level or state [89]. Efforts to delineate the neuroanatomy of the sensory gating network long have yielded inconsistent findings [90–93]. The recent works, relied on advanced MEG-based multi-dipole source localization, finally provide a reliable set of neural generators [60, 64, 94–96]. Moreover, our novel results revealed possible explanations concerning the problem of inconsistent reports regarding auditory gating network topology, suggesting that paired-click and oddball paradigms, which are often used to challenge sensory gating effects, evoke different gating generator topologies, even though they are both passive for the subjects [96].

2.2.6. Auditory sensory gating networks evoked by oddball and paired-click paradigm

Using the oddball paradigm, which evokes both gating-in and gating-out mechanisms, we have demonstrated that auditory gating network comprises a medial prefrontal (mPFC) generator along with the anticipated generators in the bilateral primary auditory cortices [60, 64, 96], as shown in panel A) of **Figure 1**. Our finding suggests the existence of a novel, very fast sensory processing stream (i.e., sensory gating loop), which links executive PFC to primary auditory cortex within the first 50 ms after stimulus presentation, alongside well-affirmed but slower limbic (dorsal) and somatic (ventral) sensory processing pathways [60, 96]. The existence of additional fast sensory processing stream, sensory gating loop, is anatomically supported by dense bidirectional connections between medial PFC and superior temporal cortices found in both primate and human anatomical studies [97, 98]. The mPFC possesses extensive cortico-cortical connections, including extensive local projections to and from other prefrontal regions, as well as with motor, limbic, and sensory cortices [99]. These structural properties of the connecting pathways provide the ability for localized primary auditory generators and PFC regions to work together as a large-scale neural network via fast sensory gating loop.

Our novel research provides evidence that passive paired-click and oddball paradigms activate a different prefrontal generator within the auditory gating network [60, 96]. Spatiotemporal source localization of auditory gating responses evoked by the passive paired-click paradigm revealed a different gating topology consisting of a dorsolateral PFC (dlPFC) source in addition to the sources in the bilateral primary auditory cortices [78, 96], as shown in panel B) of **Figure 1**. This result implies the existence of early rerouting within prefrontal cortex by shifting prefrontal gating activation from dorsolateral to medial prefrontal region, depending on a paradigm [60, 96], suggesting that mPFC and dlPFC regions serve different functions involved during the early sensory processing. A passive paired-click paradigm characterized

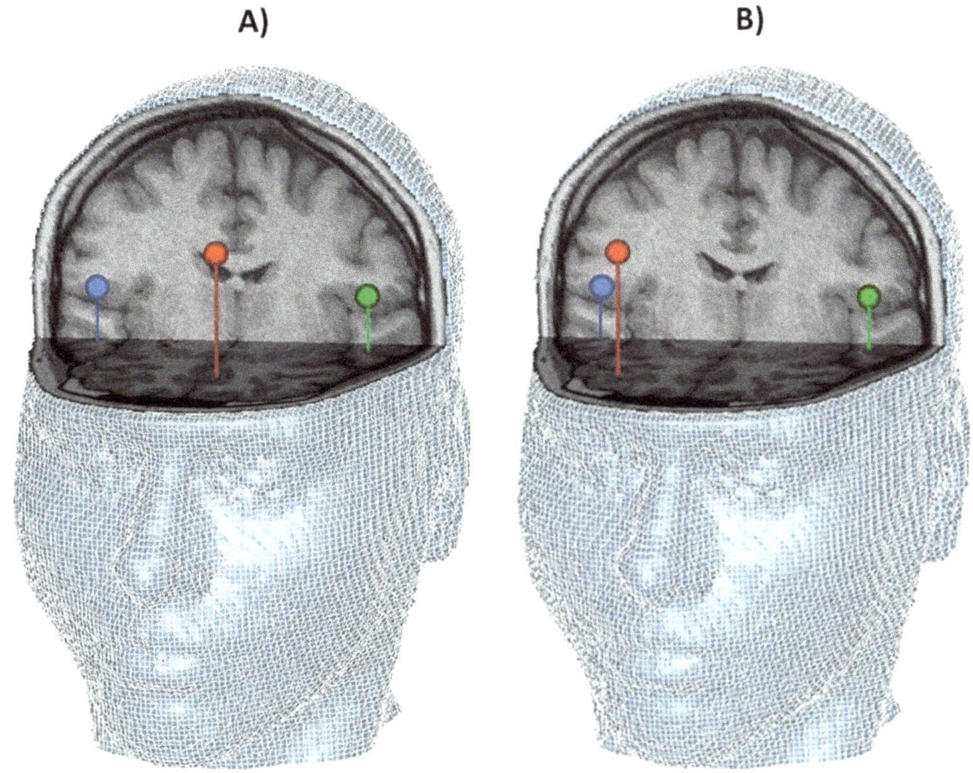

Figure 1. Auditory sensory gating network evoked by the oddball paradigm (panel A) and paired-click paradigm (panel B). The best-fitting source locations are superimposed on volumetric MRI head data to achieve a spatial (3D) rendering of the auditory gating topology. In addition to anticipated bilateral generators in primary auditory areas (blue and green dots), both paradigms evoke a prefrontal gating generator (red dot). While oddball tones provoke medial PFC activation, the tones of a paired-click paradigm activate dorsolateral PFC areas.

by the constant repetition of both short- and long-term patterns (S1–500 ms; S2–8 s) could result in long-term repetition suppression produced by the dlPFC. On the contrary, an oddball paradigm, characterized by the varying occurrence probability of a novel stimulus between a series of repeated stimuli, could put the neural network into a state of perceptual expectation (gating-in) while simultaneously suppressing redundant stimuli (gating-out). This phenomenon could be interpreted as the bottom-up, stimulus-driven initiation of attention during the very early sensory processing [100] executed by the mPFC region.

2.2.7. Functional mechanisms underlying auditory sensory gating

In addition to the spatial localization of auditory gating networks, we have disclosed the functional relation within network generators providing strong evidence of a modulatory role for the mPFC generator on bilateral superior temporal gyri (STG) sources dynamics during gating processing (**Figure 2**). This result discloses the long-sought mechanism underlying the auditory gating effect [60]. We demonstrated the complex form of estimated cortical morphology of the neural responses produced by the gating generators. In particular, gating response of STG generators is found to be composed of two consecutive cortical subcomponent, Mb1 peaking at 35–53 ms and Mb2 peaking at 75–95 ms post-stimulus, for both oddball paradigm tones [60]. We also provide the first estimates of cortical gating response produced by the mPFC generator, which has an analogous tandem form [60], as shown in **Figure 2**.

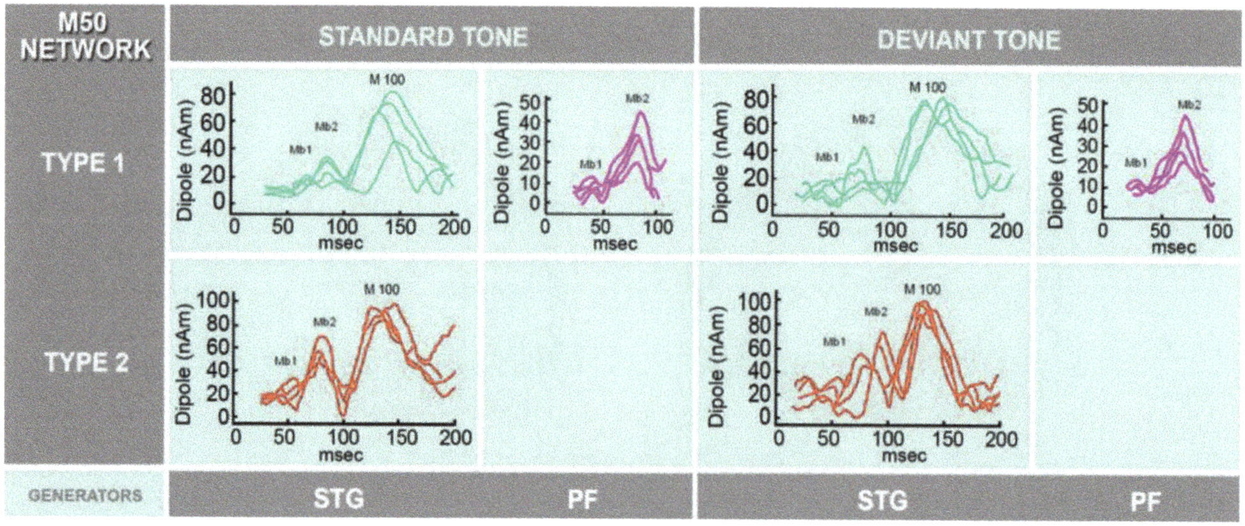

Figure 2. Estimated cortical dynamics of auditory gating network generators evoked by the oddball paradigm. Cortical dynamics of medial prefrontal (PF) and STG gating generators for both tones (standard and deviant) are shown for eight representative subjects (four of each network type). Gating network type 1 comprised bilateral STG and the PF source, while network type 2 was characterized by the absence of PF activation. The time courses of the STG activity were individually averaged across hemispheres and displayed for 30–200 ms time window to include M100, the most prominent STG response, for the amplitude comparison with earlier Mb1 and Mb2 components. Both components of STG gating response (Mb1 and Mb2) are significantly increased when PF source activation is absent.

Taking advantage of the differences in the evoked gating networks between individuals whose PFC generator was activated (Type 1 in **Figure 2**) and cognitively impaired individuals whose PFC gating generator was not activated (Type 2 in **Figure 2**) by the tones of an oddball paradigm, we have carried out a differential analysis of the functional roles for each generator. Our results show that cortical gating dynamics of STG generators evoked by both the standard and deviant tones demonstrated highly increased strength of both gating components in all subjects lacking PFC generator activity [60]. This result is of extreme clinical importance because the prevalent view of the gating-related pathologies assumes that the larger amplitude of the extracranial gating response to the standard tone (i.e., redundant stimuli) reflects impaired gating out processing of neural substrate in primary auditory areas only (i.e., STG generators) [61–63, 66–69]. Our novel results provide strong evidence of sustained inhibitory activity of the PFC generator that suppresses or modulates the activity of the STG generators as an underlying mechanism of both gating phenomena. Consequently, impaired activity of a PFC gating generator could be a primary cause of impaired extracranially measured sensory gating responses, found in numerous neurological and psychological clinical conditions.

3. Link between impaired sensory gating and AD pathology

The initial symptoms of AD include subtle decline of the ability to learn new information along with diverse amnestic disorders without present brain injuries. Clinically indicated AD signs are pointing to the existence of functional impairment of synapses that are involved in converting and forming new declarative memory [32]. Whereas longer retention of sensory memory traces derive more successful memory encoding [101], sensory gating process, conceptualized as the ability of the neural system to modulate its responses to subsequent stimuli, has a fundamental role in guiding successful encoding of new information. Impaired auditory gating processing may reduce pre-attentive signal-to-noise ratio and desynchronize synaptic consolidation in the initial phases of memory formation [58]. Augmentation of dysfunctional sensory gating process could yield to the first amnestic symptoms seen in AD neuropathology.

A range of EEG/MEG studies, measuring evoked sensory responses, have reported differences in early processing of auditory [102–104] stimuli in symptomatic AD patients, affirming the possibility of impaired inhibition of redundant information (gating-out) and processing of novel information (gating-in) in the initial phase of disease. Also, alerted connectivity among different brain regions and decline of long-distance synchronization are found to be responsible for some of the earliest cognitive changes in early phases of symptomatic AD [105]. Although the study of the extracranial neurophysiological (EEG/MEG) signals provides valuable information regarding the pathology-related changes in the amplitudes, latencies, frequency bands, spectral densities, and coherence of oscillatory brain dynamics, identified relations have received limited attention in the search for a biomarker of AD. The main reason is that classification based on the difference between group means of sensor-level measures generally cannot provide a clear individual boundary value between healthy and pathological responses and thus result in lower clinical significance. However, MEG spatiotemporal localization of cortical sources underlying extracranial magnetic field shows internal consistency and provides highly reliable and stable results of both cortical dynamics and topology of the activated network [60, 82, 84], enabling a search for an AD biomarker at the individual level.

3.1. Localization of auditory gating network generators: a topological biomarker of AD

Using MEG spatiotemporal source calculations, we have demonstrated [64] the potential of topological localization of mPFC generator within an auditory gating network as a discrete, binary, noninvasive tool for detection of AD at the individual subject level. We found three types of gating network topologies evoked by a simple auditory oddball paradigm across the research sample of elderly individuals, ranging from 63 to 87 years of age, which comprised patients with clinical diagnosis of symptomatic AD (MCI and moderate AD) and non-symptomatic elderly controls. Discrete localization/non-localization of mPFC gating generator absolutely discriminate symptomatic AD from controls confirm the indiscernibility between amnestic MCI (aMCI) and AD patients and differentiate two distinct gating network types within the elderly controls, one of which is suggested as preclinical AD. The lack of mPFC generator localization within an auditory gating network as a biomarker of symptomatic AD shows a large effect size (>0.9) and high accuracy, sensitivity, and specificity (100%) in respect of clinical diagnosis [64].

3.2. Sustained activation of mPFC gating generator: a sign of healthy cognitive aging

We have applied spectra of the multivariate analyses to disclose potentially hidden structure in complete set of our data, i.e., scores of wide neuropsychological screening and neurophysiological gating network topology results [64]. Clustering based on principal variables indicated the existence of three stable clusters across subjects as shown in **Figure 3**. Subsequent

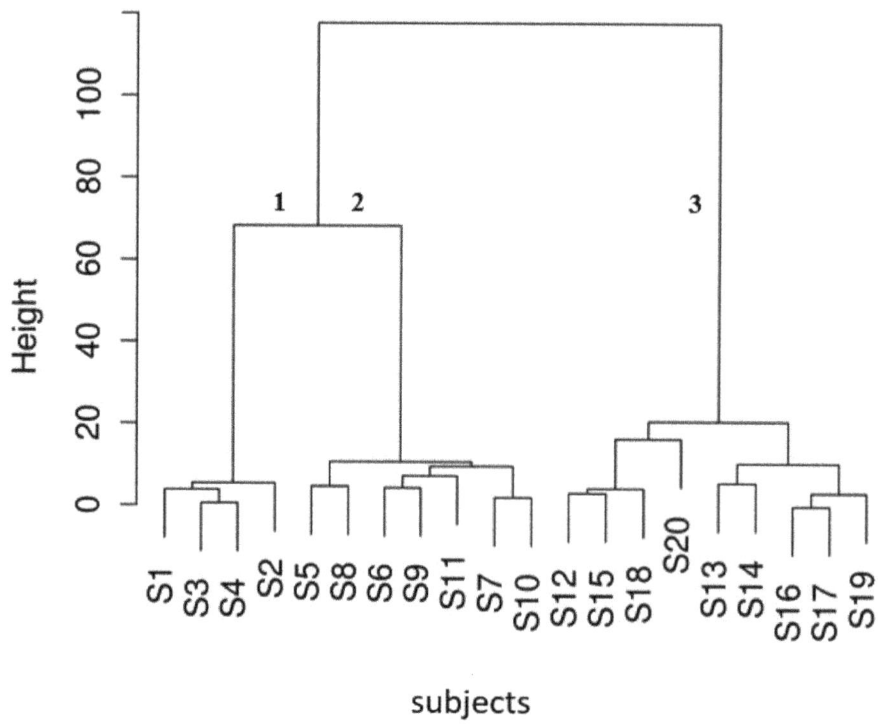

Figure 3. Dendrogram based on the neuropsychological and neurophysiological variables. Subjects were assigned numbers from 1 to 20 and grouped into clusters. Variables were normalized before using a clustering algorithm with Ward's minimum variance method as amalgamation rule and with Euclidean distance as a measure of dissimilarity. Cluster grouping disclosed three groups across two clinical categories (H-healthy subjects, MCI/AD—symptomatic AD subjects) suggesting the potential of the proposed approach to detect subgroup of control ("healthy") subjects who are in the possible preclinical phase of AD (cluster category 2).

statistical review of group differences on neuropsychological tests confirmed the low-magnitude but significant differences in Mini Mental State Exam (MMSE) and delayed Rey-Osterreith Complex Figure Test (dROCFT) scores across subjects in different cluster groups [64]. The first group of controls, characterized by sustained gating activation of mPFC generator for both oddball tones, had the highest MMSE scores and the highest performance on the dROCFT, thus considered to be cognitively healthy elderly group.

3.3. Partial activation of mPFC gating generator: a biomarker of preclinical AD

The second cluster group of controls was characterized by the first signs of neurophysiological gating alternation, which emerged as a partial activation of the mPFC gating generator to the deviant tone only, as shown in **Table 1**. The standard tone did not evoke mPFC activation, suggesting that a very early stage of impairment in sensory gating processing is manifested by an absence of mPFC gating transmission that corrupts habituation to redundant stimuli [64]. We confirmed the presence of insidious cognitive decline in this subgroup of controls, demonstrating the low-amplitude but significantly lower both MMSE and dROCFT scores in comparison with the high-functioning subgroup of controls [64]. Overall, both neuropsychological and neurophysiological impairments characteristic of an AD type of dementia found in low-functioning control group, although they did not yet meet clinical criteria for aMCI, indicate a possible preclinical AD phase. The additional weight to our speculation gave Takayama,

Subject	MMSE	dROCFT	mPFC standard	mPFC deviant	Clinical diagnosis	Cluster category
S1	30	26	1	1	H	1
S2	30	25	1	1	H	1
S3	30	23	1	1	H	1
S4	30	23	1	1	H	1
S5	30	22	0	1	H	2
S6	30	22	0	1	H	2
S7	30	17	0	1	H	2
S8	29	26	0	1	MCI	2
S9	29	25	0	1	H	2
S10	29	18	0	1	H	2
S11	26	20	0	1	H	2
S12	26	12	0	0	MCI	3
S13	26	7	0	0	MCI	3
S14	26	1.5	0	0	MCI	3
S15	25	13	0	0	MCI	3
S16	25	0	0	0	AD	3
S17	25	0	0	0	AD	3
S18	24	10.5	0	0	AD	3
S19	23	0	0	0	AD	3
S20	22	2	0	0	AD	3

Table 1. Subject scores on the MMSE, dROCFT, mPFC gating generator activation (1-activated, 0-non-activated), clinical diagnosis, and cluster group.

whose 10-year longitudinal study also discerns the dROCF test as highly assertive indicator of conversion to symptomatic phase of Alzheimer's disease, i.e., found significant sensitivity of dROCFT scores to early, possible preclinical AD pathology [106].

The possibility that partial gating activation of the mPFC generator in lower-functioning controls may be associated with preclinical AD phase is also confirmed by several recent findings. There are evidences that reduced functional connectivity affecting the PFC is associated with amyloid-β-related hypersynchronization [107] and p-tau pathology [108] in a very early phase of AD-type memory impairment. The impaired mPFC activity during endogenous brain activity or memory tasks is found in cognitively normal individuals who were AD APOE ε 4 carriers [109]. Also, evidence of decreased extracranial gating dynamics as a predictor of cerebrospinal amyloid-β reduction is demonstrated in MCI patients [65]. Alerted synaptic function along with subsequent synaptic loss and transneuronal spread of pathological tau forms [108] through PFC regions could result in the topological gating deficit that we found in a low-functioning subgroup of controls. This topological gating deficit could reflect a possible preclinical phase of AD pathology before widespread of cognitive symptoms.

3.4. Complete absence of mPFC gating generator activation: a biomarker of symptomatic AD

Subjects within the cluster group characterized by the complete absence of mPFC gating generator activation regardless of the tone condition (i.e., standard and deviant tone) had the lowest neuropsychological test results and belonged to the symptomatic AD patients with clinical diagnosis [64], as shown in **Figure 3**. Clearly, a topological deficit of mPFC gating generator activation is augmented in symptomatic AD phase, taking place during both gating out (inhibition of standard tone) and gating in (enhanced processing of novel tone), suggesting complete disruption of sensory gating process. This absolute break of a fundamental sensory process is associated with the onset of the amnestic AD symptoms. It is possible that progressive failure in sensory gating-out, found in possible preclinical phase of disease, is likely to lead to an overload of working memory due to noise accretion and consequent to the first symptoms of memory impairment.

There are numerous evidences of association between symptomatic AD pathology and alerted physiology of PFC region. Decreased frontal-parietal correlations of glucose metabolism [110], prefrontal glucose hypometabolism on 18F-fluorodeoxyglucose PET scans [111], and frontal retention of 11C-Pittsburgh compound [112] are found in AD patients. Klupp and colleagues [113] found a significant hypometabolism in PFC regions that are not loaded with amyloid plaques, suggesting that the deficit in mPFC gating activation may be related to longitudinal amyloid deposition in different but functionally connected brain regions. For instance, absence or desynchronization of mPFC gating activity could induce atrophy across fast auditory sensory gating loop, which may result in increased amyloid vulnerability of synapses terminated within primary auditory areas involved in the gating process. Inactivity of the mPFC generator during processing of repetitive stimuli (gating-out) likely impairs the ability to distinguish novel from repetitive information, which is critical for long-term memory encoding. It has been demonstrated that activation of presynaptic α-7-nAChRs, involved in gating transmission, induces long-term potentiation of the excitatory input [114]. Therefore, a topological deficit of mPFC generator activation during gating transmission could be a consequence of impaired nAChR levels found in PFC regions of AD patients. Alerted function of α-7-nAChRs could induce lower levels of intracellular calcium, consequently impairing the calcium cascade in producing synchronized postsynaptic signals required for effective both gating processing and long-term memory encoding.

4. Conclusion

Identification of a novel biomarker of AD (**Figure 4**) with the potential to detect both putative preclinical and clinical stages at the individual subject level represents significant progress toward improving diagnosis of AD and accelerating the field toward the neurobiological advantage of earlier intervention. Although the study engaged only a research sample, the very large effect size (>0.98) of proposed test, thanks to its binary nature, provides high relevance to the finding. Such a large effect size enables this study with the research sample size to yield power greater than 85%.

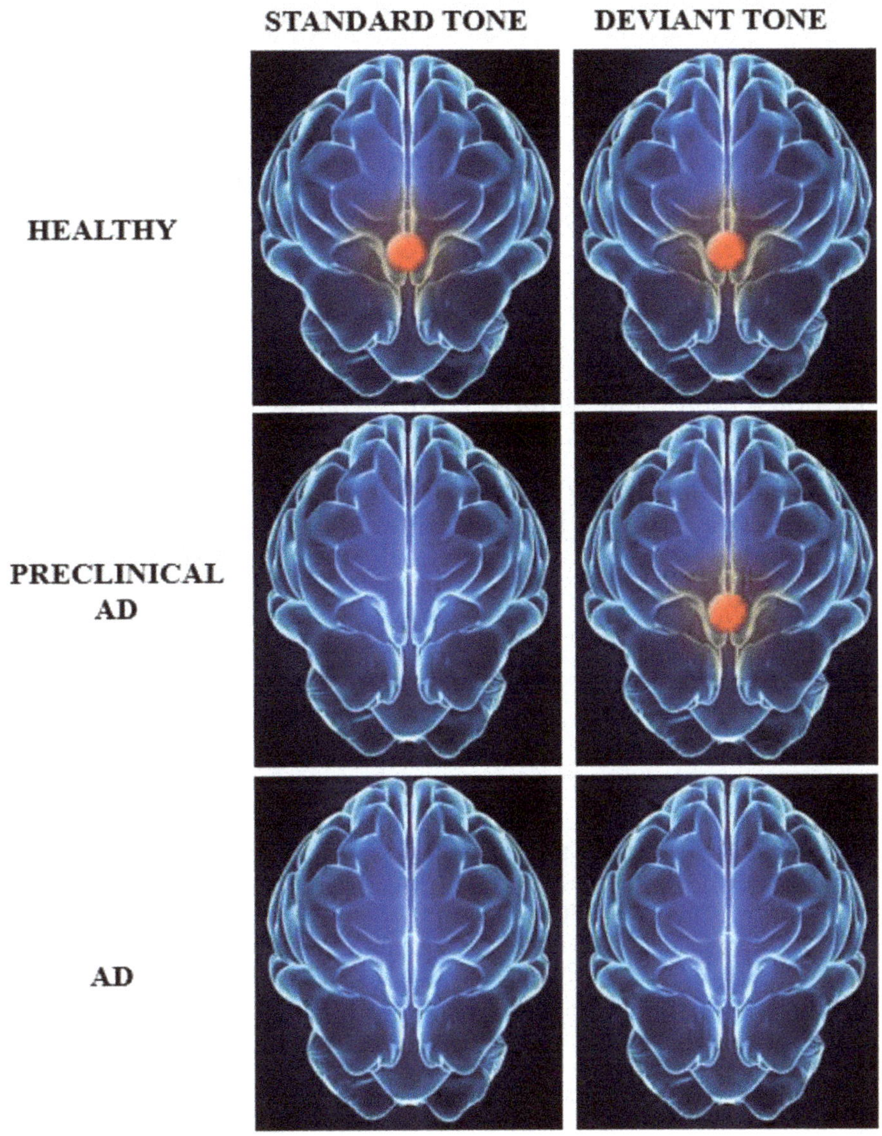

Figure 4. Proposed topological approach as biomarker of AD pathology. Three distinct types of mPFC auditory gating generator activation (red dot) were identified in healthy controls, possible preclinical AD and symptomatic AD patients. The healthy gating topology type requires mPFC activation in processing both oddball tones (standard and deviant). An altered gating topology, characterized by selective mPFC activation only by the deviant tone, presumably represents a presymptomatic phase of AD. Symptomatic AD gating topology lacks mPFC activation for both standard and deviant tones.

Novel topological biomarker, besides high accuracy, sensitivity, and specificity (100%) in identifying symptomatic AD patients in the research sample, shows the potential of following the evolution of the pathophysiological process of disease. The noninvasiveness and low sensitivity to individual heterogeneity and variability due to the discrete nature of impaired prefrontal gating activation are the most important properties of the novel biomarker. It is not based on the use of group means and is not associated with statistically significant changes in a continuous variable. The advantage of this biomarker lies in the simplicity of using a binary value, i.e., activated or not activated a prefrontal generator during gating processing of simple tones. The proposed biomarker is absolutely noninvasive; it is based on recordings of neuromagnetic fields that are produced by normal brain activity.

The new topographic tool certainly has properties, which place it within a group of high-potential biomarkers. The absolute noninvasiveness, individual detection of pathology, ability to detect the preclinical phase of the disease, discrete nature that does not require estimation of uniform cutoff levels and standardization processes, the low sensitivity to individual heterogeneity and variability, capability to follow the evolution of the pathophysiological process of AD, and finally high accuracy and sensitivity make it highly promising biomarker of AD.

However, despite mentioning highlights, the proposed biomarker requires to be tested in a large independent sample and requires assessment in longitudinal clinical MEG studies that would track nonsymptomatic elderly with partial activation of the prefrontal gating generator until the first clinical symptoms appear and finally to autopsy for confirmation of AD. It would also be necessary to investigate prefrontal gating dynamics in other dementias to determine the specificity of novel biomarker to discriminate AD from other etiologies of age-related cognitive decline.

Author details

Sanja Josef Golubic

Address all correspondence to: sanja.phy@net.hr

Department of Physics, Faculty of Science, University of Zagreb, Croatia

References

[1] Roher A, Wolfe D, Palutke M, KuKuruga D. Purification, ultrastructure, and chemical analysis of Alzheimer disease amyloid plaque core protein. Proceedings of the National Academy of Sciences of the United States of America. 1986;**83**:2662-2666

[2] Grundke-Iqbal I, Iqbal K, Quinlan M, Tung YC, Zaidi MS, Wisniewski HM. Microtubule-associated protein tau. A component of Alzheimer paired helical filaments. The Journal of Biological Chemistry. 1986;**261**:6084-6089

[3] Morris GP, Clark IA, Vissel B. Inconsistencies and controversies surrounding the amyloid hypothesis of Alzheimer's disease. Acta Neuropathologica Communications. 2014;**2**:135

[4] Braak H, Braak E. Neuropathological stageing of Alzheimer-related changes. Acta Neuropathologica. 1991;**82**:239-259

[5] Braak H, Braak E. Staging of Alzheimer's disease-related neurofibrillary changes. Neurobiology of Aging. 1995;**16**:271-278

[6] Bird TD. Genetic factors in Alzheimer's disease. The New England Journal of Medicine. 2005;**352**:862-864

[7] Corder EH, Saunders AM, Strittmatter WJ, Schmechel DE, Gaskell PC, Small GW, Roses AD, Haines JL, Pericak-Vance MA. Gene dose of apolipoprotein E type 4 allele and the risk of Alzheimer's disease in late onset families. Science. 1993;**261**:921-923

[8] Sherrington R, Rogaev EI, Liang Y, Rogaeva EA, Levesque G, et al. Cloning of a gene bearing missense mutations in early-onset familial Alzheimer's disease. Nature. 1995;**375**:754-760

[9] Rogaev EI, Sherrington R, Rogaeva EA, Levesque G, Ikeda M, et al. Familial Alzheimer's disease in kindreds with missense mutations in a gene on chromosome 1 related to the Alzheimer's disease type 3 gene. Nature. 1995;**376**:775-778

[10] Thies W, Bleiler L. Alzheimer's disease facts and figures. Alzheimer's and Dementia. 2011;**7**:208-244

[11] Rentz DM, Locascio JJ, Becker JA, Moran EK, Eng E, Buckner RL, Sperling RA, Johnson KA. Cognition, reserve, and amyloid deposition in normal aging. Annals of Neurology. 2010;**67**: 353-364

[12] Tsai J, Grutzendler J, Duff K, Gan WB. Fibrillar amyloid deposition leads to local synaptic abnormalities and breakage of neuronal branches. Nature Neuroscience. 2004;**7**: 1181-1183

[13] Schenk D, Barbour R, Dunn W, Gordon G, Grajeda H, et al. Immunization with amyloid-[beta] attenuates Alzheimer-disease-like pathology in the PDAPP mouse. Nature. 1999;**400**:173-177

[14] Lobello K, Ryan JM, Liu E, Rippon G, Black R. Targeting beta amyloid: A clinical review of immunotherapeutic approaches in Alzheimer's disease. International Journal of Alzheimer's Disease. 2012;**2012**:628070

[15] Mullane K, Williams M. Alzheimer's therapeutics: Continued clinical failures question the validity of the amyloid hypothesis-but what lies beyond? Biochemical Pharmacology. 2013;**85**:289-305

[16] Ferreira ST, Klein WL. The Aβ oligomer hypothesis for synapse failure and memory loss in Alzheimer's disease. Neurobiology of Learning and Memory. 2011;**96**:529-543

[17] Benilova I, Karran E, De Strooper B. The toxic Abeta oligomer and Alzheimer's disease: An emperor in need of clothes. Nature Neuroscience. 2012;**15**:349-357

[18] Uylings HBM, de Brabander JM. Neuronal changes in normal human aging and Alzheimer's disease. Brain and Cognition. 2002;**49**:268-276

[19] Conforti L, Adalbert R, Coleman MP. Neuronal death: Where does the end begin? Trends in Neurosciences. 2007;**30**:159-166

[20] Boncristiano S, Calhoun ME, Howard V, Bondolfi L, Kaeser SA, Wiederhold KH, Staufenbiel M, Jucker M. Neocortical synaptic Bouton number is maintained despite robust amyloid deposition in APP23 transgenic mice. Neurobiology of Aging. 2005; **26**:607-613

[21] Spires TL, Meyer-Luehmann M, Stern EA, McLean PJ, Skoch J, Nguyen PT, Bacskai BJ, Hyman BT. Dendritic spine abnormalities in amyloid precursor protein transgenic mice demonstrated by gene transfer and intravital multiphoton microscopy. The Journal of Neuroscience. 2005;**25**:7278-7287

[22] Terry RD, Masliah E, Salmon DP, Butters N, DeTeresa R, Hill R, et al. Physical basis of cognitive alternations in Alzheimer's disease: Synapse loss is the major correlate of cognitive impairment. Annals of Neurology. 1991;**30**:572-580

[23] Mesulam MM. A plasticity-based theory of the pathogenesis of Alzheimer's disease. Annals of the New York Academy of Sciences. 2000;**924**:42-24

[24] Ferreira-Vieira TH, Guimaraes IM, Silva FR, Ribeiro FM. Alzheimer's disease: Targeting the cholinergic system. Current Neuropharmacology. 2016;**14**(1):101-115

[25] Cacamo A, Oddo S, Billings LM, Green KN, Martinez-Coria H, Fisher A, LaFerla FM. M1 receptors play a central role in modulating AD-like pathology in transgenic mice. Neuron. 2006;**49**(5):671-682

[26] Kamenetz F, Tomita T, Hsieh H, Seabrook G, Borchelt D, Iwatsubo T, et al. APP processing and synaptic function. Neuron. 2003;**2003, 37**:925-937

[27] Cirrito JR, Yamada KA, Finn MB, Sloviter RS, Bales KR, May PC, et al. Synaptic activity regulates interstitial fluid amyloid-beta levels in vivo. Neuron. 2005;**48**:913-922

[28] Shankar GM, Li S, Mehta TH, Garcia-Munoz A, Shepardson NE, Smith I, et al. Amyloid-beta protein dimers isolated directly from Alzheimer's brains impair synaptic plasticity and memory. Nature Medicine. 2008;**14**:837-842

[29] Puzzo D, Privitera L, Fa M, Staniszewski A, Hashimoto G, Aziz F, et al. Endogenous amyloid-beta is necessary for hippocampal synaptic plasticity and memory. Annals of Neurology. 2011;**69**:819-830

[30] Garcia-Osta A, Alberini CM. Amyloid beta mediates memory formation. Learning & Memory. 2009;**16**:267-272

[31] Watase K, Weeber EJ, Antalffy B, Yuva-Payor L, Hashimoto K, Kano M, Atkinson R, Sun Y, Armstrong DL, Sweatt JD, Orr HT, Paylor R, Zoghby HY. A long CAG repeat in the mouse Sca1 locus replicates SCA1 features and reveals the impact of protein solubility on selective neurodegeneration. Neuron. 2002;**34**:905-919

[32] Selkoe DJ. Alzheimer's disease is a synaptic failure. Science. 2002;**298**:789-791

[33] Sperling RA, Laviolette PS, O'Keefe K, O'Brien J, Rentz DM, Pihlajamaki M. Amyloid deposition is associated with impaired default network function in older persons without dementia. Neuron. 2009;**63**:178-188

[34] Reiman EM. QuirozYT, Fleisher AS, Chen K, Velez-Pardo C, Jimenez Del-Rio M, et al. Brain imaging and fluid biomarker analysis in young adults at genetic risk for autosomal dominant Alzheimer's disease in the presenilin1 E280A kindred: Acase-control study. Lancet Neurology. 2012;**11**:1048-1056

[35] Marchetti C, Marie H. Hippocampal synaptic plasticity in Alzheimer's disease: What have we learned so far from transgenic models? Reviews in the Neurosciences. 2011;**22**:373-402

[36] Trinchese F, Liu S, Battaglia F, Walter S, Mathews PM, Arancio O. Progressive age-related development of Alzheimer-like pathology in APP/PS1 mice. Annals of Neurology. 2004;**55**:801-814

[37] Menkes-Caspi N, Yamin HG, Kellner V, Spires-Jones TL, Cohen D, Stern EA. Pathological tau disrupts ongoing network activity. Neuron. 2015;**85**:959-966

[38] Tampellini D. Synaptic activity and Alzheimer's disease: A critical update. Frontiers in Neuroscience. 2015;**9**:423

[39] Rodriguez Manzanares PA, Isoardi NA, Carrer HF, Molina VA. Previous stress facilitates fear memory, attenuates GABAergic inhibition, and increases synaptic plasticity in the rat basolateral amygdala. The Journal of Neuroscience. 2005;**25**(38):8725-8734

[40] Lee S, Kim K Zhou ZJ. Role of ACh-GABA cotransmission in detecting image motion and motion direction. Neuron. 2010;**68**:1159-1172

[41] Saunders A, Granger AJ, Sabatini BL. Corelease of acetylcholine and GABA from cholinergic forebrain neurons. eLife. 2015;**4**:e06412. DOI: 10.7554/eLife.06412

[42] Paula-Lima AC, De Felice FG, Brito-Moreira J, Ferreira ST. Activation of GABA(A) receptors by taurine and muscimol blocks the neurotoxicity of beta-amyloid in rat hippocampal and cortical neurons. Neuropharmacology. 2005;**49**:1140-1148

[43] Morris JC, Storandt M, Miller JP, McKeel DW, Price JL, Rubin EH, Berg L. Mild cognitive impairment represents early-stage Alzheimer disease. Archives of Neurology. 2001;**58**:397-405

[44] Sperling RA, Aisen PS, Beckett LA, Bennet DA, Craft D, et al. Toward definig the preclinical stages of Alzheimer's disease: Recommendetation from national institute on aging-Alzheimer's Asocciation workgroup on diagnostic guidelines for Alzheimer's disease. Alzheimer's Dementia. 2011;**7**(3):280-292

[45] Lazarczyk MJ, Hof PR, Bouras C, Giannakopoul P. Preclinical Alzheimer disease: identification of cases at risk among cognitively intact older individuals. BMC Medicine. 2012;**10**:127. doi.org/10.1186/1741-7015-10-127

[46] Dubois B, Feldman HH, Jacova C, Dekosky ST, Barberger-Gateau P. Preclinical Alzheimer disease: Identification of cases at risk among cognitively intact older individuals. BMC Medicine. 2012;**10**:127. doi.org/10.1186/1741-7015-10-1276

[47] McKhann GM, Knopman DS, Chertkow H, Hyman BT, Jack CR Jr, et al. The diagnosis of dementia due to Alzheimer's disease: Recommendations from the national institute on aging and the Alzheimer's Association Workgroup. Alzheimer's & Dementia. 2011;**7**:263-269

[48] Morris JC, Blennow K, Froelich L, Nordberg A, Soininen H, Waldemar G, Wahlund LO, Dubois B. Harmonized diagnostic criteria for Alzheimer's disease: Recommendations. Journal of Internal Medicine. 2014;**275**(3):204-213

[49] Sperling RA, Jack CR Jr, Aisen PS. Testing the right target and right drug at the right stage. Science Translational Medicine. 2011;**3**(111):111-133

[50] Holtzman DM, Morris JC, Goate AM. Alzheimer's disease: The challenge of the second century. Science Translational Medicine. 2011;**3**(77):77sr1

[51] Poulson RS, Gadbury L, Allison DB. Treatment heterogeneity and individual qualitative interaction. The American Statistician. 2012;**66**(1):16-24

[52] Jack CR Jr, Knopman DS, Jagust WJ, Petersen RC, Weiner MW, Aisen PS, Shaw LM, Vemuri P, Wiste HJ, Weigand SD, et al. Tracking pathophysiological processes in Alzheimer's disease: An updated hypothetical model of dynamic biomarkers. Lancet Neurology. 2013;**12**:207-216

[53] Adler LE, Hoffer LJ, Griffith J, Waldo MC, Freedman R. Normalization by nicotine of deficient auditory sensory gating in the relatives of schizophrenics. Biological Psychiatry. 1992;**32**:607-616

[54] Lucas-Meunier E, Fossier P, Baux G, Amar M. Cholinergic modulation of the cortical neuronal network. Pflügers Archiv. 2003;**446**:17-29

[55] Levin ED, McClernon FJ, Rezvani AH. Nicotinic effects on cognitive function: Behavioral characterization, pharmacological specification, and anatomic localization. Psychopharmacology. 2006;**184**:523-539

[56] Palop JJ, Mucke L. Amyloid-β–induced neuronal dysfunction in Alzheimer's disease: From synapses toward neural networks. Nature Neuroscience. 2010;**13**:812-818

[57] Knafo S, Sánchez-Puelles C, Palomer E, Delgado I, Draffin JE, et al. PTEN recruitment controls synaptic and cognitive function in Alzheimer's models. Nature Neuroscience. 2016;**19**(3):443-453

[58] Freedman R, Adler LE, Myles-Worsley M, Nagamoto HT, Miller C, et al. Inhibitory gating of an evoked response to repeated auditory stimuli in schizophrenic and normal subjects. Human recordings, computer simulation, and an animal model. Archives of General Psychiatry. 1996;**53**:1114-1121

[59] Gjini K, Arfken C, Boutros NN. Relationships between sensory "gating out" and sensory "gating in" of auditory evoked potentials in schizophrenia: A pilot study. Schizophrenia Research. 2010;**121**:139-145

[60] Josef Golubic S, Aine CJ, Stephen JM, Adair JC, Knoefel JE, Supek S. Modulatory role of the prefrontal generator within the auditory M50 network. NeuroImage. 2014;**92**:120-131

[61] Boutros NN, Torello MW, Barker BA, Tueting PA, Wu SC. The P50 evoked potential component and mismatch detection in normal volunteers: Implications for the study of sensory gating. Psychiatry Research. 1995;**57**:83-88

[62] Patterson JV, Hetrick WP, Boutros NN, Jin Y, Sandman C, Stern H, Potkin S, Bunney WE Jr. P50 sensory gating ratios in schizophrenics and controls: A review and data analysis. Psychiatry Research. 2008;**158**(2):226-247

[63] Yee CM, Williams TJ, White PM, Nuechterlein KH, Ames D, Subotnik KL. Attentional modulation of the P50 suppression deficit in recent-onset and chronic schizophrenia. Journal of Abnormal Psychology. 2010;**119**(1):31-39

[64] Josef Golubic S, Aine CJ, Stephen JM, Adair JC, Knoefel JE, Supek S. MEG biomarker of Alzheimer's disease: Absence of a prefrontal generator during auditory sensory gating. Human Brain Mapping. 2017;**38**(10):5180-5194

[65] Green DL, Payne L, Polikar R, Moberg PJ, Wolk D, Kounios J. P50: A candidate ERP biomarker of prodromal Alzheimer's disease. Brain Research. 2015;**624**:390-397

[66] Wang Y, Feng Y, Jia Y, Wang W, Xie Y, Guan Y, Zhong S, Zhu D, Huang L. Auditory M50 and M100 sensory gating deficits in bipolar disorder: A MEG study. Journal of Affective Disorders. 2014;**152-154**:131-138

[67] Neylan TC, Fletcher DJ, Lenoci M, McCallin K, Weiss DS, Schoenfeld FB, Fein G. Sensory gating in chronic posttraumatic stress disorder: Reduced auditory P50 suppression in combat veterans. Biological Psychiatry. 1999;**46**:1656-1664

[68] Teo C, Rasco L, al-Mefty K, Skinner RD, Boop FA, Garcia-Rill E. Decreased habituation of midlatency auditory evoked responses in Parkinson's disease. Movement Disorders. 1997;**12**(5):655-664

[69] Uc EY, Skinner RD, Rodnitzky RL, Garcia-Rill E. The midlatency auditory evoked potential P50 is abnormal in Huntington's disease. Journal of the Neurological Sciences. 2003;**212**:1-5

[70] Adler LE, Pachtman E, Franks RD, Pecevich MC, Waldo M, Freedman R. Neurophysiological evidence for a defect in neuronal mechanisms involved in sensory gating in schizophrenia. Biological Psychiatry. 1982;**17**:639-655

[71] Bramon E, Rabe-Hesketh S, Sham P, Murray RM, Frangou S. Meta-analysis of the P300 and P50 waveforms in schizophrenia. Schizophrenia Research. 2004;**70**:315-329

[72] Potter D, Summerfelt A, Gold J, Buchanan RW. Review of clinical correlates of P50 sensory gating abnormalities in patients with schizophrenia. Schizophrenia Bulletin. 2006;**32**(4):692-700

[73] Erwin RJ, Turetsky BI, Moberg P, Gur RC, Gur RE. P50 abnormalities in schizophrenia: Relationship to clinical and neuropsychological indices of attention. Schizophrenia Research. 1998;**33**:157-167

[74] Adler LE, Olincy A, Waldo M, et al. Schizophrenia, sensory gating, and nicotinic receptors. Schizophrenia Bulletin. 1998;**24**:189-202

[75] Freedman R, Leonard S, Gault JM, et al. Linkage disequilibrium for schizophrenia at the chromosome 15q13-14 locus of the alpha7-nicotinic acetylcholine receptor subunit gene (CHRNA7). American Journal of Medical Genetics. 2001;**105**:20-22

[76] Klinkenberg IPM, Blokland AAJ, Riedel WJ, Sambeth A. Cholinergic modulation of auditory processing, sensory gating and novelty detection in human participants. Psychopharmacology. 2013;**225**(4):903-921

[77] Castro NG, Albuquerque EX. Alpha-Bungarotoxin-sensitive hippocampal nicotinic receptor channel has a high calcium permeability. Biophysical Journal. 1995;**68**(2): 516-524

[78] Josef Golubic S, Susac A, Huonker R, Haueisen J, Supek S. Early attentional modulation of the neural network evoked with the auditory paired-click paradigm: An MEG study. Procedia-Social and Behavioral Sciences. 2014;**126**:195-196

[79] Freedman R, Adams CE, Adler LE, Bickford PC, Gault J, Harris J, Leonard S. Inhibitory neurophysiological deficit as a phenotype for genetic investigation of schizophrenia. American Journal of Medical Genetics. 2000;**97**:58-64

[80] Baillet S, Mosher JC, Leahy RM. Electromagnetic brain mapping. IEEE Signal Processing Magazine. 2001;**18**:14-30

[81] Barkley GL. Controversies in neurophysiology. MEG is superior to EEG in localization of interictal epileptiform activity. Pro. Clinical Neurophysiology. 2004;**115**(5):1001-1009

[82] Josef Golubic S, Susac A, Grilj V, Ranken D, Huonker R, Haueisen J, Supek S. Size matters: MEG empirical and simulation study on source localization of the earliest visual activity in the occipital cortex. Medical & Biological Engineering & Computing. 2011;**4**:545-554

[83] Michel CM, Murray MM, Lantz G, Gonzalez S, Spinelli L, Grave de Peralta R. EEG source imaging. Clinical Neurophysiology. 2004;**115**(10):2195-2222

[84] Supek S, Stingl K, Josef Golubic S, Susac A, Ranken D. Optimal spatio-temporal matrix subdivision for cortical neurodynamics estimation. In: Proceedings of the 15th International Conference on Biomagnetism (BIOMAG 2006); Vancouver. 2006. pp. 180-181

[85] Felleman DJ, Van Essen DC. Distributed hierarchical processing in the primate cerebral cortex. Cerebral Cortex. 1991;**1**:1-147

[86] Lu BY, Edgar JC, Jones AP, Smith AK, Huang MX, Miller GA, Canive JM. Improved test–retest reliability of 50 ms paired-click auditory gating using magnetoencephalopgaphy source modeling. Psychophysiology. 2007;**44**:86-90

[87] Edgar JC, Huang MX, Weisend MP, Sherwood A, Miller GA, Adler LE, Canive JM. Interpreting abnormality: An EEG and MEG study of P50 and the auditory paired-stimulus paradigm. Biological Psychology. 2003;**65**:1-20

[88] Woods DL, Knight RT, Neville HJ. Bitemporal lesions dissociate auditory evoked potentials and perception. Electroencephalography and Clinical Neurophysiology. 1984;**57**:208-220

[89] Korzyukova O, Pfliegere ME, Wagnerf M, Bowyer SM, Rosburgb T, Sundaresana K, Elgerb CE, Boutros NN. Generators of the intracranial P50 response in auditory sensory gating. NeuroImage. 2007;**35**:814-826

[90] Reite M, Teale P, Zimmerman J, Davis K, Whalen J. Source localization of a 50 msec latency auditory evoked field component. Electroencephalography and Clinical Neurophysiology. 1988;**70**:490-498

[91] Thoma RJ, Hanlon FM, Moses SN, et al. M50 sensory gating predicts negative symptoms in schizophrenia. Schizophrenia Research. 2005;**73**:311-318

[92] Grunwald T, Boutros NN, Pezer N, von Oertzen J, Fernandez G, Schaller C, Elger CE. Neuronal substrates of sensory gating within the human brain. Biological Psychiatry. 2003;**53**:511-519

[93] Boutros NN, Trautner P, Rosburg T, Korzyukov O, Grunwald T, Schaller C, Elger CE, Kurthen M. Sensory gating in the human hippocampal and rhinal regions. Clinical Neurophysiology. 2005;**116**:1967-1974

[94] Josef Golubic S, Aine C, Supek S. Lack of the neuromagnetic activity in the frontal lobe of AD subjects. In: Proceedings of the 6th znanstveni sastanak Hrvatskog fizikalnog društva. 2009; Primosten. Zagreb: HFD; 2009. pp. 156-157

[95] Supek S, Golubic SJ, Bryant J, Donahue C, Montaño R, Adair J, Hart B, Knoefel J, Stephen J, Aine CJ. Neuromagnetic auditory activity reflects differences between normal aging, MCI and AD subjects: An oddball study. Biomagnetism: Transdisciplinary Research and Exploration. 2008;**1**:34-36

[96] Josef Golubic S, Jurasic MJ, Susac A, Huonker R, Gotz T, Haueisen J. Attention modulates topology and dynamics of auditory sensory gating. (Forthcoming; In submission)

[97] Barbas H, Ghashghaei H, Dombrowski SM, Rempel-Clower NL. Medial prefrontal cortices are unified by common connections with superior temporal cortices and distinguished by input from memory-related areas in the rhesus monkey. The Journal of Comparative Neurology. 1999;**410**:343-367

[98] Croxson PL, Johansen-Berg H, Timothy EJ, Behrens M, Robson D, Pinsk MA, Gross CG, Richter W, Richter MC, Kastner S, Rushworth MPS. Quantitative investigation of connections of the prefrontal cortex in the human and macaque using probabilistic. The Journal of Neuroscience. 2005;**25**:8854-8866

[99] Cavada C, Company T, Tejedor J, Cruz-Rizzolo RJ, Reinoso-Suarez F. The anatomical connections of the macaque monkey orbitofrontal cortex. Cerebral Cortex. 2000;**10**: 220-242

[100] Summerfield C, Egner T. Expectation (and attention) in visual cognition. Trends in Cognitive Sciences. 2009;**13**:403-409

[101] Atkinson RC, Shiffrin RM. Human memory: A proposed system and its control processes. In: Spence W, Spence JT, editors. The Psychology of Learning and Motivation. Vol. 2. New York: Academic Press; 1968. pp. 89-195

[102] Irimajiri R, Golob EJ, Starr A. Auditory brain-stem, middle- and long-latency evoked potentials in mild cognitive impairment. Clinical Neurophysiology. 2005;**116**(8): 1918-1929

[103] Thomas C, VomBerg I, Rupp A, Seidl U, Schröder J, Roesch-Ely D. P50 gating deficit in Alzheimer dementia correlates to frontal neuropsychological function. Neurobiology of Aging. 2010;**31**:416-424

[104] Cheng CH, Pei-Ning W, Wan-Yu H, Yung-Yang L. Inadequate inhibition of redundant auditory inputs in Alzheimer's disease: An MEG study. Biological Psychology. 2012;**89**:365-373

[105] Bajo R, Maestú F, Nevado A, Sancho M, Gutiérrez R, et al. Functional connectivity in mild cognitive impairment during a memory task: Implications for the disconnection hypothesis. Journal of Alzheimer's Disease. 2010;**22**(1):183-193

[106] Takayama Y. A delayed recall battery as a sensitive screening for mild cognitive impairment: Follow-up study of memory clinic patients after 10 years. Journal of Medical and Dental Sciences. 2010;**57**:177-184

[107] Canuet L, Pusil S, López ME, Bajo R, Pineda-Pardo JA, et al. Network disruption and cerebrospinal fluid amyloid-beta and phospho-tau levels in mild cognitive impairment. Journal of Neuroscience. 2015;**35**(28):10325-10330

[108] Wu JW, Hussaini SA, Bastille IM, Rodriguez GA, Mrejeru A, et al. Neuronal activity enhances tau propagation and tau pathology in vivo. Nature Neuroscience. 2016;**9**(8):1085-1092

[109] Cuesta P, Garcés P, Castellanos NP, López ME, Aurtenetxe S, et al. Influence of the APOE ε4 allele and mild cognitive impairment diagnosis in the disruption of the MEG resting state functional connectivity in sources space. Journal of Alzheimer's Disease. 2015;**44**(2):493-505

[110] Rapoport SI, Horwitz B, Haxby JV, Grady CL. Alzheimer's disease: Metabolic uncoupling of associative brain regions. The Canadian Journal of Neurological Sciences. 1996;**13**(4):540-545

[111] Coleman RE. Positron emission tomography diagnosis of Alzheimer's disease. Neuroimaging Clinics of North America. 2005;**15**:837-846

[112] Klunk WE, Engler H, Nordberg A, Blomqvist G, Holt DP, et al. Imaging brain amyloid in Alzheimer's disease with Pittsburgh compound-B. Annals of Neurology. 2004;**55**:306-319

[113] Klupp E, Grimmer T, Tahmasian M, Sorg C, Yakushev I, et al. Prefrontal hypometabolism in Alzheimer disease is related to longitudinal amyloid accumulation in remote brain regions. Journal of Nuclear Medicine. 2015;**56**:399-404

[114] Sharma G, Vijayaraghavan S. Modulation of presynaptic store calcium induces release of glutamate and postsynaptic firing. Neuron. 2003;**38**(6):929-939

10

Oxidative Status Pathways: Systemic Biomarkers

Peter Zolotukhin, Viktor Chmykhalo, Anna Belanova, Alexander Dybushkin, Viktor Fedoseev and Dmitriy Smirnov

Abstract

Systemic biomarkers (i.e. biomarkers of functioning of cellular pathways) offer a broad spectrum of diagnostic capabilities. There are several approaches to using systemic biomarkers that derive from exact needs of a researcher or a clinical specialist. First, analyzing a multifunctional and multi-systemic pathway in circulating cells (e.g. leukocytes) allows to gather generalized information on functioning of the organism. Second, there are numerous pathways that, even still in circulating cells, allow to assess risks of developing or stage of development of numerous diseases, including the leaders of non-infection diseases mortality—cardiovascular diseases. Third, biopsy specimens can readily be used to assess the exact signaling type of a disease (especially cancer) thus helping in selecting the best treatment option. Due to unique properties of the human oxidative status pathways that are discussed in the present chapter, diagnostics specialists are now acquiring an all-in-one toolbox for profiling and detecting almost any non-infectious and a broad range of infectious diseases. In addition to properties of the human oxidative status pathways opening these possibilities, this chapter considers exact systemic biomarkers deriving from this approach, reveals some examples of usage of the resulting diagnostic technology and provides instances of successful clinical application of the systemic biomarker approach.

Keywords: interactomics, systems biology, personalized medicine, signaling pathways, oxidative status, systemic biomarkers

1. Introduction

The human cell is capable of receiving, processing and accordingly responding to an indefinitely wide range of stimuli [1]. These stimuli can be both exogenous and endogenous; both physical and chemical (including biochemical); both adopted to provide communication and those requiring adaptation [2, 3]. Regardless of the classification and kind of stimuli acting upon the cell, the whole chain of events—from the signal reception and to the end-point response of the cell—follows the same logic and is guided by a given signaling pathway [4].

Signaling pathways may exploit cellular machinery to a different extent. In the simplest case, a stimulus induces a cellular component capable of performing all the necessary steps from reception and to the ultimate action [5]. In the most complex instance, the reaction toward a stimulus involves complex rearrangements of cellular components, alterations in gene expression caused by epigenetic events and induction of numerous uni-directional and opposite transcription factors, translation modulation, etc. [6–9].

These different pathways confer unequal informativeness for biomedical, mostly diagnostic and follow-up, purposes. The reason is that the "shorter" a pathway, the more difficult it is to detect changes in cellular parameters due to fast turnover and lack-to-absence of signal amplification stages. In contrast, complex pathways contain signal amplification circuits, demonstrate delayed and sustained changes in cellular parameters and, moreover, interact with other pathways (i.e. respond in dependence of cellular signaling background), thus providing a researcher with a plethora of data characterized by high signal-to-noise ratio and high informativeness [10]. Superior informativeness of complex signaling pathways renders them highly promising for clinical applications. On the other hand, from analytical point of view, responses of simpler pathways are easier to interpret, while extremely complex pathways are nearly unresolvable due to ambiguity imposed by principal limitations of our knowledge of interacting components of such pathways. Thus, it is required that clinically applicable pathways be well-studied, with the triggering stimulus and characteristic effects of the pathway known in the first place.

Generally, cellular signaling pathways are specialized toward given sets of stimuli. However, there is one group of signaling pathways that, although being specialized, too, permits diagnostics of an incredibly wide range of cellular parameters. These are oxidative status signaling pathways. In humans, oxygen participates in multitudinous processes - from spontaneous reactions of auto-oxidation of small molecules, to protein folding control, multi-step electron transfer in mitochondrial and microsomal electron transport chains and to action of NADPH oxidases tightly controlled by one of the most complex pathways of the human cell [11]. Due to this deep implication of oxygen in cellular metabolism, redox processes requiring this small molecule run in all compartments of the cell and outside the cell. Since one-electron reduction is thermodynamically favorable, all processes involving oxygen are liable to generation of reactive oxygen species (ROS) [12]. Moreover, a much more safe, thus preferred and referred to as physiological two-electron reduction of molecular oxygen produces hydrogen peroxide [13]—a molecule classified as ROS as well. A significant portion of hydrogen peroxide decomposes with the formation of free radicals, including the most short-lived and dangerous hydroxyl radical [14]. On the other hand, hydrogen peroxide serves as one of key cellular messengers—and its function in this sense include direct control of transcription factors (AP-1, NFE2L2, CREB, HSF1, HIF1, TP53, NF-κB, NOTCH, SP1, etc. [15]), direct and indirect control of higher-order kinases (CAMKII, Pka, Pkb (Akt), Pkg, Mapk, Erk [16, 17]) and epigenetic machinery [18] and direct modulation of 14–3-3 proteins function [19]. Hydrogen peroxide as well as other ROS serve as primary triggers of the oxidative status pathways, while the pathways differ in signal reception compartment, signal reception mechanisms, signal intensity dependence and sets of modulating pathways. These differences confer significant specificity to triggering of the pathways and temporal characteristics of the response. Examples of such differences are given further.

With respect to the ultimate cellular effects and resulting oxidative status parameters, oxidative status pathways are rather well explored. The beginning of the extensive studying of oxidative status and pathways determining it dates back to the first half of XX century [20–22]. Over the time, due to implications of prooxidants and antioxidants in determination of quality of life, in aging (the two factors that significantly affected public attitude and mentality) and in numerous diseases, significant amount of experimental data has been collected. These data are detailed inasmuch as some pathways activation patterns have been characterized in a minutes to hours basis [23] and accounting signal intensity [24]. No less importantly, targets of the most complex and clinically relevant pathways are well known. And as it is shown further, these targets that may serve as biomarker panel candidates are not only mRNAs or proteins, but as well individual transcript variants, pre-mRNAs and miRNAs [25–28]. Consequently, although there are more data to be collected, these pathways may be utilized for developing systemic biomarkers for diagnostics of different health conditions using sets of individual RNAs, proteins and small molecules in analytically convenient combinations. For some of such pathways, this has already been done.

To sum up, oxygen-dependent redox processes participate in or modulate at least most cellular metabolic and signaling systems. Accordingly, these systems contain respective response circuits allowing the cell to adapt to changes in environmental and internal conditions or at least perceive these changes. As the above-mentioned metabolic and signaling systems of the cell strikingly differ in nature, cellular roles and even in action timeframes, the response circuits—termed oxidative status pathways—are rather specific in triggering stimulus, unique in sensing mechanism, subsequent events and the outcome. Among these events and results are changes in expression of target RNAs and proteins and fluctuations of some relatively stable biochemical parameters. Together these factors may (and do) serve as components of systemic biomarkers. And since the pathways are specific toward given stimuli or signals, the respective systemic biomarkers, i.e. panels of reporter target components of these pathways, allow for profiling of the activation status of the pathways. Consequently, as diseases originate and start to manifest at the bottom biological level - the cellular level - the cellular signaling pathways reflect the mode of cellular functioning. And since oxidative status pathways extraordinarily reflect and summarize most cellular systems functioning, these pathways are perfect for developing systemic biomarkers. However, there are several variables in selecting the sets of cellular factors to serve as systemic biomarker components that are to be accounted, and those are discussed in the next section.

2. Developing oxidative status pathways-based systemic biomarkers

Since systemic biomarkers are sets of cellular factors that may represent functioning of a given pathway, development of such biomarkers starts with interactomic data - signaling pathways maps. There are numerous available solutions, including Reactome [29], BioSystems [30],

GenAtlas [31], GeneGo [32], KEGG [33], etc. We have previously developed our own interactomic system dedicated exclusively to human oxidative status - Oxidative Status Interactome Map (OSIM) [34]. These interactomic systems differ in interface, data selection strategy and depth of interactome coverage. Importantly, quality of an interactomic map used for biomarker development significantly affects its specificity and sensitivity due to inherent biological overlap of targets control and multi-pathway signal reception.

2.1. Signal specificity

There are dozens of oxidative status signaling pathways operating in the human cell, and most of these pathways have hydrogen peroxide or other ROS as the primary triggering signal. However, as it was shown above, ROS originate in different cellular compartments in different cellular contexts, and this is one of the basic principles of disambiguation in signal reception [35, 36]. Further divergence of pathways is achieved by their signaling background dependence: different oxidative status pathways require different kinases for functioning, while these kinases are often redox-sensitive [37, 38]. Finally, oxidative status pathways are highly specialized toward various ROS-inducing agents, which can be both chemical and physical. For example, electrophilic compounds have critically distinct effects on the AP-1 and NFE2L2 sub-pathways of the NFE2L2/AP-1 pathway (often referred to as the NRF2 pathway) [39]. An example of physical signal specificity is thioredoxin 1 triggering by ionizing radiation, UV and ultrasound [40].

Although triggering signals significantly overlap for different pathways, cellular effects of these signals greatly depend on their cellular location - and these effects are mediated by compartment-specific sensors.

2.2. Sensor location and type

Protein sensors of oxidative status pathways are ample and extremely diverse. Different pathways are greatly dissimilar in mechanisms of activation by even the same basic stimulus - hydrogen peroxide. Moreover, the same pathway may have several sensors working in tandem. For example, the above-mentioned NFE2L2 sub-pathway has a primary hydrogen peroxide sensor in cytoplasm - it is KEAP1 protein. But in addition to this cytoplasmic pool of KEAP1, the same protein is also present in the nucleus, where it acts as the second-line sensor [41]. The same pathway is also characterized by a third-line sensor - BACH1 protein, a transcriptional repressor active in reduced state [36]. Thus, depending on cellular context, NFE2L2 activity may be attenuated to different extent and so as to result in activation of different sets of target genes, since BACH1, for instance, represses only a portion of NFE2L2-dependent genes.

Another peculiar example of sensor location-induced pathway functioning modulation is known from the NF-κB pathway. Under unstimulated conditions, NF-κB proteins are bound by I-κB proteins in the cytosol preventing NF-κB nuclear import. Upon ROS formation, NF-κB proteins are oxidized, change conformation and cannot be immobilized by the I-κBs. Further developments depend on nuclear redox context and cellular signaling background, since oxidized NF-κB proteins are unable to transactivate the targets [42]. Interestingly, activated NF-κB protein RELA controls nuclear import of the above considered KEAP1 protein [41].

All the events of pathways activation and subsequent signal transduction have different rates in different pathways. These temporal characteristics can be utilized to collect additional diagnostic data.

2.3. Temporal considerations

Even when oxidative status pathways are activated by the same signal, ultimate effects are achieved in different time. Moreover, even within the same pathway, targets are activated at different rate. It appears that this is dictated by the complexity of signal transduction, including presence and characteristics of signal amplification circuits. It has striking effects on pathway performance. For examples, in the above-mentioned NFE2L2 pathway, some targets are activated as early as in 5 hours, while other genes fail to increase expression rate until approximately 24 hours [23].

Another example of significantly prolonged effects of a pathway is seen in HIF1A pathway run cycle. Activated HIF1A induces expression of NF-κB genes and proteins REL, RELA and NFKB1, and DICER1. In turn, activated NF-κB (and this activation is context-dependent) transactivates genes of miRNAs *MIR-93* and *MIR-199A-5P* that are further processed by DICER1. These mature miRNAs are HIF1A suppressors that eventually block the pathway activation. Due to extremely complex chain of events, this variant of HIF1A pathway run takes considerable amount of time [25].

Temporal characteristics of the pathways analyzed should be accounted when developing and applying a systemic biomarker. This can partly be achieved by selecting appropriate analytical level.

2.4. Analytical levels

Oxidative status pathways contain numerous types of molecules that can be used as biomarkers. These are protein-coding RNAs, miRNAs, proteins, and small molecules.

Just as signal reception and transduction are multi-step processes, so is the development of the cellular reaction. Upon decoding of the stimulus by transcription factors, the first step of the cellular reaction takes place - this is preparation to transcription initiation (interactions between transcription factors [43], competition [39], nuclear import of transcription factors [44], modulation of epigenetic machinery [45], etc.). Even this first step is complex, and subsequent stages occurring in the nucleus are legion [46]: these include DNA binding by transcription factors, RNA polymerase engagement, transcription, RNA-protein interactions, splicing, RNA modification, RNA stabilization, storage, degradation and cytoplasmic export. Further, numerous cytoplasmic processes provide or accompany generation of mature protein, and another plethora of events finalize the cellular reaction (e.g. the protein is modified, re-distributed within the cell or secreted). Remarkably, all these processes, dozens of them, are affected by cellular signaling background.

Generally, it is possible to take a "snapshot" of any of these phases of the cellular reaction and use the data to decode the initial signal. However, the more elaborate the product of the cellular reaction one analyzes, the harder it is to trace back the stimulus.

Thus, most existing systemic biosensors rely on mRNA level. mRNA expression analysis is a reasonable approach to assess whether a stimulus has affected the cell or there has been a dysfunction in cellular signal transduction or decoding processes: there are only few steps between transcription factor activation (signal decoding) and mRNA maturation. However, there are still more steps that can easily be affected by the cellular functional context [47–51]. Thus, pre-mRNA might serve as a valuable alternative or addition to mRNA analysis. In one of our previous studies, we assessed whether pre-mRNAs can be used for diagnostic purposes. It appeared that two of three pre-mRNAs of single transcript variant-encoding genes had sensitivity and specificity comparable to that of the respective mRNAs [52]. Comparing such diagnostic characteristics is challenging when genes coding for more than one transcript variant are considered.

In this case, individual transcripts analysis is a great alternative to standard mRNA analysis. A pathway may control transcripts' fate individually on several levels. First, transcription factors of the pathway can directly induce individual transcripts [53]. Second, transcription factors, being central to some pathways, can attract and regulate splicing machinery themselves [54]. Third, other pathway components can easily regulate splicing machinery together with promoting target gene transcription [55]. Fourth, cellular pathways have all capabilities to individually control degradation or long-term storage of mature mRNA variants of a single gene [56–58]. Individual transcript expression-based studies are rare due to technical and interpretative difficulties [59, 60], but previously we demonstrated that this approach is highly promising in case of oxidative status pathways used for development of systemic biomarkers [28].

Proteins are also sometimes used as biomarkers in systemic diagnostics and systemic pathophysiology approaches. The drawback of this approach appears to be in decreased signal-to-noise ratio leading to significant information losses. Although our lab mostly focuses on RNAs for biomarker development, we performed several attempts to use proteome as analytical level in systemic approaches [61].

2.5. Signal amplification and autoregulatory blocking

As it was mentioned above, signaling pathways are optimal for diagnostic properties only if they contain signal amplification and abruption circuits, yet they are not too complex to hinder data interpretation, and their action rate is comparatively slow.

Human oxidative status pathways are rich in signal amplification and autoregulatory blocking circuits. In one of our previous works, we discussed 15 such experimentally proven circuits of just one of the pathways - the NFE2L2/AP-1 pathway [10].

Such circuits greatly help in interpreting data and choosing time points for sample collection in repetitive measurements that greatly improve the signal decoding procedure for diagnostic purposes.

2.6. Biomarkers quantity

Careful selection of systemic biomarkers candidates and their quantity are critical, since, on average, each gene is controlled by a great number of transcription factors (both transactivators and repressors) belonging to different signaling pathways. This implies a significant limitation—so that even some well-known targets cannot be used for diagnostic purposes involving pathway activation analysis. There are many examples of genes that are controlled by multiple and functionally opposite pathways even within the oxidative status systems [62, 63].

3. Current advances in developing systemic biomarkers

Systemic biomarkers approach is a relatively new area of biomedicine. However, over two decades of its existence [64], significant advances have been made. Great effort spent in this area not only improved analytical algorithms, but also underlined the importance of personalized approach. For example, many prognostic markers have been suggested for breast cancer in the literature, in particular for predicting survival. But data collected in separate studies led to striking discovery of the lack of overlap of the predictive genes in most of these studies. This emphasized the need of personalized approach even within tumor groups that share the same histomorphology [65]. The reason for discrepancies is debatable—divergent patterns of expression profiles might have been due to several analytical factors considered in the present chapter, but the solution holds the same: systemic biomarkers are only informative when patterns of pathways activation, rather than changes in individual genes expression, are analyzed. This idea led foundation to development of several analytical tools and panels. Our lab developed an NFE2L2/AP-1 pathway-based systemic biomarker for assessing slight changes in physiological parameters of the human organism using peripheral blood leukocytes as the preferred sample type [66]. The same systemic approach utilizing another set of oxidative status markers was successfully used for unveiling features of uterine cervical incompetence patients [67]. Other labs also successfully apply pathway activation-based technologies in various field and other sample types, with special attention paid to fresh solid tumors samples and paraffin blocks [68]. Of note, Oncofinder technology [69, 70] and Oncotype DX assay [71] are among the most effective interactomics/multi-gene analysis-based tests in oncology.

In **Table 1**, some examples of suitable NFE2L2/AP-1 targets and complex markers are given along with their diagnostic properties (only area under the curve (AUC) is given, please see details in the cited publications).

As seen from **Table 1**, not only the markers may highly vary in nature, but they have different receiver operator characteristics. Notably, for each model to be studied, it is possible to choose or find a set of markers having extremely high AUCs that are hardly achievable using the traditional biomarker approaches.

Marker	ROC indices		Model	Reference
	AUC	p-value		
AKR1B1 mRNA (normalized to reference)	1.0	<0.0001	*In vitro*, HeLa cells, 24 h 400 uM hydrogen peroxide	[52]
AKR1B10 mRNA	1.0	<0.0001		
AKR1B1 mRNA/pre-mRNA ratio	0.984	<0.0001		
GSTP1 pre-mRNA	0.984	<0.0001		
AKR1B10 mRNA/pre-mRNA ratio	0.946	<0.0001		
AKR1B10 pre-mRNA	0.781	0.0284		
BACH1 tv2/*NFE2L2* mRNAs ratio	0.965	<0.0001	*In vivo*, 19–22 y.o. females, repetitive measurements, self-reported analogue-scaled psychological stress	[66]
SRXN1/*NFE2L2* mRNAs ratio	0.922	<0.0001		
NQO1/*NFE2L2* mRNAs ratio	0.902	<0.0001		
HMOX1/NFE2L2 mRNAs ratio	0.879	<0.0001		
KEAP1/*NFE2L2* mRNAs ratio	0.867	<0.0001		
PRDX6/*NFE2L2* mRNAs ratio	0.687	0.0586		
TXN tv1/*NFE2L2* mRNAs ratio	0.609	0.2891		

Table 1. The NFE2L2/AP-1 pathway functioning markers used in two in vitro and in vivo studies, with AUC in descending order within each study.

4. Conclusions

Oxidative status pathways-based interactomic profiling using the expression analysis-based methods promises a lot to the field of development of the novel diagnostic approaches and has already demonstrated great results in various areas of biomedicine. In this branch of personalized medicine, interactomics serves as a tool to select factors to be analyzed (systemic biomarkers), to suggest a method of analysis and to further account for data collected. Expression profiling then serves as the immediate molecular biological procedure used to collect biological data in the interactomic diagnostics.

Current advances in molecular biology have led to creation of numerous interactomic maps and analytical systems that can readily be used for developing novel diagnostics assays. Fast evolution of oxidative status cell biology and emerging molecular biology suggestions on cellular factors to be considered as systemic biomarkers candidate complement and promote this field. Despite the complexity of development of systemic biomarker-based assays, this novel type of diagnostic technologies appears to be inextricably intertwined with the personalized medicine era.

Acknowledgements

The chapter preparation was funded by Biomedical Innovations LLC, a part of Evolution corporate group.

Conflict of interest

The authors claim that there were no financial or other conflicts of interests related to the present chapter.

Author details

Peter Zolotukhin*, Viktor Chmykhalo, Anna Belanova, Alexander Dybushkin, Viktor Fedoseev and Dmitriy Smirnov

*Address all correspondence to: p.zolotukhin@icloud.com

Biomedical Innovations LLC, Rostov-on-Don, Russia

References

[1] Kiel C, Yus E, Serrano L. Engineering signal transduction pathways. Cell. 2010;**140**:33-47. DOI: 10.1016/j.cell.2009.12.028

[2] Keyse SM, Tyrrell RM. Heme oxygenase is the major 32-kDa stress protein induced in human skin fibroblasts by UVA radiation, hydrogen peroxide, and sodium arsenite. Proceedings of the National Academy of Sciences of the United States of America. 1989;**86**:99-103

[3] Dent P, Yacoub A, Contessa J, Caron R, Amorino G, Valerie K, Hagan MP, Grant S, Stress S-UR. Radiation-induced activation of multiple intracellular signaling pathways. Radiation Research. 2003;**159**:283-300

[4] An JY, Zhou LL, Sun P, Pang HG, Li DD, Li Y, Zhang M, Song JN. Role of the AMPK signaling pathway in early brain injury after subarachnoid hemorrhage in rats. Acta Neurochirurgica. 2015;**157**:781-792. DOI: 10.1007/s00701-015-2370-3

[5] Li WG. Miller FJ Jr, Zhang HJ, Spitz DR, Oberley LW, Weintraub NL. H(2)O(2)-induced O(2) production by a non-phagocytic NAD(P)H oxidase causes oxidant injury. Journal of Biological Chemistry. 2001;**276**:29251-29256

[6] Liu GH, Qu J, Shen X. NF-kappaB/p65 antagonizes Nrf2-ARE pathway by depriving CBP from Nrf2 and facilitating recruitment of HDAC3 to MafK. Biochimica et Biophysica Acta. 2008;**1783**:713-727. DOI: 10.1016/j.bbamcr.2008.01.002

[7] Imberti B, Morigi M, Zoja C, Angioletti S, Abbate M, Remuzzi A, Remuzzi G. Shear stress-induced cytoskeleton rearrangement mediates NF-kappaB-dependent endothelial expression of ICAM-1. Microvascular Research. 2000;**60**:182-188

[8] Herdy B, Jaramillo M, Svitkin YV, Rosenfeld AB, Kobayashi M, Walsh D, Alain T, Sean P, Robichaud N, Topisirovic I, Furic L, Dowling RJO, Sylvestre A, Rong L, Colina R, Costa-Mattioli M, Fritz JH, Olivier M, Brown E, Mohr I, Sonenberg N. Translational control of the activation of transcription factor NF-κB and production of type I interferon by phosphorylation of the translation factor eIF4E. Nature Immunology. 2012;**13**:543-550. DOI: 10.1038/ni.2291

[9] Hariri F, Arguello M, Volpon L, Culjkovic-Kraljacic B, Nielsen TH, Hiscott J, Mann KK, Borden KL. The eukaryotic translation initiation factor eIF4E is a direct transcriptional target of NF-κB and is aberrantly regulated in acute myeloid leukemia. Leukemia. 2013;**27**:2047-2055. DOI: 10.1038/leu.2013.73

[10] Zolotukhin PV, Belanova AA. Feed-Forward and Feed-back circuits of the NRF2/AP-1 composite pathway. In: A Master Regulator of Oxidative Stress—The Transcription Factor Nrf2. Rijeka, Croatia: InTech; 2016. pp. 65-90. DOI: 10.5772/65216

[11] Sarniak A, Lipińska J, Tytman K, Lipińska S. Endogenous mechanisms of reactive oxygen species (ROS) generation. Postepy Higieny I Medycyny Doswiadczalnej (Online). 2016;**70**:1150-1165

[12] Starkov AA. The role of mitochondria in reactive oxygen species metabolism and signaling. Annals of the New York Academy of Sciences. 2008;**1147**:37-52. DOI: 10.1196/annals.1427.015

[13] Komarov DA, Slepneva IA, Glupov VV, Khramtsov VV. Superoxide and hydrogen peroxide formation during enzymatic oxidation of DOPA by phenoloxidase. Free Radical Research. 2005;**39**:853-858

[14] Marinho HS, Real C, Cyrne L, Soares H, Antunes F. Hydrogen peroxide sensing, signaling and regulation of transcription factors. Redox Biology. 2014;**2**:535-562. DOI: 10.1016/j.redox.2014.02.006

[15] Gough DR, Cotter TG. Hydrogen peroxide: A Jekyll and Hyde signalling molecule. Cell Death & Disease. 2011;**2**:e213. DOI: 10.1038/cddis.2011.96

[16] Burgoyne JR, Oka S, Ale-Agha N, Eaton P. Hydrogen peroxide sensing and signaling by protein kinases in the cardiovascular system. Antioxidants & Redox Signaling. 2013;**18**:1042-1052. DOI: 10.1089/ars.2012.4817

[17] Blanc A, Pandey NR, Srivastava AK. Synchronous activation of ERK 1/2, p38mapk and PKB/Akt signaling by H2O2 in vascular smooth muscle cells: Potential involvement in vascular disease (review). International Journal of Molecular Medicine. 2003;**11**:229-234

[18] Zhang W, Ji W, Yang L, Yao L, Wang G, Xuan A, Zhuang Z. The involvement of epigenetic silencing of Foxa2 in cellular replicative and premature senescence induced by hydrogen peroxide. Free Radical Research. 2013;**47**:325-332. DOI: 10.3109/10715762.2013.773589

[19] Jeon YH, Ko KY, Lee JH, Park KJ, Jang JK, Kim IY. Identification of a redox-modulatory interaction between selenoprotein W and 14-3-3 protein. Biochimica et Biophysica Acta. 2016;**1863**:10-18. DOI: 10.1016/j.bbamcr.2015.10.006

[20] Sirotkina RG, Vitamin C. Metabolism in the second half of complicated pregnancy. Akush Ginekol (Mosk). 1945;**1945**:19-21

[21] Levine R, Wolfson WQ, Huddlestun B. A purine metabolite in plasma, which gives the same color reaction as uric acid. Proceedings of American Federation for Clinical Research. 1945;**2**:56

[22] Stadie WC, Riggs BC, Haugaard N. Oxygen poisoning; the effect of high oxygen pressure upon enzymes; pepsin, catalase, cholinesterase, and carbonic anhydrase. The Journal of Biological Chemistry. 1945;**161**:175-180

[23] Marrot L, Jones C, Perez P, Meunier JR. The significance of Nrf2 pathway in (photo)-oxidative stress response in melanocytes and keratinocytes of the human epidermis. Pigment Cell & Melanoma Research. 2008;**21**:79-88. DOI: 10.1111/j.1755-148X.2007.00424.x

[24] Fratta Pasini A, Albiero A, Stranieri C, Cominacini M, Pasini A, Mozzini C, Vallerio P, Cominacini L, Garbin U. Serum oxidative stress-induced repression of Nrf2 and GSH depletion: A mechanism potentially involved in endothelial dysfunction of young smokers. PLoS One. 2012;**7**:e30291. DOI: 10.1371/journal.pone.0030291

[25] Jiang Y, Zhu Y, Wang X, Gong J, Hu C, Guo B, Zhu B, Li Y. Temporal regulation of HIF-1 and NF-κB in hypoxic hepatocarcinoma cells. Oncotarget. 2015;**6**:9409-9419

[26] Yang M, Yao Y, Eades G, Zhang Y, Zhou Q. MiR-28 regulates Nrf2 expression through a Keap1-independent mechanism. Breast Cancer Research and Treatment. 2011;**129**:983-991. DOI: 10.1007/s10549-011-1604-1

[27] Papp D, Lenti K, Módos D, Fazekas D, Dúl Z, Türei D, Földvári-Nagy L, Nussinov R, Csermely P, Korcsmáros T. The NRF2-related interactome and regulome contain multifunctional proteins and fine-tuned autoregulatory loops. FEBS Letters. 2012;**586**:1795-1802. DOI: 10.1016/j.febslet.2012.05.016

[28] Belanova AA, Smirnov DS, Makarenko MS, Belousova MM, Mashkina EV, Aleksandrova AA, Soldatov AV, Zolotukhin PV. Individual expression features of GPX2, NQO1 and SQSTM1 transcript variants induced by hydrogen peroxide treatment in HeLa cells. Genetics and Molecular Biology. 2017;**40**:515-524. DOI: 10.1590/1678-4685-GMB-2016-0005

[29] Haw R, Stein L. Using the reactome database. Current Protocols in Bioinformatics. 2012;Chapter 8:Unit8.7. DOI: 10.1002/0471250953.bi0807s38

[30] Sayers EW, Barrett T, Benson DA, Bolton E, Bryant SH, Canese K, Chetvernin V, Church DM, Dicuccio M, Federhen S, Feolo M, Fingerman IM, Geer LY, Helmberg W, Kapustin Y, Krasnov S, Landsman D, Lipman DJ, Lu Z, Madden TL, Madej T, Maglott DR,

Marchler-Bauer A, Miller V, Karsch-Mizrachi I, Ostell J, Panchenko A, Phan L, Pruitt KD, Schuler GD, Sequeira E, Sherry ST, Shumway M, Sirotkin K, Slotta D, Souvorov A, Starchenko G, Tatusova TA, Wagner L, Wang Y, Wilbur WJ, Yaschenko E, Ye J. Database resources of the National Center for Biotechnology Information. Nucleic Acids Research. 2012;**40**(Database issue):D13-D25. DOI:10.1093/nar/gkr1184

[31] Frézal J. Genatlas database, genes and development defects. Comptes Rendus de l'Académie des Sciences—Series III. 1998 Oct;**321**(10):805-817

[32] Bureeva S, Nikolsky Y. Quantitative knowledge-based analysis in compound safety assessment. Expert Opinion on Drug Metabolism & Toxicology. 2011;**7**:287-298. DOI: 10.1517/17425255.2011.553191

[33] Ogata H, Goto S, Fujibuchi W, Kanehisa M. Computation with the KEGG pathway database. Bio Systems. 1998;**47**:119-128

[34] Zolotukhin P, Kozlova Y, Dovzhik A, Kovalenko K, Kutsyn K, Aleksandrova A, Shkurat T. Oxidative status interactome map: Towards novel approaches in experiment planning, data analysis, diagnostics and therapy. Molecular BioSystems. 2013;**9**(8):2085-2096. DOI: 10.1039/c3mb70096h

[35] Ramana CV, Boldogh I, Izumi T, Mitra S. Activation of apurinic/apyrimidinic endonuclease in human cells by reactive oxygen species and its correlation with their adaptive response to genotoxicity of free radicals. Proceedings of the National Academy of Sciences of the United States of America. 1998;**95**(9):5061-5066

[36] Ishikawa M, Numazawa S, Yoshida T. Redox regulation of the transcriptional repressor Bach1. Free Radical Biology & Medicine. 2005;**38**:1344-1352

[37] Clark J, Simon DK. Transcribe to survive: Transcriptional control of antioxidant defense programs for neuroprotection in Parkinson's disease. Antioxidants & Redox Signaling. 2009;**11**:509-528. DOI: 10.1089/ARS.2008.2241

[38] Sonderegger S, Haslinger P, Sabri A, Leisser C, Otten JV, Fiala C, Knöfler M. Wingless (Wnt)-3A induces trophoblast migration and matrix metalloproteinase-2 secretion through canonical Wnt signaling and protein kinase B/AKT activation. Endocrinology. 2010;**151**:211-220. DOI: 10.1210/en.2009-0557

[39] Yoshioka K, Deng T, Cavigelli M, Karin M. Antitumor promotion by phenolic antioxidants: Inhibition of AP-1 activity through induction of Fra expression. Proceedings of the National Academy of Sciences of the United States of America. 1995;**92**:4972-4976

[40] Wei SJ, Botero A, Hirota K, Bradbury CM, Markovina S, Laszlo A, Spitz DR, Goswami PC, Yodoi J, Gius D. Thioredoxin nuclear translocation and interaction with redox factor-1 activates the activator protein-1 transcription factor in response to ionizing radiation. Cancer Research. 2000;**60**:6688-6695

[41] Yu M, Li H, Liu Q, Liu F, Tang L, Li C, Yuan Y, Zhan Y, Xu W, Li W, Chen H, Ge C, Wang J, Yang X. Nuclear factor p65 interacts with Keap1 to repress the Nrf2-ARE pathway. Cellular Signalling. 2011;**23**:883-892. DOI: 10.1016/j.cellsig.2011.01.014

[42] Kim HJ, Jung KJ, Yu BP, Cho CG, Choi JS, Chung HY. Modulation of redox-sensitive transcription factors by calorie restriction during aging. Mechanisms of Ageing and Development. 2002;**123**:1589-1595

[43] Kaspar JW, Niture SK, Jaiswal AK. Nrf2:INrf2 (Keap1) signaling in oxidative stress. Free Radical Biology and Medicine. 2009;**47**:1304-1309. DOI: 10.1016/j.freeradbiomed.2009.07.035

[44] Sykiotis GP, Bohmann D. Stress-activated cap'n'collar transcription factors in aging and human disease. Science Signaling. 2010;**3**:re3. DOI: 10.1126/scisignal.3112re3

[45] Jin C, Li H, Ugai H, Murata T, Yokoyama KK. Transcriptional regulation of the c-Jun gene by AP-1 repressor protein JDP2 during the differentiation of F9 cells. Nucleic Acids Research. Supplement (2001). 2002;**2**:97-98

[46] Morris DP, Lei B, Longo LD, Bomsztyk K, Schwinn DA, Michelotti GA. Temporal dissection of rate limiting transcriptional events using pol II ChIP and RNA analysis of adrenergic stress gene activation. PLoS One. 2015;**10**:e0134442. DOI: 10.1371/journal.pone.0134442

[47] Eulalio A, Behm-Ansmant I, Izaurralde E. P bodies: At the crossroads of post-transcriptional pathways. Nature Reviews. Molecular Cell Biology. 2007;**8**:9-22

[48] Takemura R, Takeiwa T, Taniguchi I, McCloskey A, Ohno M. Multiple factors in the early splicing complex are involved in the nuclear retention of pre-mRNAs in mammalian cells. Genes to Cells. 2011;**16**:1035-1049. DOI: 10.1111/j.1365-2443.2011.01548.x

[49] Änkö ML, Müller-McNicoll M, Brandl H, Curk T, Gorup C, Henry I, Ule J, Neugebauer KM. The RNA-binding landscapes of two SR proteins reveal unique functions and binding to diverse RNA classes. Genome Biology. 2012;**13**:R17. DOI: 10.1186/gb-2012-13-3-r17

[50] Koga M, Satoh T, Takasaki I, Kawamura Y, Yoshida M, Kaida D. U2 snRNP is required for expression of the 3′ end of genes. PLoS One. 2014;**9**:e98015. DOI: 10.1371/journal.pone.0098015

[51] Lareau LF, Brenner SE. Regulation of splicing factors by alternative splicing and NMD is conserved between kingdoms yet evolutionarily flexible. Molecular Biology Evolution. 2015;**32**:1072-1079. DOI: 10.1093/molbev/msv002

[52] Belanova AA, Makarenko MS, Lyangasova OV, Belousova MM, Kurbatov SV, Zolotukhin PV. Pre-mRNAs vs mRNAs as biomarkers of pathway activation: an NFE2L2/AP-1 pathway example. Cell Biochemistry and Biophysics. 2018. In press (Tentatively accepted pending appropriate revision)

[53] Jyrkkänen HK, Kuosmanen S, Heinäniemi M, Laitinen H, Kansanen E, Mella-Aho E, Leinonen H, Ylä-Herttuala S, Levonen AL. Novel insights into the regulation of antioxidant-response-element-mediated gene expression by electrophiles: Induction of the transcriptional repressor BACH1 by Nrf2. The Biochemical Journal. 2011;**440**:167-174

[54] Pan J, Jin C, Murata T, Yokoyama KK. Sequence specific transcription factor, JDP2 interacts with histone and inhibits p300-mediated histone acetylation. Nucleic Acids Research. Supplement (2001). 2003;**2003**:305-306

[55] Yadav AK, Vashishta V, Joshi N, Taneja P. AR-A 014418 used against GSK3beta Down-regulates expression of hnRNPA1 and SF2/ASF splicing factors. Journal of Oncology. 2014;**2014**:695325. DOI: 10.1155/2014/695325

[56] Shim J, Karin M. The control of mRNA stability in response to extracellular stimuli. Molecules and Cells. 2002;**14**:323-331

[57] Rattenbacher B, Bohjanen PR. Evaluating posttranscriptional regulation of cytokine genes. Methods in Molecular Biology. 2012;**820**:71-89. DOI: 10.1007/978-1-61779-439-1_5

[58] Kurinna S, Werner S. NRF2 and microRNAs: New but awaited relations. Biochemical Society Transactions. 2015;**43**:595-601. DOI: 10.1042/BST20140317

[59] Arseneau JR, Laflamme M, Lewis SM, Maïcas E, Ouellette RJ. Multiple isoforms of PAX5 are expressed in both lymphomas and normal B-cells. British Journal of Haematology. 2009;**147**:328-338. DOI: 10.1111/j.1365-2141.2009.07859.x

[60] Boudreau LH, Bertin J, Robichaud PP, Laflamme M, Ouellette RJ, Flamand N, Surette ME. Novel 5-lipoxygenase isoforms affect the biosynthesis of 5-lipoxygenase products. The FASEB Journal. 2011;**25**:1097-1105. DOI: 10.1096/fj.10-173856

[61] Kit OI, Vodolazhsky DI, Kutilin DS, Enin YS, Gevorkyan YA, Zolotukhin PV, Boumber Y, Kharin LV, Panina SB. A proteomics analysis reveals 9 up-regulated proteins associated with altered cell signaling in colon cancer patients. The Protein Journal. 2017;**36**:513-522. DOI: 10.1007/s10930-017-9746-6

[62] Manea A, Manea SA, Gafencu AV, Raicu M, Simionescu M. AP-1-dependent transcriptional regulation of NADPH oxidase in human aortic smooth muscle cells: Role of p22phox subunit. Arteriosclerosis, Thrombosis, and Vascular Biology. 2008;**28**:878-885. DOI: 10.1161/ATVBAHA.108.163592

[63] Cevik MO, Katsuyama M, Kanda S, Kaneko T, Iwata K, Ibi M, Matsuno K, Kakehi T, Cui W, Sasaki M, Yabe-Nishimura C. The AP-1 site is essential for the promoter activity of NOX1/NADPH oxidase, a vascular superoxide-producing enzyme: Possible involvement of the ERK1/2-JunB pathway. Biochemical and Biophysical Research Communications. 2008;**374**:351-355. DOI: 10.1016/j.bbrc.2008.07.027

[64] Perou CM, Sørlie T, Eisen MB, van de Rijn M, Jeffrey SS, Rees CA, Pollack JR, Ross DT, Johnsen H, Akslen LA, Fluge O, Pergamenschikov A, Williams C, Zhu SX, Lønning PE, Børresen-Dale AL, Brown PO, Botstein D. Molecular portraits of human breast tumours. Nature 2000;**406**:747-752

[65] Sørlie T. Molecular classification of breast tumors: Toward improved diagnostics and treatments. Methods in Molecular Biology. 2007;**360**:91-114

[66] Zolotukhin PV, Dovzhik AD, Lebedeva UA, Kuzminova ON, Mashkina EV, Aleksandrova AA, Shkurat TP. Testing the concept of the interatomic status of the NFE2L2/AP1 pathway as a systemic biomarker for examination stress. Molecular Diagnosis & Therapy. 2014;**18**:355-369

[67] Zolotukhin P, Aleksandrova A, Goncharova A, Shestopalov A, Rymashevskiy A, Shkurat T. Oxidative status shifts in uterine cervical incompetence patients. Systems Biology in Reproductive Medicine. 2014;**60**:98-104

[68] Xin L, Liu YH, Martin TA, Jiang WG. The era of multigene panels comes? The clinical utility of Oncotype DX and MammaPrint. World Journal of Oncology. 2017;**8**:34-40. DOI: 10.14740/wjon1019w

[69] Borisov NM, Terekhanova NV, Aliper AM, Venkova LS, Smirnov PY, Roumiantsev S, Korzinkin MB, Zhavoronkov AA, Buzdin AA. Signaling pathways activation profiles make better markers of cancer than expression of individual genes. Oncotarget. 2014;**5**:10198-10205

[70] Lezhnina K, Kovalchuk O, Zhavoronkov AA, Korzinkin MB, Zabolotneva AA, Shegay PV, Sokov DG, Gaifullin NM, Rusakov IG, Aliper AM, Roumiantsev SA, Alekseev BY, Borisov NM, Buzdin AA. Novel robust biomarkers for human bladder cancer based on activation of intracellular signaling pathways. Oncotarget. 2014;**5**:9022-9032

[71] Cobleigh MA, Tabesh B, Bitterman P, Baker J, Cronin M, Liu ML, Borchik R, Mosquera JM, Walker MG, Shak S. Tumor gene expression and prognosis in breast cancer patients with 10 or more positive lymph nodes. Clinical Cancer Research. 2005;**11**:8623-8631

11

Ovarian Reserve Markers: An Update

Harold Moreno-Ortiz, Iván Darío Acosta,
Elkin Lucena-Quevedo, Luis Alejandro Arias-Sosa,
Alix Eugenia Dallos-Báez, Maribel Forero-Castro and
Clara Esteban-Pérez

Abstract

Ovarian reserve (OR) is defined as the pool of follicles available to provide eggs cells throughout the fertile age in each woman and define the potential of fertility to predict the reproductive lifespan of women. Several studies have focused on the clinical use in order to identify women with a decreased ovarian function and to improve the clinical approach to these patients. In this chapter we will describe different OR markers such as antimullerian hormone (AMH) and follicle stimulating hormone (FSH), count by ultrasound of antral follicles (AFC) and ovarian volume. The measure of OR markers has been reported as an effective test to predict a possible failure of reproductive capacity and important tool in the primary prevention of infertility and other related problems. Therefore, we will show the clinical use of these markers in both healthy and infertile women studies. Additionally, we describe the most recent and promising progress in the OR evaluation by construction of algorithms.

Keywords: ovarian reserve markers, infertility, potential of fertility

1. Introduction

Ovarian reserve (OR) is defined as the pool of follicles available to provide eggs cells throughout the fertile age in each woman [1, 2]. In reproductive medicine, OR reflects the potential of fertility and also predicts the length of reproductive lifespan on female patients [1, 2]. The evaluation of OR allows to identify cases of premature ovarian insufficiency and provide the opportunity to design programs for egg freezing preservation and egg donation. In addition,

OR can predicts the success of the assisted reproductive techniques, oncofertility programs, and infertility counseling programs [3–5].

Some patients with spontaneous follicle depletion show a decrease of OR. A diminished OR (DOR) is related to the decline of the potential of female fertility that accompanies the normal ovarian aging [6].In some cases OR declines before 40 years which is a condition previously known as premature menopause, premature ovarian failure, or early menopause characterized by amenorrhea, hipoestrogenism, and elevated levels serum gonadotropins levels [6]. The decreasing of OR gives rise lower pregnancy rates, repetitive implantation failure, and high risk of miscarriages [3, 7–10]. The negative impact of DOR forces to organize early programs of detection that prevents numerous cases of woman infertility [6, 11, 12]. Additionally, early detection of DOR cases grants a better comprehension of the woman reproductive status to impede expensive assisted treatments and also generates strategies to ameliorate negative effects on emotional condition [6, 11, 12].

Today, the loss of fertility has been related with an increase use of assisted reproductive techniques (ART) [11]. One of the main factors is the delay of the motherhood to advanced age due to social, academic, familiar, economic, and demographic reasons [6, 13]. Unfortunately, mostly cases of advanced maternal age did not receive any medical advice in reproduction and they accept the age as a remarkable reference for fertility [6, 13]. It is known that the female age is not enough fact to determine and predict the individual fertility [6, 13]. Women have wide variations on their reproductive potential and the cessation of fertility can occur in an unexpected way [11, 14–18]. As a consequence, the use of predictive markers that reflects the reproductive status is remarkable and important [11, 14–18]. On the basis of fertility evaluation, health providers can improve plans for counseling for infertile patients and modify the management guides for prevention and promotion of sexual and reproductive health.

In clinical practice, the evaluation of OR can be assessed by blood markers and ultrasound markers. Antimullerian hormone, basal follicle-stimulating hormone, and basal estradiol are the blood markers whilst antral follicular count (AFC) and the ovarian volume are the ultrasound markers [13]. The use of above-mentioned markers permits the categorization and the assessment of fertility potential in female patients [14, 17] and brings the opportunity to design mathematical formulas for further evaluations for each patient.

2. Ovarian reserve

Ovarian reserve (OR) is defined as the pool of follicles available to provide eggs cells throughout the fertile age on female patients. The OR is considered as the biological and reproductive clock and it is a clinical term used to determine the capacity of the ovary to supply eggs for fertilization and resulting in a healthy and successful pregnancy [2].

OR is assured during the embryo development period starting with a cluster of 100 of primordial germinal cells (PGC) in the primary ectoderm (epiblast). In the third week of gestation, PGCs migrate from the primary ectoderm into the yolk sac wall and collect near the exit of the allantois and proliferate colonizing the gonadal ridge to develop the female gonad. At the 20th week of gestation the proliferation of PGCs reaches 6–7 million of oogonias decreasing in a unexplained manner to 1 million of oogonias at the time of birth [19, 20]. The number of follicles continues to decrease and reaching approximately a number of 300000 - 500000 at the puberty time and later 25,000 follicles are identified at age of 35 years [19, 20]. Once the menopause time appears the number of follicles drops to 1000 at age of 51 years [19, 20].

Ovarian reserve assessment is the first step in determining the fertile potential of the ovary. In an effort to predict the status of OR, markers and tests described in the literature for OR evaluation includes: basal follicle-stimulating hormone (FSH), basal estradiol (measured on day 3 of the menstrual cycle), serum antimullerian hormone (AMH), and antral follicular count (AFC) assessed by transvaginal ultrasound [11, 21].

2.1. Ovarian reserve blood markers

Follicle-stimulating hormone (FSH) is a gonadotropin secreted by the anterior pituitary in response to gonadotropin release hormone (GnRH). FSH is responsible for growth and maturation of ovarian follicles and also for estrogen ovarian production [22]. Basal FSH is the most widely marker used for evaluation of OR. Regardless of age, high blood levels of FSH (>10 mUI/ml) at day 3 of the menstrual cycle are related with DOR and reduced fertility. However, there are some concerns about the use of FSH as marker of OR as result of inter and intramenstrual variations, the use of oral contraceptives, and some gynecological pathologies [11, 21].

Antimullerian Hormone (AMH) is a homodimeric glycoprotein secreted by granulose cells (GC) from the ovary. AMH blood levels reflects de overall amount of GC in the antral follicular pool. GCs surround early antral follicles and antral follicles, however AMH expression is found in follicles from primary follicles to 4-mm sized antral follicles [21]. In addition, AMH secreted by 5–8 mm-sized follicles is known to account for 60% of all blood AMH. The AMH level is not affected by the menstrual cycle and it is strongly correlated with the antral follicular count assessed with transvaginal ultrasound at day 1 of menstrual bleeding. AMH indirectly represents the ovarian reserve due to it is well-characterized throughout the female lifespan with increases levels in early childhood, a peak in the early 20s, and subsequently declines gradually with age toward menopause [21, 23–28]. Currently, the blood level of AMH is considered an effective and informative biomarker to evaluate fertility ovarian conditions.

2.2. Potential blood markers in ovarian reserve

Luteinizing hormone (LH) is a pituitary hormone that plays a critical role in folliculogenesis, follicular antrum formation, and development of the thecal vasculature. Additionally, LH is fundamental for supporting steroidogenesis via theca cells-LH receptors [22]. Whilst LH is essential for oocyte maturation, oocyte release, follicular rupture, and embryo implantation, follicles exposed to high concentrations of LH can compromise the normal oocyte development. Basal LH levels in blood rise during reproductive life and peak at the menopause. Although LH levels remain consistent throughout reproductive life, studies have found low predictive value as a marker of ovarian reserve [21]. Currently, in the clinical practice serum LH level is a non-routine marker for OR evaluation.

In the other hand, estradiol is an ovarian steroid involved in the regulation of the menstrual reproductive cycle. Blood levels of estradiol should be measured in the early follicular phase of the menstrual cycle to determine the status of OR [21]. Additionally, basal estradiol has been used to evaluate menopause cases, amenorrhea, and follicular response in ART cases [21]. However, published literature is still controversial in regards to its use of OR marker due to low predictive value and the differences in results from various studies [11, 21, 33]. Therefore, it is recommended that estradiol levels should not be used as an individual marker of OR but also with other markers such as AMH [11, 21, 29].

2.3. Ultrasound markers of OR

Antral Follicle count (AFC) is a conducted transvaginal ultrasound study that assesses the number of antral follicles during the early follicular period. Studies have confirmed that this method of evaluating OR is noninvasive and easy to perform [30]. The number of small antral follicles between 2 and 8 mm of size is closely related to the ovarian function. This number declines with age and the recognition of antral follicles has a significant predictive value in cases of OR conditions, ovarian aging, and reproductive lifespan status. Additionally, AFC is related to ovarian response in cases of controlled ovarian stimulation and it is strongly correlated with AMH levels [31, 32].

Ovarian volume is an indirect ultrasound marker that indicates the condition of individual OR. Calculation of ovarian volume is operator dependent, and has to be studied at the early days of the menstrual cycle [33, 34]. Ovarian volume is the result of follicular size, ovarian stroma and the vascular tissue. Likewise, ovarian volume is affected by age, gynecological conditions, and menstrual cycle phase leading to some limitations for this marker [35]. For this reason, some authors have proposed the use of antral follicular count and ovarian volume as strategy for further evaluation of OR [11, 35].

2.4. Evaluation of ovarian reserve markers in women with no reproductive failure

Research in the field of reproductive medicine is required and is important providing to infertility patients with answers about their behavior of OR markers to establish the fertility condition in normo-ovulatory women and identify patients with poor ovarian reserve. Bentzen et al. [36] described different markers of OR such as antimullerian hormone (AMH), AFC, and the ovarian volume in Danish patients throughout the natural ovarian aging. This research has identified the inverse relationship between age and the ovarian reserve markers showing an average decreasing of 5.6% of AMH levels, 4.4% of AFC, and 1.1% of ovarian volume each year [36]. In 2011 and 2016, two studies evaluated levels of AMH, FSH, and AFC and they found levels of AMH have a high predictive value for menopause individually, however the predictive capacity of AMH levels decrease with age requiring further studies [14, 16]. Different studies showed AMH levels and AFC are critical markers that reflect decreasing of reproductive capacity through the years and the high predictive value for evaluation of menopause [17]. Additionally, La Marca et al. and Grisendi et al. identified the reference levels for AMH, FSH, estradiol and AFC over the fertile life in healthy Italian women [2, 30, 37, 38].

Similarly, Rosen et al. [15] evaluated blood levels of AMH, FSH, estradiol, inhibin B and AFC in a North American population with no reproductive deficiencies. This study confirms that AMH and the AFC are the accurate noninvasive markers for ovarian reserve evaluation due to a significant progressive decline to age while FSH, estradiol and inhibin B did not exhibit significant correlation between age and ovarian reserve [15].

Du et al. [39] established the age-specific reference serum levels for AMH in healthy Chinese women and they found a positive correlation of AMH levels with AFC, testosterone, LH, progesterone, and prolactin levels but a negative correlation with FSH serum levels [39]. Similarly, Tehrani et al. [40] identified the age reference normograms for AMH in a large Iranian population to facilitate the individual clinic interpretation for assessment of ovarian reserve [40].

Okunola et al. [41] evaluated serum levels of AMH and FSH in fertile and subfertile women. They reported significant differences between groups of population related to low ovarian reserve in subfertile women and suggesting that early ovarian aging is associated to decreased number of follicles [41].

Additionally, studies of AMH levels in different ethnicity groups (Caucasians, Hispanics, Afro-Americans, and Asiatic) have shown significant variations. Bleil et al. [42] has shown that Hispanics and Chinese groups exhibit consistent low levels of AMH across all ages compared to Caucasian group supporting possibly a high risk of premature ovarian insufficiency. Similarly, African American group show low levels of AMH at younger ages but less reduction of AMH with advanced age [42], however further studies are needed to validate these results.

Kelsey et al. [33] established a normative validated model of ovarian volume using a systematic review in healthy women. This study found that the ovarian volume has a maximum peak (7.7 mL) at 20 years of age and smaller volumes thereafter leading to generate normal values and ranges for ovarian volume that help to clinicians in the evaluation of fertility conditions [33].

2.5. Evaluation of ovarian reserve markers in women with reproductive failure

Studies have shown the importance of the OR in the reproductive field because of its correlation with infertile patients [43, 44]. Furthermore, researches have been focused in the clinical use of OR to improve the possibility of pregnancy, delay maternity and prevent infertility in young women. Dayal et al. [45] studied the predictive capacity of AMH, FSH, LH, inhibin B, and estradiol with the evaluation of ovarian function from Indian infertile women. They found that AMH has strong correlation to ovarian reserve supporting the association between the number of follicles and AMH blood levels [45]. Similarly, Barbakadze et al. [13] evaluated the correlations between the markers used for OR evaluation such as AMH, FSH, and AFC in 112 infertile women. This study has shown that the use of AMH is best reliable marker for OR evaluation compared to FSH blood levels and the combination of AMH and AFC may improve the assessment of fertility conditions in patients with infertile factors [13].

Likewise, several studies have established reference values of markers as a tool for fertility counseling. Moon et al. [46] developed normograms for AMH, FSH and AFC to predict the ovarian response (number of retrieved oocytes) to the use of exogenous gonadotropins in IVF cycles. Interestingly, they concluded that these normograms might be applied to both high and poor responders [46]. Likewise, Almog et al. [47] showed the data distribution and percentiles were constructed for AMH values of infertile women from Europe and North America [47]. Similarly, Castro et al. [48] developed AFC normograms in Brazilian infertile women as a reference guide to the clinician for individual evaluation in Latin American patients [48].

Interest in research on prediction of ovarian response in assisted reproductive techniques has increased in recent years. Lee et al. [49] studied variations of AMH FSH, LH hormones in Korean women. This study described that basal LH/FSH ratio and AMH level has a valuable clinical meaning as an important predictor of ovarian response in IVF patients [49]. Furthermore, Cohen et al. [10], Keane et al. [50], Zebitay et al. [51], Zheng et al. [52], Goswami et al. [53] and Spressão et al. [54] have shown the important clinical application of AMH and AFC in the fertility counseling on infertile women correlated with pregnancy rates, live birth rates, number of retrieved eggs, fertilization rates and embryo development rates [10, 50–54].

Satwik et al. [55] reported the use of specific markers such as AMH has high predictive value for poor ovarian response compared to age and FSH [55]. Similarly, Mutlu et al. [32] compared AMH, FSH, age, and AFC for prognosis of success in TRA. They found AFC and AMH have significant predictive value of poor ovarian response in IVF patients, however age has significant predictive value of live births [32].

2.6. Proposed algorithm for reproductive determination

Recently, integration of different ovarian reserve markers with high significant statistical value has been proposed by a math equation to calculate reproductive units in Hispanic healthy young women with no signs of reproductive failure [56].

Reproductive units (RU) = (AMH [ng/ml] × total AFC × Ovarian volume [cc])/Chronological age

Calculation of the RU reflects the individual reproductive condition as a tool to prevent reproductive failure from early ages through advanced maternal age. Additionally, RU allows to clinicians provide individual counseling of birth control programs, postpone maternity by egg freeze programs, determine possible ovarian response to exogenous gonadotropins in ART, and prognosis of pregnancy success [56].

3. Discussion and conclusions

Ovarian reserve (OR) is characterized by the number of eggs cells available to be fertilized throughout the female reproductive lifespan. OR is related with the capacity of female fertility suggesting that the clinical potential of measuring different biomarkers is a perfect tool to predict infertility cases. This has led to research to determine the high predictive value of different biomarkers and to increase treatment factors and to prevent new cases of infertility.

Recent studies have investigated biomarkers such as AMH levels and AFC considered first line tests for counseling patients who desire future fertility due to high predictive value. The relevance of FSH, LH, estradiol, ovarian volume, and inhibin B as biomarkers of OR is considered of low potential for clinical evaluation because predictive superiority of other metrics have emerged with robust studies. Nevertheless, recent studies have constructed algorithms to integrate different biomarkers and approach individualized and reliable evaluations to establish with confidence the risk factors of infertility.

Acknowledgements

This work was supported by a grant from the Universidad Pedagógica y Tecnológica de Colombia—Vicerrectoría de Investigación y Extensión (Grupo de Investigación en Ciencias Biomédicas UPTC—GICBUPTC, Escuela de Ciencias Biológicas).

Conflict of interest

The authors have no conflict of interest.

Author details

Harold Moreno-Ortiz[1], Iván Darío Acosta[2], Elkin Lucena-Quevedo[1], Luis Alejandro Arias-Sosa[2], Alix Eugenia Dallos-Báez[2], Maribel Forero-Castro[2]* and Clara Esteban-Pérez[2]

*Address all correspondence to: maribel.forero@uptc.edu.co

1 Department of Reproductive Genetics, Fertility and Sterility Colombian Center (CECOLFES), Bogotá, Colombia

2 Escuela de Ciencias Biológicas, Grupo de Investigación en Ciencias Biomédicas (GICBUPTC). Universidad Pedagógica y Tecnológica de Colombia, Tunja, Colombia

References

[1] Maheshwari A, Fowler P, Bhattacharya S. Assessment of ovarian reserve: Should we perform tests of ovarian reserve routinely? Human Reproduction Oxford University Press. 2006;**21**(11):2729-2735

[2] Grisendi V, Spada E, Argento C, Plebani M, Milani S, Seracchioli R, et al. Age-specific reference values for serum FSH and estradiol levels throughout the reproductive period. Gynecological Endocrinology. 2014;**30**(6):451-455. Available from: http://www.ncbi.nlm.nih.gov/pubmed/24805832

[3] Dua M, Bhatia V, Malik S, Prakash V. ART outcome in young women with premature ovarian aging. Journal of Mid-Life Health [Internet]. Medknow Publications. 2013;**4**(4):230-232. Available from: http://www.ncbi.nlm.nih.gov/pubmed/24381465

[4] Martyn F, O'Brien YM, Wingfield M. Review of clinical indicators, including serum anti-Müllerian hormone levels, for identification of women who should consider egg freezing. International Journal of Gynecology and Obstetrics. 2017;**138**(1):37-41. Available from: http://www.ncbi.nlm.nih.gov/pubmed/28378324

[5] Guzy L, Demeestere I. Assessment of ovarian reserve and fertility preservation strategies in children treated for cancer. Minerva Ginecologica [Internet]. 2017;**69**(1):57-67. Available from: http://www.ncbi.nlm.nih.gov/pubmed/27787477

[6] Bozkurt B, Erdem M, Mutlu MF, Erdem A, Guler I, Mutlu I, et al. Comparison of age-related changes in anti-Müllerian hormone levels and other ovarian reserve tests between healthy fertile and infertile population. Human Fertility. 2016;**19**(3):192-198. Available from: http://www.ncbi.nlm.nih.gov/pubmed/27499425

[7] Lin S, Yang R, Chi H, Lian Y, Wang J, Huang S, et al. Increased incidence of ectopic pregnancy after in vitro fertilization in women with decreased ovarian reserve. Oncotarget. 2017;**8**(9):14570-14575

[8] Kumbak B, Oral E, Kahraman S, Karlikaya G, Karagozoglu H. Young patients with diminished ovarian reserve undergoing assisted reproductive treatments: A preliminary report. Reproductive BioMedicine Online. 2005;**11**(3):294-299. Available from: http://www.ncbi.nlm.nih.gov/pubmed/16176667

[9] Sunkara SK, Khalaf Y, Maheshwari A, Seed P, Coomarasamy A. Association between response to ovarian stimulation and miscarriage following IVF: An analysis of 124 351 IVF pregnancies. Human Reproduction. 2014;**29**(6):1218-1224

[10] Cohen J, Mounsambote L, Prier P. Mathieu d'Argent E, Selleret L, Chabbert-buffet N, et al. outcomes of first IVF/ICSI in young women with diminished ovarian reserve. Minerva Ginecologica. 2017;**69**(4):315-321

[11] de Carvalho BR, Rosa e Silva ACJ de S, Rosa e Silva JC, dos Reis RM, Ferriani RA, Silva de Sá MF. Ovarian reserve evaluation: State of the art. Journal of Assisted Reproduction and Genetics, Springer. 2008;**25**(7):311-322. Available from: http://www.ncbi.nlm.nih.gov/pubmed/18679790

[12] Qin Y, Jiao X, Simpson JL, Chen Z-J. Genetics of primary ovarian insufficiency: New developments and opportunities. Human Reproduction Update. 2015;**21**(6):787-808

[13] Barbakadze L, Kristesashvili J, Khonelidze N, Tsagareishvili G. The correlations of anti-mullerian hormone, follicle-stimulating hormone and antral follicle count in different age groups of infertile women. International Journal of Fertility and Sterility. 2015; **8**(4):393-398. Available from: http://www.ncbi.nlm.nih.gov/pubmed/25780521

[14] Broer SL, Eijkemans MJC, Scheffer GJ, van Rooij IAJ, de Vet A, Themmen APN, et al. Anti-Müllerian hormone predicts menopause: A long-term follow-up study in normoovulatory women. Journal of Clinical Endocrinology and Metabolism, Endocrine

Society Chevy Chase MD. 2011;**96**(8):2532-2539. Available from: http://press.endocrine.org/doi/10.1210/jc.2010-2776

[15] Rosen MP, Johnstone E, McCulloch CE, Schuh-Huerta SM, Sternfeld B, Reijo-Pera RA, et al. A characterization of the relationship of ovarian reserve markers with age. Fertility and Sterility, NIH Public Access. 2012;**97**(1):238-243. Available from: http://www.ncbi.nlm.nih.gov/pubmed/22130324

[16] Depmann M, Eijkemans MJC, Broer SL, Scheffer GJ, van Rooij IAJ, Laven JSE, et al. Does anti-Müllerian hormone predict menopause in the general population? Results of a prospective ongoing cohort study. Human Reproduction. 2016;**31**(7):1579-1587

[17] van Rooij IAJ, Broekmans FJM, Scheffer GJ, Looman CWN, Habbema JDF, de Jong FH, et al. Serum antimullerian hormone levels best reflect the reproductive decline with age in normal women with proven fertility: A longitudinal study. Fertility and Sterility. 2005;**83**(4):979-987. Available from: http://www.ncbi.nlm.nih.gov/pubmed/15820810

[18] te Velde ER, Pearson PL.The variability of female reproductive ageing. Human Reproduction Update. Oxford University Press. 2002;**8**(2):141-154. Available from: http://www.ncbi.nlm.nih.gov/pubmed/12099629

[19] Faddy MJ, Gosden RG, Gougeon A, Richardson SJ, Nelson JF. Accelerated disappearance of ovarian follicles in mid-life: Implications for forecasting menopause. Human Reproduction. 1992;**7**(10):1342-1346. Available from: http://www.ncbi.nlm.nih.gov/pubmed/1291557

[20] Fleming R, Seifer DB, Frattarelli JL, Ruman J. Assessing ovarian response: Antral follicle count versus anti-Müllerian hormone. Reproductive BioMedicine Online. 2015; **31**:486-496

[21] Jamil Z, Fatima SS, Ahmed K, Malik R, Jamil Z, Fatima SS, et al. Anti-Mullerian hormone: Above and beyond conventional ovarian reserve markers. Disease Markers, Hindawi Publishing Corporation. 2016;**2016**:1-9. Available from: http://www.hindawi.com/journals/dm/2016/5246217/

[22] Raju GAR, Chavan R, Deenadayal M, Gunasheela D, Gutgutia R, Haripriya G, et al. Luteinizing hormone and follicle stimulating hormone synergy: A review of role in controlled ovarian hyper-stimulation. Journal of Human Reproductive Sciences. Medknow Publications. 2013;**6**(4):227-234. Available from: http://www.ncbi.nlm.nih.gov/pubmed/24672160

[23] Kucera R, Ulcova-Gallova Z, Topolcan O. Effect of long-term using of hormonal contraception on anti-Müllerian hormone secretion. Gynecological Endocrinology. 2016; **32**(5):383-385. Available from: http://www.ncbi.nlm.nih.gov/pubmed/26651155

[24] Deb S, Campbell BK, Pincott-Allen C, Clewes JS, Cumberpatch G, Raine-Fenning NJ. Quantifying effect of combined oral contraceptive pill on functional ovarian reserve as measured by serum anti-Müllerian hormone and small antral follicle count using three-dimensional ultrasound. Ultrasound in Obstetrics and Gynecology. 2012; **39**(5):574-580. Available from: http://www.ncbi.nlm.nih.gov/pubmed/21997961

[25] Li HWR, Wong CYG, Yeung WSB, Ho PC, Ng EHY. Serum anti-müllerian hormone level is not altered in women using hormonal contraceptives. Contraception. 2011;**83**(6):582-585

[26] Streuli I, Fraisse T, Pillet C, Ibecheole V, Bischof P, de Ziegler D. Serum antimüllerian hormone levels remain stable throughout the menstrual cycle and after oral or vaginal administration of synthetic sex steroids. Fertility and Sterility. 2008;**90**(2):395-400. Available from: http://www.ncbi.nlm.nih.gov/pubmed/17919608

[27] van Disseldorp J, Lambalk CB, Kwee J, Looman CWN, Eijkemans MJC, Fauser BC, et al. Comparison of inter- and intra-cycle variability of anti-Mullerian hormone and antral follicle counts. Human Reproduction. 2010;**25**(1):221-227. Available from: http://www.ncbi.nlm.nih.gov/pubmed/19840990

[28] Overbeek A, Broekmans FJ, Hehenkamp WJ, Wijdeveld ME, van Disseldorp J, van Dulmen-den Broeder E, et al. Intra-cycle fluctuations of anti-Müllerian hormone in normal women with a regular cycle: A re-analysis. Reproductive BioMedicine Online. 2012; **24**(6):664-669. Available from: http://www.ncbi.nlm.nih.gov/pubmed/22503280

[29] Broekmans FJ, Kwee J, Hendriks DJ, Mol BW, Lambalk CB. A systematic review of tests predicting ovarian reserve and IVF outcome. Human Reproduction Update. 2006; **12**(6):685-718. Available from: http://www.ncbi.nlm.nih.gov/pubmed/16891297

[30] La Marca A, Spada E, Sighinolfi G, Argento C, Tirelli A, Giulini S, et al. Age-specific nomogram for the decline in antral follicle count throughout the reproductive period. Fertility and Sterility. 2011;**95**(2):684-688. Available from http://www.ncbi.nlm.nih.gov/pubmed/20797717

[31] Hsu A, Arny M, Knee AB, Bell C, Cook E, Novak AL, et al. Antral follicle count in clinical practice: analyzing clinical relevance. Fertility and Sterility. 2011;**95**(2):474-479. Available from: http://www.ncbi.nlm.nih.gov/pubmed/20434151

[32] Mutlu MF, Erdem M, Erdem A, Yildiz S, Mutlu I, Arisoy O, et al. Antral follicle count determines poor ovarian response better than anti-müllerian hormone but age is the only predictor for live birth in in vitro fertilization cycles. Journal of Assisted Reproduction and Genetics. 2013;**30**(5):657-665

[33] Kelsey TW, Dodwell SK, Wilkinson AG, Greve T, Andersen CY, Anderson RA, et al. Kim S, editor. Ovarian Volume throughout Life: A Validated Normative Model. PLoS One. Public Library of Science; 2013;**8**(9):e71465. Available from: http://dx.plos.org/10.1371/journal.pone.0071465

[34] Chen Y, Li L, Chen X, Zhang Q, Wang W, Li Y, et al. Ovarian volume and follicle number in the diagnosis of polycystic ovary syndrome in Chinese women. Ultrasound in Obste trics and Gynecology. 2008;**32**(5):700-703. Available from http://www.ncbi.nlm.nih.gov/pubmed/18773451

[35] Parry JP, Moran T, Koch CA. Ovarian Reserve Testing [Internet]. Endotext. MDText.com, Inc.; 2000. Available from: http://www.ncbi.nlm.nih.gov/pubmed/25905286

[36] Bentzen JG, Forman JL, Johannsen TH, Pinborg A, Larsen EC, Andersen AN. Ovarian antral follicle subclasses and anti-mullerian hormone during normal reproductive aging. Journal of Clinical Endocrinology and Metabolism. 2013;**98**(4):1602-1611. Available from: http://www.ncbi.nlm.nih.gov/pubmed/23463653

[37] La Marca A, Sighinolfi G, Giulini S, Traglia M, Argento C, Sala C, et al. Normal serum concentrations of anti-Müllerian hormone in women with regular menstrual cycles. Reproductive Biomedicine Online. 2010;**21**(4):463-469

[38] La Marca A, Spada E, Grisendi V, Argento C, Papaleo E, Milani S, et al. Normal serum anti-Müllerian hormone levels in the general female population and the relationship with reproductive history. European Journal of Obstetrics and Gynecology and Reproductive Biology. 2012;**163**(2):180-184. Available from: http://www.ncbi.nlm.nih.gov/pubmed/22579227

[39] Du X, Ding T, Zhang H, Zhang C, Ma W, Zhong Y, et al. Age-specific normal reference range for serum anti-Müllerian hormone in healthy chinese han women: A nationwide population-based study. Reproductive Sciences. 2016;**23**(8):1019-1027. Available from: http://www.ncbi.nlm.nih.gov/pubmed/26763552

[40] Tehrani FR, Mansournia MA, Solaymani-Dodaran M, Azizi F. Age-specific serum anti-Müllerian hormone levels: estimates from a large population-based sample. Climacteric. 2014;**17**(5):591-597. Available from: http://www.ncbi.nlm.nih.gov/pubmed/24716733

[41] Okunola T, Olusegun Ajenifuja K, Morebise Loto O, Salawu A, Omitinde SO. Follicle stimulating hormone and anti-Müllerian hormone among fertile and infertile women in Ile-Ife, Nigeria: Is there a difference? International Journal of Fertility and Sterility, Royan Institute. 2017;**11**(1):33-39. Available from: http://www.ncbi.nlm.nih.gov/pubmed/28367303

[42] Bleil ME, Gregorich SE, Adler NE, Sternfeld B, Rosen MP, Cedars MI. Race/ethnic disparities in reproductive age: An examination of ovarian reserve estimates across four race/ethnic groups of healthy, regularly cycling women. Fertility and Sterility. 2014;**101**(1):199-207

[43] Raeissi A, Torki A, Moradi A, Mousavipoor SM, Pirani MD. Age-specific serum anti-mullerian hormone and follicle stimulating hormone concentrations in infertile Iranian women. International Journal of Fertility and Sterility. 2015;**9**(1):27-32. Available from: http://www.ncbi.nlm.nih.gov/pubmed/25918589

[44] Agarwal A, Verma A, Agarwal S, Shukla RC, Jain M, Srivastava A. Antral follicle count in normal (fertility-proven) and infertile Indian women. Indian Journal of Radiology and Imaging, Medknow Publications. 2014;**24**(3):297-302. Available from: http://www.ncbi.nlm.nih.gov/pubmed/25114395

[45] Dayal M, Sagar S, Chaurasia A, Singh U. Anti-Mullerian hormone: A new marker of ovarian function. Journal of Obstetrics and Gynecology of India, Springer. 2013;**64**(2):130-133

[46] Moon KY, Kim H, Lee JY, Lee JR, Jee BC, Suh CS, et al. Nomogram to predict the number of oocytes retrieved in controlled ovarian stimulation. Clinical and Experimental Reproductive Medicine. 2016;**43**(2):112-118. Available from http://www.ncbi.nlm.nih.gov/pubmed/27358830

[47] Almog B, Shehata F, Suissa S, Holzer H, Shalom-Paz E, La Marca A, et al. Age-related normograms of serum antimüllerian hormone levels in a population of infertile women: A multicenter study. Fertility and Sterility. 2011;**95**(7):2359-2363, 2363.e1. Available from: http://www.ncbi.nlm.nih.gov/pubmed/21457958

[48] de Castro EC, Florêncio R de S, Monteiro Filho G, do Amaral WN. Correlação entre a idade e a contagem dos fol'{\i}culos antrais em mulheres inférteis. Rev Bras Ginecol e Obs. Federação Brasileira das Sociedades de Ginecologia e Obstetricia; 2012;**34**(4):184-188. Available from: http://www.scielo.br/scielo.php?script=sci_arttext&pid=S0100-72032012000400008&lng=pt&nrm=iso&tlng=en

[49] Lee JE, Yoon SH, Kim HO, Min EG. Correlation between the serum luteinizing hormone to folliclestimulating hormone ratio and the anti-Müllerian hormone levels in normo-ovulatory women. Journal of Korean Medical Science. 2015;**30**(3):296-300

[50] Keane K, Cruzat VF, Wagle S, Chaudhary N, Newsholme P, Yovich J. Specific ranges of anti-Mullerian hormone and antral follicle count correlate to provide a prognostic indicator for IVF outcome. Reproductive Biology. 2017;**17**(1):51-59. Available from: http://www.ncbi.nlm.nih.gov/pubmed/28132758

[51] Zebitay AG, Cetin O, Verit FF, Keskin S, Sakar MN, Karahuseyinoglu S, et al. The role of ovarian reserve markers in prediction of clinical pregnancy. Journal of Obstetrics and G ynaecology (Lahore). 2017;**37**(4):492-497. Available from: http://www.ncbi.nlm.nih.gov/pubmed/28421902

[52] Zheng H, Chen S, Du H, Ling J, Wu Y, Liu H, et al. Ovarian response prediction in controlled ovarian stimulation for IVF using anti-Müllerian hormone in Chinese women: A retrospective cohort study. Medicine (Baltimore). Wolters Kluwer Health. 2017;**96**(13):e6495

[53] Goswami M, Nikolaou D. Is AMH level, independent of age, a predictor of live birth in IVF? Journal of Human Reproductive Sciences, Medknow Publications. 2017;**10**(1):24-30. Available from: http://www.ncbi.nlm.nih.gov/pubmed/28479752

[54] Spressão M, Oliani A, Oliani D. Value of the ultrasound in the study of ovarian reserve for prediction of oocyte recovery. Rev Bras Ginecol e Obs/RBGO Gynecology and Obstetrics. 2016;**38**(10):499-505

[55] Satwik R, Kochhar M, Gupta SM, Majumdar A. Anti-mullerian hormone cut-off values for predicting poor ovarian response to exogenous ovarian stimulation in in-vitro fertilization. Journal of Human Reproductive Sciences, Wolters Kluwer – Medknow Publications. 2012;**5**(2):206-212

[56] Acosta ID, Arias Sosa LA. Evaluation of Ovarian Reserve Markers in a Sample of Young Women without Signs of Reproductive Failure. Research thesis. School of Biological Sciences, Universidad Pedagógica y Tecnológica de Colombia; 2017. pp. 57-72

12

Biomarkers in Breast Cancer

Serena Bertozzi, Ambrogio P Londero, Luca Seriau,
Roberta Di Vora, Carla Cedolini and Laura Mariuzzi

Abstract

Breast cancer is the most common cancer in women and its incidence experienced an important increase, thanks to the introduction of a systematic screening. The increased incidence of early breast cancer has led to debates on its over-treatment, which may cause unnecessary harm to patients with favorable prognosis. Therefore, modern research is in the quest of finding the perfect prognostic marker to avoid overtreatment in patients with a favorable prognosis. In this perspective, many molecular markers have been studied in the last decades in order to provide both a useful prognostic tool, able to determine whether the cancer is likely to be indolent or aggressive, and a possible therapeutic target. In this chapter, we review the current knowledge about the principal biomarkers, which are usually immunohistochemically tested on breast surgical specimens, including ER and PR, Mib1/Ki-67 and HER2/neu expression. Furthermore, we will analyze other possible prognostic markers which may have in the future a key role in breast cancer management, such as several multigene panels (OncotypeDX, Mammaprint, NanoString Prosigma). Finally, we will discuss the role of genetic tests for some know genetic mutations associated with higher breast cancer susceptibility (BRCA1 and 2 genes).

Keywords: breast cancer, biomolecular markers, biohumoral markers, therapy target, prognostic factors

1. Introduction

Breast cancer is the most common cancer in women, accounting for about one-third of cancer cases in women and more than 10% of all cancers worldwide [1], and its incidence experienced an important increase, thanks to the introduction at the beginning of this century of a systematic mammographic screening in the most developed countries, and the subsequent successful detection of an always greater number of early breast cancers [2–4]. The incidence of breast cancer is also rapidly rising in developing countries, so that it will become in the next decades a major health burden in both developed and developing countries.

Improvement in the adjuvant chemotherapy and endocrine therapy decreased breast cancer mortality by approximately 50%. However, the increased incidence of early breast cancer has led to debates on its overtreatment, which not only increases social and family burden, but may also cause unnecessary harm to patients with a favorable prognosis [5, 6]. Therefore, the research is focusing on the development of new adjuvant therapies with a more precise target and fewer side effects. In this perspective, many molecular markers have been studied in the last decades in order to provide both a useful prognostic tool, able to determine whether the cancer is likely to be indolent or aggressive [7, 8], and a possible therapeutic target.

Breast cancer includes a heterogeneous group of tumors with a wide spectrum of morphologically and molecularly different subtypes, resulting in different biological behaviors, presentation, and prognosis. Along with the disease stage and the patient performance, the molecular pattern of the tumor is fundamental to identify patients who will particularly benefit from a given treatment. Among the molecular markers associated with breast cancer, the estrogen receptor (ER), the progesterone receptor (PR), the human epidermal growth factor receptor (HER2) and the Mib1/Ki-67 proliferation index are the most important ones and are firmly established in the standard care of all primary, recurrent, and metastatic breast cancer patients.

In this chapter, we review the clinical relevance of the principal biomarkers, which are usually immunohistochemically tested on breast surgical specimens. We discuss about their implication in the prognosis and treatment of breast cancer patients, and thus how this information is translated to treatment decision-making, the valid assays for these markers, and the guidelines for testing them. Furthermore, we analyze other possible prognostic markers which may have in the future a key role in breast cancer management, such as several multigene panels, which have been developed to predict the possibility of distant metastasis in the hormonal receptor-positive disease [9–11]. Finally, we discuss the role of genetic tests for some know genetic mutations associated with higher breast cancer susceptibility in the screening and follow-up of women at high risk.

2. Estrogen and progesterone receptor: Prognosis prediction and treatment planning

Human breast cancer usually depends on sexual hormones for its growth, as it arises from breast tissue that normally responds to endogenous hormones [12]. As in 1896 was firstly noticed that bilteral oophorectomy could induce a significant regression in breast cancer in the fertile age [13], endocrine therapy became quickly a standard of care in the treatment of breast cancer, but only one-third of patients responded.

Then, as in the early 1960s, radiolabeled estrogens were observed to concentrate on specific target organs, the existence of an estrogen receptor (ER) was hypothesized, which could be a predictive factor for the endocrine responsiveness of breast cancer to ovarian ablation [14, 15].

In fact, about 60% of ER-positive tumors, but only about 8% of ER-negative ones showed an objective response to endocrine therapy. The small proportion of patients who respond to hormone therapy with ER-negative disease may be mostly due to false-negative receptor assay results.

The identification of the estrogen receptor has not only proved to be a successful therapeutic target for the treatment and prevention of breast cancer, but has also represented a selective molecular model for all subsequent efforts to design oncological targeted therapies. Estrogen and progesterone receptor (PR), together with the HER2 status represent the most important molecular markers in the standard care of all primary, recurrent, and metastatic breast cancer patients, and the standardized assessment of the ER/PR/HER2 status is crucial in the evaluation of every newly diagnosed breast cancer.

Hormonal receptor-positive disease represents usually an indolent and slowly growing tumor with longer time to recurrence. The responsiveness of a tumor to hormone therapy is an important parameter in breast cancer management in both adjuvant and metastatic settings. The clinical aspects of anti-hormonal treatments are exposed in the following sections.

2.1. Biology of hormone receptors

The ER is a ligand-regulated, cytoplasmic receptor that belongs to the steroid nuclear receptor family, which in the ER-positive breast disease, promotes cell proliferation, survival, and invasion. The key components of ER are the DNA-binding domain, which binds with high affinity and specificity to estrogen response elements (ERE sequence) of DNA to regulate the transcription rates of target genes, and the ligand-binding domain, which binds estrogens [16]. The binding of estrogen to its receptor is essential for its translocation into the nucleus, where it functions as a transcription factor and transduces hormonal signals into a large variety of physiological responses in various target organs.

Two forms of ER, *ERα* and *ERβ*, are encoded by two separate genes that are differentially expressed in tissues. In the normal mammary gland, both *ERα* and *ERβ* bind estradiol to control cell proliferation and differentiation [17, 18]. *ERα* is also responsible for estrogen-induced mitogenic signaling in epithelial cells in breast, uterine, and ovarian tissues [19] and is prevalently expressed by breast cancer cells [20], whereas *ERβ* is usually associated with less aggressive tumors, as it inhibits both *ERα*-mediated transcription and estradiol-induced proliferation in various types of cancer cells [21]. The *ERα*/*ERβ* ratio may play a critical role in the regulation of estradiol activity in breast cancer cells [22].

Estradiol binding to ER activates the receptor through phosphorylation, which undergoes conformational changes and dissociates proteins which usually tightly wrap the DNA [23]. Thereafter, ER binds to the ERE sequence within the gene promoter, and dynamically and sequentially recruits various regulatory protein complexes that contribute to chromatin remodeling and enhance transcriptional activity [24].

ER-mediated transcription involves also other multiple coregulatory proteins, which coordinately act to influence gene transcription, cell cycle regulation, cell differentiation and apoptosis.

Nuclear receptors coactivators of ER include the ubiquitary general transcription factor P300/CBP, some methyltransferases such as CARM1 and PRMT1, some members of the p160 protein family such as the steroid receptor coactivators (SRC1, SRC2, and SRC3) [25, 26].

The regulation of ER and PR function can occur at three levels: differential translation of exons, splicing of their mRNA, and post-translational modifications. These lasts include phosphorylation, ubiquitylation, acetylation, and methylation. Among the multiple kinases that can phosphorylate *ERα* are p38 mitogen-activated protein kinase (MAPK), cyclin A-CDK2, CDK7, c-Src, pp90rsk1, extracellular regulated kinase (Erk) 1 and 2, protein kinase A (PKA) and B (Akt) [27–35]. The effects of this phosphorylation involve receptor turnover, cellular localization, and transcriptional activity and are complex and interdependent. The PR can be phosphorylated at different sites coordinately regulated by ligands or kinases [36].

Few mutations of the *ERα* gene have been reported in the literature, resulting in a receptor with hypersensitivity to the estrogen-mediated growth-promoting effects. These mutations in breast cancer correlate with older age, larger tumor size, nodal involvement, and poor prognosis [37–39].

Along with their classical genomic activity, ER and PR exhibit also a more rapid, nongenomic activity, which occurs within seconds to minutes independently of gene transcription, by mediating signaling cascades originating from the membrane or the cytoplasm through direct interaction with signal-transduction mediators [40, 41]. ER may establish a cross talk with other signal transduction pathways, such as that of growth factors, using its membrane and cytoplasmic receptors to transmit their signals through kinase cascades, triggering the phosphorylation and activation of the epidermal growth factor receptors (EGFR), insulin-like growth factor-1R (IGF-1R), transforming growth factor (TGF)α, Src kinase, Shc adaptor protein, and phosphatidylinositol 3-kinase (PI3K), and the inhibition of TGFβ and tyrosine phosphatases [20, 42–45]. Finally, ER may also use calcium, cyclic adenosine monophosphate (cAMP), and other second messengers for signal transduction.

2.2. Clinical relevance of hormone receptors

Hormone receptors are expressed by about two-thirds of invasive breast cancers in women younger than 50 and approximately 80% of tumors in women older than 50 [46]. Measurement of hormone receptors has become a routine part of the evaluation of breast cancers, as they represent a predictive factor for hormone therapy responsiveness. Both ER and PR increasing levels directly correlate with better response, longer time to treatment failure, and longer survival [47, 48].

Hormone receptor expression represents also an important favorable prognostic factor, being an important marker of growth rate, rather than metastatic potential. In particular, patients with ER+/PR+ tumors have a better prognosis than patients with ER+/PR- tumors, who in turn have a better prognosis than patients with ER-/PR- tumors [49]. ER expression is significantly associated with some favorable prognostic indicators, such as older age, low grading, lower fraction of dividing cells, lower genetic mutation, but not with nodal involvement [46, 50–53].

Adjuvant hormone therapy can halve the recurrence rate of patients with ER-positive breast cancer [54] and, due to its quite limited side effects, it can be administered with success also in the elderly or in the presence of comorbidities, and responses can last for many years in some patients with metastatic disease. Patients with stage I ER-positive breast cancer, who receive no systemic therapy, have a 5–10% lower probability of recurrence at 5 years in comparison with ER-negative patients [55]. On the other hand, in ER-negative tumors are unlikely to respond to hormone therapy and respond better to cytotoxic chemotherapy.

The literature demonstrates that the benefit of 5 years of adjuvant tamoxifen treatment depends on the tumor ER and PR status [54, 56], and the efficacy of tamoxifen in reducing local, contralateral and distant relapse or death was strongly confirmed by more recent large prospective trials [57, 58]. A marginally significant relationship between ER level and time to recurrence was observed also in patients treated with aromatase inhibitors [59]. However, studies about adjuvant tamoxifen in early breast cancers did not show any benefit of PR expression among ER-positive patients, but only a benefit among ER-negative patients [54, 60, 61]. Definitely, ER+/PR+ tumors had a 15–30% lower risk of recurrence and death than ER+/PR- ones [49].

Hormone therapy may be an interesting option also in the advanced disease, as the level of ER expression is associated with good responses in the ER-positive disease, and provides good palliation, better quality of life, and improved survival [62]. In fact, approximately 30–40% of patients with ER-positive metastatic disease will respond to first-line hormone therapies, another 20% will experience disease stabilization, and despite a gradual efficacy decline, about 20–30% will respond to subsequent lines of hormone therapy [63]. ER status is also prognostic for the site of metastasis, metastasizing ER-positive tumors more frequently to the bone, soft tissue, or the reproductive and genital tracts, and ER-negative ones to visceral organs or the brain [64].

As the hormone receptor status of the metastases should be more predictive than that of the primary tumor, before making treatment decisions, the molecular markers of breast cancer should be retested in the metastatic lesions when possible, due to the risk of discordance between the hormone receptor status between the relapse/metastases and the primary tumor. In fact, a conversion rate of 20–30% has been reported from ER-positive to ER-negative status, related with a poorer prognosis, while less frequent conversion has been reported from ER-negative to ER-positive status [65–68]. The same happens for what concerns PR expression in metastatic lesions, which often converts from PR-positive to PR-negative [66, 67].

Beyond the probable technical causes of false-negative or false-positive results, possible explanations for the hormone status changes include the tumor dedifferentiation over time and the intratumoral heterogeneity, leading to clonal selection of hormone receptor negative and more resistant clones, as an adaptive mechanism to prior treatments [68]. Apart from the hormon status change, the resistance to endocrine therapy may be explained by the modulation of many cellular signaling networks, which usually provide alternative mitogenic and survival stimuli for the cells. Therefore, multigene predictive scores have been developed to predict tumors hormonal responsiveness, such as the Oncotype DX 21 gene assay, which includes several downstream ER-regulated genes and several proliferation genes in addition to ER mRNA, and will be discussed in another section [11].

The results of adjuvant chemotherapy trials support that ER-negative tumors derive more benefit from chemotherapy than ER-positive ones, as well as luminal A (ER/PR+/HER2-) tumors [54, 69]. A study comparing adjuvant TAC (docetaxel-adriamycin-cyclophosphamide) with FAC (fluorouracil-adriamycin-cyclophosphamide) showed a benefit of adding taxanes regardless of ER status, as they exhibit endocrine effects by inducing amenorrhea in premenopausal women [70]. On the other hand, as expected, the ovarian ablative effects of chemotherapy are not observed in postmenopausal patients. Neoadjuvant chemotherapy trials have also shown the effect of ER status in pathologic complete response (pCR) rates, which result significantly higher in the ER-positive group than in ER-negative one [71].

2.3. Methods for measuring hormone receptors

Various assay methods have been used to measure ER expression in breast cancer specimens, which is fundamental for the therapeutic planning. The dextran-coated charcoal/ligand-binding assay (DCC/LBA) was the first available standard inked immunosorbent assay (ELISA). Thereafter, since 1990s, immunohistochemistry (IHC) of formalin-fixed paraffin-embedded specimens began to replace the DCC assay because it needs smaller tissue amounts, does not require fresh/frozen tissue, correlates staining with histology, and allows the storage and retrieval of archived slides for later testing [72].

The last guidelines for hormone receptor testing, reported by the Society of Clinical Oncology (ASCO)/Collage of American Pathologists (CAP) in 2010, establish mandatory proficiency testing and inspection criteria to improve the accuracy of these tests [73]. Breast resection specimens should be fixed as quickly as possible (within 1 h from reesection) in an adequate volume of fixative (optimally 10-fold greater than the volume of the specimen). After being received in the pathology laboratory, specimens should be oriented and carefully inked for surgical margin assessment, sectioned at 5 mm intervals, and placed in 10% neutral (phosphate) buffered formalin for no less than 6 h and for not more than 72 h before processing.

After treatment for antigen retrieval, the tissue sections are incubated with a primary antibody directed against the ER or PR, and subsequently with a secondary detection systems that are conjugated to an enzyme to amplify the chromogenic signal, and finally microscopically evaluated. External and internal controls can be used to ensure the proper performance of IHC test. The percentage of cells with nuclear staining is reported by either estimation or quantitation, which may be performed either manually or by image analysis. Both the average intensity (weak, moderate, strong) and extent of staining (as a percentage) are reported. ER or PR expression is considered positive or negative in case of immunoreaction in respectively ≥1 or <1% of tumor cell nuclei [73].

3. HER2/neu testing: Prognosis prediction and targeted therapies

3.1. Biology of HER2/neu

The human epidermal growth factor receptor 2 (HER2/neu) gene, localized on chromosome 17, encodes a a 185 kDa, transmembrane member of the tyrosine kinase epidermal growth factor receptors, which are normally expressed at low levels in all epithelial cells in normal fetal and adult tissues, but are also essential for cancer proliferation and survival [74]. HER2 gene amplification has been associated with increased levels of expression of HER2 mRNA and protein product, which lead to oncogenic signaling and resultant self-sufficiency in growth signals, uncontrolled proliferation, sustained angiogenesis, survival, enhanced invasion, and metastasis processes, which are drivers of carcinogenesis [75–77]. The HER2/neu gene results amplified in a variable percentage of breast [77, 78], ovarian [77], bladder, endometrial [79], salivary gland [80], and gastric cancer [81].

The human epidermal growth factor receptor (HER) family consists of four members: EGFR/ErbB1, HER2/ErbB2, HER3/ErbB3, and HER4/ErbB4. The structure of these receptors consists of a ligand-binding extracellular domain, a transmembrane domain, and a cytoplasmic catalytic kinase domain that drives downstream signaling pathways, such as the PI3K/Akt/mTOR and RAS/RAF/MEK/ERK ones [82]. HER heterodimers are more potent in signal transduction than are homodimers. HER2 is the preferred partner for dimerization, triggering with its overexpression breast cancer progression with a poor prognosis, and the HER2-HER3 heterodimer is known to be the most potent oncogenic combination in breast cancer.

HER2 overexpression ultimately activates ligand-independent HER2/HER3/PI3K complex formation and kinase activity in tumor cells, so that the resistance to trastuzumab can be circumvented through PI3K inhibition, as well as gain-of-function mutations of PI3K and the loss of PTEN. Furthermore, the upregulation of insulin-like growth factor receptor 1 (IGF-1R) results in sustained activation of the PI3K/Akt pathway, thereby leading to resistance to anti-hormonal and HER2-targeted therapies.

3.2. Clinical relevance of HER2/neu

Having a look at the currrent literature, HER2 results amplified in approximately 15–30% of breast cancers [75, 83]. HER2 overexpression, in the absence of adjuvant treatment, correlates with a poor prognosis in terms of both overall and disease-free survival, independent of tumor size, grade and hormone receptor status [84]. However, HER2 is also an important predictive marker for responsiveness to HER2-targeted therapies, in both metastatic and adjuvant settings [85, 86].

Trastuzumab, the most famous humanized monoclonal antibody against HER2, significantly improves response rates, time to progression and survival when used alone or added to chemotherapy in both early stage and metastatic breast cancer [87]. Other HER2-targeted drugs, including the tyrosine kinase inhibitor lapatinib, the antibody pertuzumab, and the antibody drug conjugate adotrastuzumab emtansine (T-DM1), improve outcomes in HER2-positive metastatic breast cancer [88–90].

A controversial association exists between HER2 positivity and resistance to hormone therapies, but randomized trials in either adjuvant or metastatic settings failed to provide supporting evidence. [91]. This probably happens due to a physiological cross talk between the HER2 and ER signal transduction pathways, but other mechanisms of hormone independent endocrine resistance of HER2-expressing cells have been described, such as phosphorylation of the ER, ligand-independent ER activation, and regulation of hormone receptor expression [92]. Moreover, some data suggest that endocrine resistance may be specific to selective estrogen modulator (SERM) therapy such as tamoxifen and perhaps not to estrogen depletion therapies such as aromatase inhibitors [59, 93]. Furthermore, the response to ligand-depleting therapies such as ovarian ablation or aromatase inhibitors is not affected by HER2 overexpression.

HER2 may be associated with either sensitivity or resistance to some chemotherapeutic agents. For example, HER2 positivity is associated with better outcomes in response to adjuvant anthracycline containing regimens in most studies, probably due to the coamplification of HER2 with topoisomerase II, which is the direct target of anthracyclines [94]. Anyway, the combination of trastuzumab and anthracycline has cardiotoxicity concerns, so that an accurate determination of HER2 alterations in breast carcinomas is mandatory. On the other hand, data about the possibile correlation of HER2 positivity with responsiveness to paclitaxel containing chemotherapy are still contradictory [95].

3.3. Methods for measuring HER2/neu

HER2 gene amplification is directly correlated with its mRNA expression and protein levels, and HER2 status can potentially be evaluated at any of these levels. A great number of commercially available testing kits are approved from FDA for the assessment of patients suitable for the treatment whit trastuzumab (humanized mouse 4D5 monoclonal antibody) may be a suitable treatment. Overexpression of the HER2 protein product may be evaluated by Western blotting, ELISA or IHC; overexpression of its mRNA by Northern blotting or RT-PCR, and its gene amplification by fluorescence (FISH), chromogenic (CISH) or silver-enhanced in situ hybridization (SISH) [96].

FISH is more accurate, reproducible, and robust than IHC [97], but IHC has been more widely used as the primary test for HER2 status because it results quicker, is viewed using a conventional bright-field microscope, permits parallel viewing of tumor morphological features, and stained tissues do not degrade over time [98]. Moreover, automated IHC techniques may enable more rapid testing.

Recommendations for tissue handling as well as preanalytic, analytic, and postanalytic factors in ER/PR testing are also suitable for HER2 testing. Laboratories performing these tests should follow all accreditation requirements, which conform to the 2010 ASCO/CAP recommendations for ER/PR testing, one of which is the initial testing validation [83]. Laboratories are responsible for ensuring the reliability and accuracy of their testing results and should review and document external and internal controls with each test and each batch of tests.

The final IHC result is classified as 3+ in the case of a complete circumferential membrane staining in >10% of neoplastic cells, 2+ in the presence of moderate circumferential membrane staining of >10% of neoplastic cells, 1+ or 0 if there is incomplete membrane staining or no staining in >10% of neoplastic cells. A positive result includes the 3+ and the 2+ in the presence of a ISH confirmation [83].

4. Mib1/Ki-67: Prognosis prediction and treatment planning

Numerous measures of tumor cell proliferation have been studied over time, including thymidine labeling index, flow cytometry and S-phase fraction, thymidine kinase, cyclins D and E and their inhibitors p27 and p21, topoisomerase $II\alpha$, p53, bax, bcl-2, and Ki67, but methodological shortcomings precluded attribution of prognostic or predictive significance to any of these potential markers [99].

The mitotic index, which is one of the three components of the tumor grading assessment, results the strongest prognostic discriminant in node-negative breast cancer, being the most significant predictor of survival, and rendering less significant the other two elements of tumor grading evaluation, pleomorphism and tubular formation [100]. In particular, patients with mitotic index ≥10 should be considered at high risk and be offered adjuvant therapy.

Mib1/Ki-67 is a proliferation index used as both a prognostic and predictive marker, although its widespread use is limited by the lack of standardization of the assay and its interpretation [99, 101]. This marker of proliferation results an independent prognostic factor for DFS, is significantly predictive for responsiveness to both adjuvant chemotherapy and endocrine therapy, and is predictive for pathological complete response in the neoadjuvant setting [102, 103]. In fact, the Mib1/Ki-67 decrease in the post-treatment samples of women who underwent neoadjuvant therapies is a strong independent predictor of better clinical outcomes [104].

5. Genomic markers, prognosis, and personalized treatment

In the past, breast cancers were simply treated based on some clinicopathological features, such as tumor size, lymph node status, patients age and menopausal status, and tumor biomarkers such as ER, PR, and HER2/neu. Then, systemic chemotherapy was applied nearly universally to locally advanced breast cancers regardless of their biomolecular profile, and to about 60% of early breast cancers, but often without any significant effect on women prognosis [105]. As a consequence, a great debate has emerged about quality-of-life issues, acute and long-term side effects of systemic therapies, and the cost of unnecessary treatments [54, 106]. Therefore, in the last decades, quantitative approaches for prognosis prediction and treatment individualization have been developed, and genomic and molecular technologies are routinely applied to prevent overtreatments.

Recently, thanks to the increased level of knowledge regarding the molecular pathways and underlying genetic changes in breast cancer, the molecular signatures of gene expression have been correlated with breast cancer recurrence risk [7, 107, 108]. Anyway, their current clinical application is still limited due to reproducibility questions and the need for fresh or frozen tissue.

In this section, we discuss about susceptibility genes, the carriers of which results to have an increased breast cancer risk and consequently deserve a more frequent and specific screening, and about some signatures, which are usually used to predict breast cancer responsiveness to adjuvant and neoadjuvant therapies.

5.1. BRCA1 and BRCA2

Inherited susceptibility to breast cancer has been hypothesized due to the discovery and characterization of a number of high-risk, relatively uncommon genes responsible for the clustering of breast cancer in certain families, which thereafter had a significantly increased risk in comparison with the general population [109, 110]. Many studies suggest that breast cancer susceptibility is transmitted in an autosomal dominant mendelian way [111], but the actual risk of developing breast cancer in a mutation carrier is based on the penetrance of the gene, which consists in the likelihood that the effect (phenotype) of a mutation (genotype) will become clinically apparent.

The BRCA1 gene was firstly identified in 1994 [112] and is localized on the 17th chromosome, whereas the BRCA2 gene was found some years after and is localized on the 13th chromosome [113]. The big size of these genes is important in the context of genetic testing because of the increased probability of mutations and the consequent technically demanding and costly mutations testing, but fortunately the use of modern next generation DNA sequencing is already overcoming these technical and cost issues. Moreover, the BRCA1 gene contains a large number of repetitive elements that facilitate the generation of large deletions and duplications.

BRCA1 is a nuclear protein with two important regions of sequence similarity with known functional motifs: a 42–amino-acid RING (Really Interesting New Gene) domain at the beginning of BRCA1 which binds zinc and is essential in cell growth and differentiation, and the BRCT (breast cancer-1 terminus) motif at the carboxyl terminus, which acts as a phosphoprotein docking motif and a transcriptional activation domain [114, 115]. BRCA2 is also a nuclear protein composed of the following major structural motifs: the eight tandem BRC repeats in the central portion of the protein, which mediates the critical interaction of BRCA2 and RAD51, the TR2 at the carboxyl terminus, which binds RAD51 exists, a single-strand and double-strand DNA binding domain in the C-terminus [113, 116].

Both BRCA1 and BRCA2 genes encode large proteins with multiple functions, which act mainly as tumor suppressor gene products, affecting transcription, cell cycle regulation, genome stability maintenance, and repair of doublestranded DNA breaks for protection of the genome during replication [117, 118]. In particular, BRCA1 prevents replication of damaged DNA by altering chromatin structure and nucleosome organization at the local site of damage, facilitates access by repair complexes, and promotes the use of the error-free repair pathway of homologous recombination-mediated repair rather than the error-prone process of nonhomologous end joining [118]. BRCA2 affects the choice between the two homologous recombination pathways in favor of the error-free one, by interacting with RAD51 [118]. When the wild-type BRCA1 or BRCA2 allele is lost, mutated, or silenced, a high degree of chromosome instability is observed and defective DNA repair may occur, with the consequent accumulation of additional mutations during replication and promotion of carcinogenesis [119].

Mutations in BRCA1 and BRCA2 genes are the most frequent hereditary genetic aberrations in breast cancer and account for approximately half of all hereditary breast cancers. Initial estimates found BRCA1 mutations to be responsible for 45–90% of breast cancer cases in families with apparent autosomal dominant transmission of breast cancer, and this percentage rises if the median age at onset of breast cancer is younger than 45 years [120, 121]. Estimates of BRCA1 and BRCA2 mutation prevalence in unselected patients with breast cancer are in the range of 2–3% [122].

Among BRCA1 mutation carriers, the estimated breast cancer risk is about 65%, the estimated risk of contralateral breast cancer occurrence results 60%, the cumulative risk of ovarian cancer varies between 27 and 45%, and there is also a significantly increased risk of fallopian tube, uterine and cervical cancer, as well as of male breast cancer, stomach, pancreatic, colon and testicular cancer [123–126].

Among BRCA2 mutation carriers, the estimated lifetime breast cancer risk ranges between 45 and 84%, and that of ovarian cancer between 10 and 20% [123, 127]. There is an increased male breast cancer risk of about 6%, as well as an increased risk of prostate, pancreatic, stomach, gallbladder and bile duct cancers, and malignant melanoma [122, 128].

More than 500 coding region sequence variations have been detected in BRCA1 and 250 in BRCA2. Most unequivocally confirmed mutations reported to date are truncating mutations, adding little in the way of clues for defining functional regions. Although few mutations have been identified in either gene in sporadic breast cancers, a phenotype termed "BRCAness" exist, in which the BRCA1 and BRCA2 proteins act may be somehow disrupted also in sporadic cancer [129]. Finally, there are also some syndromes characterized by an increased breast cancer susceptibility, which are discussed in the following section.

Although germline mutations in BRCA1 and BRCA2 confer a high risk of breast cancer, a great deal of variability has been observed in cancer risk among individuals, both between and within families, as many environmental or genetic factors can modify the penetrance of BRCA1 and BRCA2 mutations. The Consortium of Investigators of Modifiers of BRCA1 and BRCA2 (CIMBA), analyzing DNA and clinical data from approximately 10,000 BRCA1 and 5000 BRCA2 mutation carriers, demonstrated the role of a number of gene variants in affecting the penetrance in mutation carriers [130].

The most important prognostic modifiers of BRCA1 and BRCA2 mutation carriers are prophylactic oophorectomy and the use of tamoxifen for chemoprevention, which approximately halve the breast cancer risk and decrease the risk of ovarian cancer by about 95% [131, 132].

In comparison with sporadic breast cancers, those related with high-penetrance susceptibility genes correlate with younger age at diagnosis, more aggressive tumor biological behavior, bilaterality, and the eventual coexistence of other cancers in the same individual or in other individuals of the same family, including ovarian, colon, prostate, pancreatic, and endometrial cancers, as well as sarcomas and male breast cancer [133].

Breast cancers arising in BRCA1 mutation carriers are frequently, although not exclusively, basal-like and ER-negative, probably because BRCA1 plays a crucial role in the transcriptional regulation of ER [129, 134]. On the other hand, breast cancer originated in BRCA2 mutation carriers are typically much more similar to sporadic cases, despite with higher grading, higher frequency of ER-positivity and lower frequency of HER2/neu overexpression [135].

Breast cancer prognosis in BRCA1 and BRCA2 mutation carriers is still controversial, and if some authors describe a worse prognosis even in classically low-risk node-negative disease [136], other exclude any significant difference if compared to the general breast cancer population [137]. Furthermore, BRCA1 and BRCA2 mutation carriers result to have an increased risk of contralateral breast cancer occurrence [138].

New drugs have been purposed as a promising therapeutic strategy in BRCA defective tumor cells, such as the inhibitors of the poly(adenosine diphosphate-ribose) polymerase-1 (PARP1), which is an enzyme involved in the single-stranded DNA repair that use base excision repair.

Other breast cancer susceptibility genes have been described, which can be divided into three categories in terms of mutation risk and the frequency of mutation. Along with BRCA1 and BRCA2 gene mutation, the first category includes PTEN and TP53 gene mutations, which are classified as high-penetrance, low-frequency predisposition genes, and the occurrence of even one of these mutations can increase the risk of breast cancer to 25% [139, 140]. The second category includes the CHEK2, ATM, PALB and BRIP1 2 genes, which are moderate-penetrance, low-frequency predisposition genes, and lead to an increased risk of cancer of twofold to fourfold [110]. Finally, the third category consists of the FGFR2, MAP3K1,and TGFB1 gene mutations, which are low-penetrance, high-frequency predisposition genes [141].

5.2. Multigene signatures

In the last decades, many genomic and molecular classification have been described with a prognostic intent. The most famous divides breast cancers into the following subtypes: luminal A, luminal B, HER2-enriched, basal-like, and normal-like [142]. Luminal subtypes express high levels of ER, they usually have an indolent clinical course, with a low distant recurrence rate, which anyway persists even up to 15 years after the diagnosis. Luminal B subtypes express fewer ER-related genes, have a higher proliferation rate and may overexpress HER2/neu, so that they usually require to be treated with both hormonal therapy and chemotherapy. HER2-enriched subtype exhibits HER2/neu gene amplification but does not express ER-related genes, they have an aggressive natural clinical course but fortunately respond very well to HER2-targeted therapy. The basal-like or triple-negative subtype does not express ER, PR, and HER2/neu but expresses basal cytokeratins 5/6 and 17, they have a poor prognosis and a high recurrence rate.

The first molecular signature of breast cancer was determined in 2000 by the expression of a set of genes within the tumor, which were able to predict the clinical outcome [143]. The main limitations of gene signature profiling include difficulties in reproducing the specific gene sets, testing expense, and reporting standardization. However, gene signature cannot be substituted by IHC surrogates which have significant discordances with genetic profiling [144].

The three multigene tests for breast cancer which are commercially available and currently used in the clinical practice are the Oncotype DX test (Genomic Health, Redwood, CA, USA), the MammaPrint test (Netherlands Cancer Institute™ and Agendia™, Netherland), and the Prosigma one (NanoString Technologies, Seattle, WA, USA). The Oncotype DX test is the most widely used molecular test in the therapeutic decision-making, is strongly predictive for endocrine responsiveness in hormone receptor-positive breast cancers with 0–3 positive nodes, and is recommended by both the National Comprehensive Cancer Network (NCCN) and the St. Gallen Consensus [7, 145, 146].

The Oncotype DX is a real-time reverse transcriptase chain reaction (RT-PCR) assay, which measures the expression of a panel of 21 genes in formalin-fixed paraffin-embedded samples, including 16 cancer-related genes (ER, PR, Bcl2, SCUBE2, HER2, GRB7, Ki-67, STK15, survivin, cyclin B1, MYBL2, stromelysin 3, cathepsin L2, GSTM1, CD68, and BAG1) and 5 housekeeping control genes (beta-actin, GAPDH, RPLPO, GUS, and TFRC), to generate a recurrence score to stratify breast cancer patients into three risk groups. The low risk group (score < 18), the intermediate (score 18–30), and the high risk one (score ≥ 31) have a 10-year distant recurrence rate of respectively 6.8, 14.3, and 30.5% [144].

The MammaPrint assay is the second most commonly ordered molecular test approved by the US-FDA and measure the expression of 70 genes involved in the cell cycle, invasion, proliferation, angiogenesis, metastasis, and signal transduction, none of which is tested by the Oncotype DX assay. The MammaPrint customized microarray contains a reduced set of 1900 probes suitable for high-throughput processing, and allows the use of less RNA and a short processing time of 5 days. This assay can be applied in both node-positive and node-negative and both hormone-positive and hormone-negative cancers, it is predictive for responsiveness to chemotherapy and prognostic for early distant recurrence within the first 10 years after diagnosis, which results 13 and 56% respectively in the low- and high-risk group [147–149].

The Prosigna test is an assay approved by the US-FDA which measures the expression of 50 target genes and 5 constitutively expressed normalization genes, using a proprietary technology called the "nCounter Dx Analysis System." The assay is highly sensitive and precise and uses 250 ng of RNA from formalin-fixed paraffine-embadded tumor tissue, and generates a risk of recurrence score, which assesses the 10-year risk of distant recurrence for hormone receptor-positive stage I–III breast cancers to be treated with adjuvant endocrine therapy, and correlates to one of the five molecular subtypes previously described [143, 150]. The Prosigna assay results superior to the Oncotype DX test in predicting late distant recurrence after 5–10 years [9, 151].

Acknowledgements

The authors would like to thank the whole collaborating staff of the Universitât dal Friûl, and the support from Ennergi research non-profit association.

Author details

Serena Bertozzi[1*†], Ambrogio P Londero[2†], Luca Seriau[1], Roberta Di Vora[1], Carla Cedolini[1] and Laura Mariuzzi[3]

*Address all correspondence to: ambrogio.londero@gmail.com

1 Breast Unit, Clinic of Surgery, DAME, University of Udine, University Hospital of Udine, Udine, Italy

2 Clinic of Obstetrics and Gynecology, University Hospital of Udine, Udine, Italy

3 Institute of Pathologic Anatomy, DAME, University of Udine, University Hospital of Udine, Udine, Italy

† These authors contributed equally.

References

[1] Jemal A, Center MM, De Santis C, Ward EM. Global patterns of cancer incidence and mortality rates and trends. Cancer Epidemiology Biomarkers and Prevention. 2010;**19**: 1893-1907. DOI: 10.1158/1055-9965.epi-10-0437

[2] Bleyer A, Welch HG. Effect of three decades of screening mammography on breast-cancer incidence. The New England Journal of Medicine. 2012;**367**:1998-2005. DOI: 10.1056/NEJMoa1206809

[3] Driul L, Bernardi S, Bertozzi S, Schiavon M, Londero AP, Petri R. New surgical trends in breast cancer treatment: Conservative interventions and oncoplastic breast surgery. Minerva Ginecologica. 2013;**65**:289-296

[4] Cedolini C, Bertozzi S, Londero AP, Bernardi S, Seriau L, Concina S, et al. Type of breast cancer diagnosis, screening, and survival. Clinical Breast Cancer. 2014;**14**:235-240. DOI: 10.1016/j.clbc.2014.02.004

[5] Esserman LJ, Thompson IM, Reid B. Overdiagnosis and overtreatment in cancer: An opportunity for improvement. Journal of the American Medical Association. 2013;**310**: 797-798. DOI: 10.1001/jama.2013.108415

[6] Katz SJ, Morrow M. Addressing overtreatment in breast cancer: The doctors' dilemma. Cancer. 2013;**119**:3584-3588. DOI: 10.1002/cncr.28260

[7] van't Veer LJ, Dai H, van de Vijver MJ, He YD, Hart AAM, Mao M, et al. Gene expression profiling predicts clinical outcome of breast cancer. Nature2002; **415**:530–536. DOI: 10.1038/415530a

[8] Wang Y, Klijn JGM, Zhang Y, Sieuwerts AM, Look MP, Yang F, et al. Gene-expression profiles to predict distant metastasis of lymph-node-negative primary breast cancer. Lancet (London, England). 2005;**365**:671-679. DOI: 10.1016/S0140-6736(05)17947-1

[9] Naoi Y, Noguchi S. Multi-gene classifiers for prediction of recurrence in breast cancer patients. Breast cancer (Tokyo, Japan). 2016;**23**:12-18. DOI: 10.1007/s12282-015-0596-9

[10] Harris LN, Ismaila N, McShane LM, Andre F, Collyar DE, Gonzalez-Angulo AM, et al. Use of biomarkers to guide decisions on adjuvant systemic therapy for women with early-stage invasive breast cancer: American Society of Clinical Oncology clinical practice guideline. Journal of Clinical Oncology : Official Journal of the American Society of Clinical Oncology. 2016;**34**:1134-1150. DOI: 10.1200/JCO.2015.65.2289

[11] Sparano JA, Gray RJ, Makower DF, Pritchard KI, Albain KS, Hayes DF, et al. Prospective validation of a 21-gene expression assay in breast cancer. The New England Journal of Medicine. 2015;**373**:2005-2014. DOI: 10.1056/NEJMoa1510764

[12] Zumoff B, Fishman J, Bradlow HL, Hellman L. Hormone profiles in hormone-dependent cancers. Cancer Research. 1975;**35**:3365-3373

[13] Stockwell S. Classics in oncology. George Thomas Beatson, M.D. (1848–1933). CA: A Cancer Journal for Clinicians. 1983;**33**:105-121

[14] Jensen EV, Jordan VC. The estrogen receptor: a model for molecular medicine. Clinical Cancer Research: An Official Journal of the American Association for Cancer Research. 2003;**9**:1980-1989

[15] McGuire WL. Current status of estrogen receptors in human breast cancer. Cancer. 1975; **36**:638-644

[16] Klinge CM. Estrogen receptor interaction with estrogen response elements. Nucleic Acids Research. 2001;**29**:2905-2919

[17] Helguero LA, Faulds MH, Gustafsson JA, Haldosén LA. Estrogen receptors alfa (ERalpha) and beta (ERbeta) differentially regulate proliferation and apoptosis of the normal murine mammary epithelial cell line HC11. Oncogene. 2005;**24**:6605-6616. DOI: 10.1038/sj.onc.1208807

[18] Grober OMV, Mutarelli M, Giurato G, Ravo M, Cicatiello L, De Filippo MR, et al. Global analysis of estrogen receptor beta binding to breast cancer cell genome reveals an extensive interplay with estrogen receptor alpha for target gene regulation. BMC Genomics. 2011;**12**:36. DOI: 10.1186/1471-2164-12-36

[19] Ali S, Coombes RC. Estrogen receptor alpha in human breast cancer: Occurrence and significance. Journal of Mammary Gland Biology and Neoplasia. 2000;**5**:271-281

[20] Renoir JM, Marsaud V, Lazennec G. Estrogen receptor signaling as a target for novel breast cancer therapeutics. Biochemical Pharmacology. 2013;**85**:449-465. DOI: 10.1016/j.bcp.2012.10.018

[21] Paruthiyil S, Parmar H, Kerekatte V, Cunha GR, Firestone GL, Leitman DC. Estrogen receptor beta inhibits human breast cancer cell proliferation and tumor formation by causing a G2 cell cycle arrest. Cancer Research. 2004;**64**:423-428

[22] Matthews J, Gustafsson JA. Estrogen signaling: A subtle balance between ER alpha and ER beta. Molecular Interventions. 2003;**3**:281-292. DOI: 10.1124/mi.3.5.281

[23] Osborne CK, Schiff R. Estrogen-receptor biology: Continuing progress and therapeutic implications. Journal of Clinical Oncology: Official Journal of the American Society of Clinical Oncology. 2005;**23**:1616-1622. DOI: 10.1200/JCO.2005.10.036

[24] Métivier R, Penot G, Hübner MR, Reid G, Brand H, Kos M, et al. Estrogen receptor-alpha directs ordered, cyclical, and combinatorial recruitment of cofactors on a natural target promoter. Cell. 2003;**115**:751-763

[25] Lonard DM, O'malley BW. Nuclear receptor coregulators: Judges, juries, and executioners of cellular regulation. Molecular Cell. 2007;**27**:691-700. DOI: 10.1016/j. molcel.2007. 08.012

[26] Heger Z, Guran R, Zitka O, Beklova M, Adam V, Kizek R. In vitro interactions between 17β-estradiol and DNA result in formation of the hormone-DNA complexes. International Journal of Environmental Research and Public Health. 2014;**11**:7725-7739. DOI: 10.3390/ijerph110807725

[27] Arnold SF, Obourn JD, Jaffe H, Notides AC. Phosphorylation of the human estrogen receptor by mitogen-activated protein kinase and casein kinase II: Consequence on DNA binding. The Journal of Steroid Biochemistry and Molecular Biology. 1995;**55**:163-172

[28] Rogatsky I, Trowbridge JM, Garabedian MJ. Potentiation of human estrogen receptor alpha transcriptional activation through phosphorylation of serines 104 and 106 by the cyclin A-CDK2 complex. The Journal of Biological Chemistry. 1999;**274**:22296-22302

[29] Chen D, Washbrook E, Sarwar N, Bates GJ, Pace PE, Thirunuvakkarasu V, et al. Phosphorylation of human estrogen receptor alpha at serine 118 by two distinct signal transduction pathways revealed by phosphorylation-specific antisera. Oncogene. 2002;**21**: 4921-4931. DOI: 10.1038/sj.onc.1205420

[30] Lee H, Bai W. Regulation of estrogen receptor nuclear export by ligand-induced and p38-mediated receptor phosphorylation. Molecular and Cellular Biology. 2002;**22**:5835-5845

[31] Joel PB, Smith J, Sturgill TW, Fisher TL, Blenis J, Lannigan DA. pp90rsk1 regulates estrogen receptor-mediated transcription through phosphorylation of Ser-167. Molecular and Cellular Biology. 1998;**18**:1978-1984

[32] Chen D, Pace PE, Coombes RC, Ali S. Phosphorylation of human estrogen receptor alpha by protein kinase a regulates dimerization. Molecular and Cellular Biology. 1999;**19**:1002-1015

[33] Cui Y, Zhang M, Pestell R, Curran EM, Welshons WV, Fuqua SAW. Phosphorylation of estrogen receptor alpha blocks its acetylation and regulates estrogen sensitivity. Cancer Research. 2004;**64**:9199-9208. DOI: 10.1158/0008-5472.CAN-04-2126

[34] Wang RA, Mazumdar A, Vadlamudi RK, Kumar R. P21-activated kinase-1 phosphorylates and transactivates estrogen receptor-alpha and promotes hyperplasia in mammary epithelium. The EMBO Journal. 2002;**21**:5437-5447

[35] Likhite VS, Stossi F, Kim K, Katzenellenbogen BS, Katzenellenbogen JA. Kinase-specific phosphorylation of the estrogen receptor changes receptor interactions with ligand, deoxyribonucleic acid, and coregulators associated with alterations in estrogen and tamoxifen activity. Molecular Endocrinology (Baltimore, Md). 2006;**20**:3120–3132. DOI: 10.1210/me.2006-0068

[36] Daniel AR, Qiu M, Faivre EJ, Ostrander JH, Skildum A, Lange CA. Linkage of progestin and epidermal growth factor signaling: Phosphorylation of progesterone receptors mediates transcriptional hypersensitivity and increased ligand-independent breast cancer cell growth. Steroids. 2007;**72**:188-201. DOI: 10.1016/j.steroids.2006.11.009

[37] Herynk MH, Parra I, Cui Y, Beyer A, Wu MF, Hilsenbeck SG, et al. Association between the estrogen receptor alpha A908G mutation and outcomes in invasive breast cancer. Clinical Cancer Research: An Official Journal of the American Association for Cancer Research. 2007;**13**:3235-3243. DOI: 10.1158/1078-0432.CCR-06-2608

[38] Conway K, Parrish E, Edmiston SN, Tolbert D, Tse CK, Geradts J, et al. The estrogen receptor-alpha A908G (K303R) mutation occurs at a low frequency in invasive breast tumors: Results from a population-based study. Breast Cancer Research: BCR. 2005;**7**: R871-R880. DOI: 10.1186/bcr1315

[39] Conway K, Parrish E, Edmiston SN, Tolbert D, Tse CK, Moorman P, et al. Risk factors for breast cancer characterized by the estrogen receptor alpha A908G (K303R) mutation. Breast Cancer Research : BCR. 2007;**9**:R36. doi:10.1186/bcr1731

[40] Wehling M, Lösel R. Non-genomic steroid hormone effects: Membrane or intracellular receptors? The Journal of Steroid Biochemistry and Molecular Biology. 2006;**102**:180-183. DOI: 10.1016/j.jsbmb.2006.09.016

[41] Boonyaratanakornkit V, McGowan E, Sherman L, Mancini MA, Cheskis BJ, Edwards DP. The role of extranuclear signaling actions of progesterone receptor in mediating progesterone regulation of gene expression and the cell cycle. Molecular Endocrinology (Baltimore, Md). 2007;**21**:359–375. DOI:10.1210/me.2006-0337

[42] Levin ER, Pietras RJ. Estrogen receptors outside the nucleus in breast cancer. Breast Cancer Research and Treatment. 2008;**108**:351-361. DOI: 10.1007/s10549-007-9618-4

[43] Song RXD, Zhang Z, Chen Y, Bao Y, Santen RJ. Estrogen signaling via a linear pathway involving insulin-like growth factor I receptor, matrix metalloproteinases, and epidermal growth factor receptor to activate mitogen-activated protein kinase in MCF-7 breast cancer cells. Endocrinology. 2007;**148**:4091-4101. DOI: 10.1210/en.2007-0240

[44] Stoica GE, Franke TF, Moroni M, Mueller S, Morgan E, Iann MC, et al. Effect of estradiol on estrogen receptor-alpha gene expression and activity can be modulated by the ErbB2/PI 3-K/Akt pathway. Oncogene. 2003;**22**:7998-8011. DOI: 10.1038/sj.onc.1206769

[45] Schiff R, Massarweh SA, Shou J, Bharwani L, Mohsin SK, Osborne CK. Cross-talk between estrogen receptor and growth factor pathways as a molecular target for overcoming

endocrine resistance. Clinical Cancer Research: An Official Journal of the American Association for Cancer Research. 2004;**10**:331S-336S

[46] Anderson WF, Chatterjee N, Ershler WB, Brawley OW. Estrogen receptor breast cancer phenotypes in the surveillance, epidemiology, and end results database. Breast Cancer Research and Treatment. 2002;**76**:27-36

[47] Buzdar AU, Vergote I, Sainsbury R. The impact of hormone receptor status on the clinical efficacy of the new-generation aromatase inhibitors: A review of data from first-line metastatic disease trials in postmenopausal women. The Breast Journal. 2004;**10**:211-217. DOI: 10.1111/j.1075-122X.2004.21320.x

[48] Ravdin PM, Green S, Dorr TM, McGuire WL, Fabian C, Pugh RP, et al. Prognostic significance of progesterone receptor levels in estrogen receptor-positive patients with metastatic breast cancer treated with tamoxifen: Results of a prospective southwest oncology group study. Journal of Clinical Oncology : Official Journal of the American Society of Clinical Oncology. 1992;**10**:1284-1291. DOI: 10.1200/JCO.1992.10.8.1284

[49] Bardou VJ, Arpino G, Elledge RM, Osborne CK, Clark GM. Progesterone receptor status significantly improves outcome prediction over estrogen receptor status alone for adjuvant endocrine therapy in two large breast cancer databases. Journal of Clinical Oncology: Official Journal of the American Society of Clinical Oncology. 2003;**21**:1973-1979. DOI: 10.1200/JCO.2003.09.099

[50] Nadji M, Gomez-Fernandez C, Ganjei-Azar P, Morales AR. Immunohistochemistry of estrogen and progesterone receptors reconsidered: Experience with 5,993 breast cancers. American Journal of Clinical Pathology. 2005;**123**:21-27

[51] Wenger CR, Beardslee S, Owens MA, Pounds G, Oldaker T, Vendely P, et al. DNA ploidy, S-phase, and steroid receptors in more than 127,000 breast cancer patients. Breast Cancer Research and Treatment. 1993;**28**:9-20

[52] Elledge RM, Fuqua SA, Clark GM, Pujol P, Allred DC, McGuire WL. Prognostic significance of p53 gene alterations in node-negative breast cancer. Breast Cancer Research and Treatment. 1993;**26**:225-235

[53] Arisio R, Sapino A, Cassoni P, Accinelli G, Cuccorese MC, Mano MP, et al. What modifies the relation between tumour size and lymph node metastases in T1 breast carcinomas? Journal of Clinical Pathology. 2000;**53**:846-850

[54] Early Breast Cancer Trialists' Collaborative Group (EBCTCG). Effects of chemotherapy and hormonal therapy for early breast cancer on recurrence and 15-year survival: An overview of the randomised trials. Lancet (London, England). 2005;**365**:1687-1717. DOI: 10.1016/S0140-6736(05)66544-0

[55] Fisher B, Redmond C, Fisher ER, Caplan R. Relative worth of estrogen or progesterone receptor and pathologic characteristics of differentiation as indicators of prognosis in node negative breast cancer patients: Findings from National Surgical Adjuvant Breast

and bowel project protocol B-06. Journal of Clinical Oncology: Official Journal of the American Society of Clinical Oncology. 1988;**6**:1076-1087. DOI: 10.1200/JCO.1988.6.7. 1076

[56] Rakha EA, El-Sayed ME, Green AR, Paish EC, Powe DG, Gee J, et al. Biologic and clinical characteristics of breast cancer with single hormone receptor positive phenotype. Journal of Clinical Oncology: Official Journal of the American Society of Clinical Oncology. 2007; **25**:4772-4778. DOI: 10.1200/JCO.2007.12.2747

[57] Hutchins LF, Green SJ, Ravdin PM, Lew D, Martino S, Abeloff M, et al. Randomized, controlled trial of cyclophosphamide, methotrexate, and fluorouracil versus cyclophosphamide, doxorubicin, and fluorouracil with and without tamoxifen for high-risk, node-negative breast cancer: Treatment results of intergroup protocol INT-0102. Journal of Clinical Oncology: Official Journal of the American Society of Clinical Oncology. 2005; **23**:8313-8321. DOI: 10.1200/JCO.2005.08.071

[58] Fisher B, Anderson S, Tan-Chiu E, Wolmark N, Wickerham DL, Fisher ER, et al. Tamoxifen and chemotherapy for axillary node-negative, estrogen receptor-negative breast cancer: Findings from National Surgical Adjuvant Breast and bowel project B-23. Journal of Clinical Oncology: Official Journal of the American Society of Clinical Oncology. 2001; **19**:931-942. DOI: 10.1200/JCO.2001.19.4.931

[59] Dowsett M, Allred C, Knox J, Quinn E, Salter J, Wale C, et al. Relationship between quantitative estrogen and progesterone receptor expression and human epidermal growth factor receptor 2 (HER-2) status with recurrence in the Arimidex, Tamoxifen, alone or in combination trial. Journal of Clinical Oncology: Official Journal of the American Society of Clinical Oncology. 2008;**26**:1059-1065. DOI: 10.1200/JCO.2007.12. 9437

[60] Early Breast Cancer Trialists' Collaborative Group. Tamoxifen for early breast cancer: An overview of the randomised trials. Early breast cancer Trialists' collaborative group. Lancet (London England). 1998;**351**:1451-1467

[61] Goss PE, Ingle JN, Martino S, Robert NJ, Muss HB, Piccart MJ, et al. Efficacy of letrozole extended adjuvant therapy according to estrogen receptor and progesterone receptor status of the primary tumor: National Cancer Institute of Canada clinical trials group MA.17. Journal of Clinical Oncology: Official Journal of the American Society of Clinical Oncology. 2007;**25**:2006-2011. DOI: 10.1200/JCO.2006.09.4482

[62] Reinert T, Debiasi M, Bines J, Barrios CH. Trends in progression-free survival (PFS) and time to progression (TTP) over time within first-line aromatase inhibitors trials in hormone receptor-positive advanced breast cancer. Breast Cancer Research and Treatment. 2017. DOI: 10.1007/s10549-017-4593-x

[63] Mouridsen H, Gershanovich M, Sun Y, Perez-Carrion R, Boni C, Monnier A, et al. Phase III study of letrozole versus tamoxifen as first-line therapy of advanced breast cancer in postmenopausal women: Analysis of survival and update of efficacy from the international Letrozole breast cancer group. Journal of Clinical Oncology: Official Journal of the American Society of Clinical Oncology. 2003;**21**:2101-2109. DOI: 10.1200/JCO.2003.04.194

[64] Hess KR, Pusztai L, Buzdar AU, Hortobagyi GN. Estrogen receptors and distinct patterns of breast cancer relapse. Breast Cancer Research and Treatment. 2003;**78**:105-118

[65] Kuukasjärvi T, Kononen J, Helin H, Holli K, Isola J. Loss of estrogen receptor in recurrent breast cancer is associated with poor response to endocrine therapy. Journal of Clinical Oncology: Official Journal of the American Society of Clinical Oncology. 1996;**14**:2584-2589. DOI: 10.1200/JCO.1996.14.9.2584

[66] Lower EE, Glass EL, Bradley DA, Blau R, Heffelfinger S. Impact of metastatic estrogen receptor and progesterone receptor status on survival. Breast Cancer Research and Treatment. 2005;**90**:65-70. DOI: 10.1007/s10549-004-2756-z

[67] Sari E, Guler G, Hayran M, Gullu I, Altundag K, Ozisik Y. Comparative study of the immunohistochemical detection of hormone receptor status and HER-2 expression in primary and paired recurrent/metastatic lesions of patients with breast cancer. Medical Oncology (Northwood, London, England). 2011;**28**:57-63. DOI: 10.1007/s12032-010-9418-2

[68] Arslan C, Sari E, Aksoy S, Altundag K. Variation in hormone receptor and HER-2 status between primary and metastatic breast cancer: Review of the literature. Expert Opinion on Therapeutic Targets. 2011;**15**:21-30. DOI: 10.1517/14656566.2011.537260

[69] Henry NL, Hayes DF. Can biology trump anatomy? Do all node-positive patients with breast cancer need chemotherapy. Journal of Clinical Oncology: Official Journal of the American Society of Clinical Oncology. 2007;**25**:2501-2503. DOI: 10.1200/JCO.2007.11. 3290

[70] Martin M, Pienkowski T, Mackey J, Pawlicki M, Guastalla JP, Weaver C, et al. Adjuvant docetaxel for node-positive breast cancer. The New England Journal of Medicine. 2005; **352**:2302-2313. DOI: 10.1056/NEJMoa043681

[71] Mazouni C, Kau SW, Frye D, Andre F, Kuerer HM, Buchholz TA, et al. Inclusion of taxanes, particularly weekly paclitaxel, in preoperative chemotherapy improves pathologic complete response rate in estrogen receptor-positive breast cancers. Annals of Oncology : Official Journal of the European Society for Medical Oncology. 2007;**18**:874-880. DOI: 10.1093/annonc/mdm008

[72] Nofech-Mozes S, Vella ET, Dhesy-Thind S, Hagerty KL, Mangu PB, Temin S, et al. Systematic review on hormone receptor testing in breast cancer. Applied Immunohistochemistry and Molecular Morphology: AIMM. 2012;**20**:214-263. DOI: 10.1097/PAI.0b013e318234aa12

[73] Hammond MEH, Hayes DF, Dowsett M, Allred DC, Hagerty KL, Badve S, et al. American Society of Clinical Oncology/college of American pathologists guideline recommendations for immunohistochemical testing of estrogen and progesterone receptors in breast cancer. Journal of Clinical Oncology: Official Journal of the American Society of Clinical Oncology. 2010;**28**:2784-2795. DOI: 10.1200/JCO.2009.25.6529

[74] Press MF, Cordon-Cardo C, Slamon DJ. Expression of the HER-2/neu proto-oncogene in normal human adult and fetal tissues. Oncogene. 1990;**5**:953-962

[75] Yarden Y, Pines G. The ERBB network: At last, cancer therapy meets systems biology. Nature Reviews Cancer. 2012;**12**:553-563. DOI: 10.1038/nrc3309

[76] Oh JJ, Grosshans DR, Wong SG, Slamon DJ. Identification of differentially expressed genes associated with HER-2/neu overexpression in human breast cancer cells. Nucleic Acids Research. 1999;**27**:4008-4017

[77] Slamon DJ, Godolphin W, Jones LA, Holt JA, Wong SG, Keith DE, et al. Studies of the HER-2/neu proto-oncogene in human breast and ovarian cancer. Science (New York, N.Y.). 1989; **244**:707-712

[78] Slamon DJ, Clark GM, Wong SG, Levin WJ, Ullrich A, McGuire WL. Human breast cancer: Correlation of relapse and survival with amplification of the HER-2/neu oncogene. Science (New York, N.Y.). 1987;**235**:177-182

[79] Saffari B, Jones LA, el Naggar A, Felix JC, George J, Press MF. Amplification and overexpression of HER-2/neu (c-erbB2) in endometrial cancers: Correlation with overall survival. Cancer Research. 1995;**55**:5693-5698

[80] Press MF, Pike MC, Hung G, Zhou JY, Ma Y, George J, et al. Amplification and overexpression of HER-2/neu in carcinomas of the salivary gland: Correlation with poor prognosis. Cancer Research. 1994;**54**:5675-5682

[81] Park JB, Rhim JS, Park SC, Kimm SW, Kraus MH. Amplification, overexpression, and rearrangement of the erbB-2 protooncogene in primary human stomach carcinomas. Cancer Research. 1989;**49**:6605-6609

[82] Sorkin A, Goh LK. Endocytosis and intracellular trafficking of ErbBs. Experimental Cell Research. 2008;**314**:3093-3106. DOI: 10.1016/j.yexcr.2008.08.013

[83] Wolff AC, Hammond MEH, Hicks DG, Dowsett M, McShane LM, Allison KH, et al. Recommendations for human epidermal growth factor receptor 2 testing in breast cancer: American Society of Clinical Oncology/College of American Pathologists clinical practice guideline update. Archives of Pathology and Laboratory Medicine. 2014;**138**: 241-256. DOI: 10.5858/arpa.2013-0953-SA

[84] Press MF, Bernstein L, Thomas PA, Meisner LF, Zhou JY, Ma Y, et al. HER-2/neu gene amplification characterized by fluorescence in situ hybridization: Poor prognosis in node-negative breast carcinomas. Journal of Clinical Oncology : Official Journal of the American Society of Clinical Oncology. 1997;**15**:2894-2904. DOI: 10.1200/JCO.1997.15.8. 2894

[85] Mass RD, Press MF, Anderson S, Cobleigh MA, Vogel CL, Dybdal N, et al. Evaluation of clinical outcomes according to HER2 detection by fluorescence in situ hybridization in women with metastatic breast cancer treated with trastuzumab. Clinical Breast Cancer. 2005;**6**:240-246. DOI: 10.3816/CBC.2005.n.026

[86] Seidman AD, Berry D, Cirrincione C, Harris L, Muss H, Marcom PK, et al. Randomized phase III trial of weekly compared with every-3-weeks paclitaxel for metastatic breast

cancer, with trastuzumab for all HER-2 overexpressors and random assignment to trastuzumab or not in HER-2 nonoverexpressors: Final results of cancer and leukemia group B protocol 9840. Journal of Clinical Oncology: Official Journal of the American Society of Clinical Oncology. 2008;**26**:1642-1649. DOI: 10.1200/JCO.2007.11.6699

[87] Slamon D, Eiermann W, Robert N, Pienkowski T, Martin M, Press M, et al. Adjuvant Trastuzumab in HER2-positive breast cancer. The New England Journal of Medicine. 2011;**365**:1273-1283. DOI: 10.1056/NEJMoa0910383

[88] Geyer CE, Forster J, Lindquist D, Chan S, Romieu CG, Pienkowski T, et al. Lapatinib plus Capecitabine for HER2-positive advanced breast cancer. The New England Journal of Medicine. 2006;**355**:2733-2743. DOI: 10.1056/NEJMoa064320

[89] Baselga J, Cortés J, Kim SB, Im SA, Hegg R, Im YH, et al. Pertuzumab plus Trastuzumab plus docetaxel for metastatic breast cancer. The New England Journal of Medicine. 2012; **366**:109-119. DOI: 10.1056/NEJMoa1113216

[90] Verma S, Miles D, Gianni L, Krop IE, Welslau M, Baselga J, et al. Trastuzumab Emtansine for HER2-positive advanced breast cancer. The New England Journal of Medicine. 2012; **367**:1783-1791. DOI: 10.1056/NEJMoa1209124

[91] Dati C, Antoniotti S, Taverna D, Perroteau I, De Bortoli M. Inhibition of c-erbB-2 oncogene expression by estrogens in human breast cancer cells. Oncogene. 1990;**5**:1001-1006

[92] Pietras RJ, Arboleda J, Reese DM, Wongvipat N, Pegram MD, Ramos L, et al. HER-2 tyrosine kinase pathway targets estrogen receptor and promotes hormone-independent growth in human breast cancer cells. Oncogene. 1995;**10**:2435-2446

[93] Ellis MJ, Coop A, Singh B, Mauriac L, Llombert-Cussac A, Jänicke F, et al. Letrozole is more effective neoadjuvant endocrine therapy than tamoxifen for ErbB-1- and/or ErbB-2-positive, estrogen receptor-positive primary breast cancer: Evidence from a phase III randomized trial. Journal of Clinical Oncology: Official Journal of the American Society of Clinical Oncology. 2001;**19**:3808-3816. DOI: 10.1200/JCO.2001.19.18.3808

[94] Gennari A, Sormani MP, Pronzato P, Puntoni M, Colozza M, Pfeffer U, et al. HER2 status and efficacy of adjuvant anthracyclines in early breast cancer: A pooled analysis of randomized trials. Journal of the National Cancer Institute. 2008;**100**:14-20. DOI: 10.1093/jnci/djm252

[95] Hayes DF, Thor AD, Dressler LG, Weaver D, Edgerton S, Cowan D, et al. HER2 and response to paclitaxel in node-positive breast cancer. The New England Journal of Medicine. 2007;**357**:1496-1506. DOI: 10.1056/NEJMoa071167

[96] Wolff AC, Hammond MEH, Schwartz JN, Hagerty KL, Allred DC, Cote RJ, et al. American Society of Clinical Oncology/College of American pathologists guideline recommendations for human epidermal growth factor receptor 2 testing in breast cancer. Archives of Pathology and Laboratory Medicine. 2007;**131**:18-43. DOI: 10.1043/1543-2165(2007)131[18:ASOCCO]2.0.CO;2

[97] Press MF, Slamon DJ, Flom KJ, Park J, Zhou JY, Bernstein L. Evaluation of HER-2/neu gene amplification and overexpression: Comparison of frequently used assay methods in a molecularly characterized cohort of breast cancer specimens. Journal of Clinical Oncology: Official Journal of the American Society of Clinical Oncology. 2002;**20**:3095-3105. DOI: 10.1200/JCO.2002.09.094

[98] Penault-Llorca F, Bilous M, Dowsett M, Hanna W, Osamura RY, Rüschoff J, et al. Emerging technologies for assessing HER2 amplification. American Journal of Clinical Pathology. 2009;**132**:539-548. DOI: 10.1309/AJCPV2I0HGPMGBSQ

[99] Colozza M, Azambuja E, Cardoso F, Sotiriou C, Larsimont D, Piccart MJ. Proliferative markers as prognostic and predictive tools in early breast cancer: Where are we now? Annals of Oncology: Official Journal of the European society for Medical Oncology. 2005; **16**:1723-1739. DOI: 10.1093/annonc/mdi352

[100] Baak JPA, van Diest PJ, Janssen EAM, Gudlaugsson E, Voorhorst FJ, van der Wall E, et al. Proliferation accurately identifies the high-risk patients among small, low-grade, lymph node-negative invasive breast cancers. Annals of Oncology: Official Journal of the European Society for Medical Oncology. 2008;**19**:649-654. DOI: 10.1093/annonc/mdm535

[101] Harris L, Fritsche H, Mennel R, Norton L, Ravdin P, Taube S, et al. American Society of Clinical Oncology 2007 update of recommendations for the use of tumor markers in breast cancer. Journal of Clinical Oncology: Official Journal of the American Society of Clinical Oncology. 2007;**25**:5287-5312. DOI: 10.1200/JCO.2007.14.2364

[102] Dowsett M, Smith IE, Ebbs SR, Dixon JM, Skene A, A'Hern R, et al. Prognostic value of Ki67 expression after short-term presurgical endocrine therapy for primary breast cancer. Journal of the National Cancer Institute. 2007;**99**:167-170. DOI: 10.1093/jnci/djk020

[103] Fasching PA, Heusinger K, Haeberle L, Niklos M, Hein A, Bayer CM, et al. Ki67, chemotherapy response, and prognosis in breast cancer patients receiving neoadjuvant treatment. BMC Cancer. 2011;**11**:486. DOI: 10.1186/1471-2407-11-486

[104] Ellis MJ, Suman VJ, Hoog J, Lin L, Snider J, Prat A, et al. Randomized phase II neoadjuvant comparison between letrozole, anastrozole, and exemestane for postmenopausal women with estrogen receptor-rich stage 2 to 3 breast cancer: Clinical and biomarker outcomes and predictive value of the baseline PAM50-based intrinsic subtype–ACOSOG Z1031. Journal of Clinical Oncology: Official Journal of the American Society of Clinical Oncology. 2011; **29**:2342-2349. DOI: 10.1200/JCO.2010.31.6950

[105] Fisher B, Dignam J, Wolmark N, DeCillis A, Emir B, Wickerham DL, et al. Tamoxifen and chemotherapy for lymph node-negative, estrogen receptor-positive breast cancer. Journal of the National Cancer Institute. 1997;**89**:1673-1682

[106] Bedard PL, Cardoso F. Can some patients avoid adjuvant chemotherapy for early-stage breast cancer? Nature Reviews Clinical Oncology. 2011;**8**:272-279. DOI: 10.1038/nrclinonc. 2011.19

[107] Golub TR. Molecular classification of cancer: Class discovery and class prediction by gene expression monitoring. Science. 1999;**286**:531-537. DOI: 10.1126/science.286.5439. 531

[108] van de, Vijver MJ, He YD, van't Veer LJ, Dai H, Hart AAM, Voskuil DW, et al. A gene-expression signature as a predictor of survival in breast cancer. The New England Journal of Medicine. 2002;**347**:1999-2009. DOI: 10.1056/NEJMoa021967

[109] Williams WR, Anderson DE. Genetic epidemiology of breast cancer: Segregation analysis of 200 Danish pedigrees. Genetic Epidemiology. 1984;**1**:7-20. DOI: 10.1002/gepi. 1370010104

[110] Stratton MR, Rahman N. The emerging landscape of breast cancer susceptibility. Nature Genetics. 2008;**40**:17-22. DOI: 10.1038/ng.2007.53

[111] Newman B, Austin MA, Lee M, King MC. Inheritance of human breast cancer: Evidence for autosomal dominant transmission in high-risk families. Proceedings of the National Academy of Sciences of the United States of America. 1988;**85**:3044-3048

[112] Miki Y, Swensen J, Shattuck-Eidens D, Futreal PA, Harshman K, Tavtigian S, et al. A strong candidate for the breast and ovarian cancer susceptibility gene BRCA1. Science (New York, NY). 1994;**266**:66-71

[113] Wooster R, Bignell G, Lancaster J, Swift S, Seal S, Mangion J, et al. Identification of the breast cancer susceptibility gene BRCA2. Nature. 1995;**378**:789-792. DOI: 10.1038/378789a0

[114] Kerr P, Ashworth A. New complexities for BRCA1 and BRCA2. Current Biology: CB. 2001;**11**:R668-R676

[115] Leung CCY, Glover JNM. BRCT domains: Easy as one, two, three. Cell Cycle (Georgetown, Tex). 2011;**10**:2461-2470. DOI: 10.4161/cc.10.15.16312

[116] Esashi F, Galkin VE, Yu X, Egelman EH, West SC. Stabilization of RAD51 nucleoprotein filaments by the C-terminal region of BRCA2. Nature Structural and Molecular Biology. 2007;**14**:468-474. DOI: 10.1038/nsmb1245

[117] Venkitaraman AR. Cancer susceptibility and the functions of BRCA1 and BRCA2. Cell. 2002;**108**:171-182

[118] Lord CJ, Ashworth A. The DNA damage response and cancer therapy. Nature. 2012;**481**: 287-294. DOI: 10.1038/nature10760

[119] Tutt ANJ, Lord CJ, McCabe N, Farmer H, Turner N, Martin NM, et al. Exploiting the DNA repair defect in BRCA mutant cells in the design of new therapeutic strategies for cancer. Cold Spring Harbor Symposia on Quantitative Biology. 2005;**70**:139-148. DOI: 10. 1101/sqb.2005.70.012

[120] Narod SA, Feunteun J, Lynch HT, Watson P, Conway T, Lynch J, et al. Familial breast-ovarian cancer locus on chromosome 17q12-q23. Lancet (London, England). 1991;**338**:82-83

[121] Easton DF, Bishop DT, Ford D, Crockford GP. Genetic linkage analysis in familial breast and ovarian cancer: Results from 214 families. The breast cancer linkage consortium. American Journal of Human Genetics. 1993;**52**:678-701

[122] Wooster R, Weber BL. Breast and ovarian cancer. The New England Journal of Medicine. 2003;**348**:2339-2347. DOI: 10.1056/NEJMra012284

[123] Antoniou A, Pharoah PDP, Narod S, Risch HA, Eyfjord JE, Hopper JL, et al. Average risks of breast and ovarian cancer associated with BRCA1 or BRCA2 mutations detected in case series unselected for family history: A combined analysis of 22 studies. American Journal of Human Genetics. 2003;**72**:1117-1130. DOI: 10.1086/375033

[124] Brose MS, Rebbeck TR, Calzone KA, Stopfer JE, Nathanson KL, Weber BL. Cancer risk estimates for BRCA1 mutation carriers identified in a risk evaluation program. Journal of the National Cancer Institute. 2002;**94**:1365-1372

[125] Whittemore AS, Gong G, Itnyre J. Prevalence and contribution of BRCA1 mutations in breast cancer and ovarian cancer: Results from three U.S. population-based case-control studies of ovarian cancer. American Journal of Human Genetics. 1997;**60**:496-504

[126] Ford D, Easton DF, Bishop DT, Narod SA, Goldgar DE. Risks of cancer in BRCA1-mutation carriers. Breast Cancer Linkage Consortium. Lancet (London, England). 1994; **343**:692-695

[127] Ford D, Easton DF, Stratton M, Narod S, Goldgar D, Devilee P, et al. Genetic heterogeneity and penetrance analysis of the BRCA1 and BRCA2 genes in breast cancer families. The Breast Cancer Linkage Consortium. American Journal of Human Genetics. 1998;**62**: 676-689

[128] Breast Cancer Linkage Consortium. Cancer risks in BRCA2 mutation carriers. Journal of the National Cancer Institute. 1999;**91**:1310-1316

[129] Turner N, Tutt A, Ashworth A. Hallmarks of 'BRCAness' in sporadic cancers. Nature Reviews Cancer. 2004;**4**:814-819. DOI: 10.1038/nrc1457

[130] Chenevix-Trench G, Milne RL, Antoniou AC, Couch FJ, Easton DF, Goldgar DE, et al. An international initiative to identify genetic modifiers of cancer risk in BRCA1 and BRCA2 mutation carriers: The consortium of investigators of modifiers of BRCA1 and BRCA2 (CIMBA). Breast Cancer Research: BCR. 2007;**9**:104. DOI: 10.1186/bcr1670

[131] Gronwald J, Tung N, Foulkes WD, Offit K, Gershoni R, Daly M, et al. Tamoxifen and contralateral breast cancer in BRCA1 and BRCA2 carriers: An update. International Journal of Cancer. 2006;**118**:2281-2284. DOI: 10.1002/ijc.21536

[132] Domchek SM, Friebel TM, Neuhausen SL, Wagner T, Evans G, Isaacs C, et al. Mortality after bilateral salpingo-oophorectomy in BRCA1 and BRCA2 mutation carriers: A prospective cohort study. The Lancet Oncology. 2006;**7**:223-229. DOI: 10.1016/S1470-2045(06) 70585-X

[133] Lakhani SR, Gusterson BA, Jacquemier J, Sloane JP, Anderson TJ, van de, Vijver MJ, et al. The pathology of familial breast cancer: Histological features of cancers in families not attributable to mutations in BRCA1 or BRCA2. Clinical Cancer Research: An Official Journal of the American Association for Cancer Research. 2000;**6**:782-789

[134] Hosey AM, Gorski JJ, Murray MM, Quinn JE, Chung WY, Stewart GE, et al. Molecular basis for estrogen receptor alpha deficiency in BRCA1-linked breast cancer. Journal of the National Cancer Institute. 2007;**99**:1683-1694. DOI: 10.1093/jnci/djm207

[135] Bane AL, Beck JC, Bleiweiss I, Buys SS, Catalano E, Daly MB, et al. BRCA2 mutation-associated breast cancers exhibit a distinguishing phenotype based on morphology and molecular profiles from tissue microarrays. The American Journal of Surgical Pathology. 2007;**31**:121-128. DOI: 10.1097/01.pas.0000213351.49767.0f

[136] Moller P, Evans DG, Reis MM, Gregory H, Anderson E, Maehle L, et al. Surveillance for familial breast cancer: Differences in outcome according to BRCA mutation status. International Journal of Cancer. 2007;**121**:1017-1020. DOI: 10.1002/ijc.22789

[137] Rennert G, Bisland-Naggan S, Barnett-Griness O, Bar-Joseph N, Zhang S, Rennert HS, et al. Clinical outcomes of breast cancer in carriers of BRCA1 and BRCA2 mutations. The New England Journal of Medicine. 2007;**357**:115-123. DOI: 10.1056/NEJMoa070608

[138] Liebens FP, Carly B, Pastijn A, Rozenberg S. Management of BRCA1/2 associated breast cancer: A systematic qualitative review of the state of knowledge in 2006. European Journal of Cancer (Oxford, England: 1990). 2007;**43**:238-257. DOI: 10.1016/j.ejca.2006.07.019

[139] Gayther SA, Pharoah PD, Ponder BA. The genetics of inherited breast cancer. Journal of Mammary Gland Biology and Neoplasia. 1998;**3**:365-376

[140] Nathanson KL, Wooster R, Weber BL, Nathanson KN. Breast cancer genetics: What we know and what we need. Nature Medicine. 2001;**7**:552-556. DOI: 10.1038/87876

[141] Hirshfield KM, Rebbeck TR, Levine AJ. Germline mutations and polymorphisms in the origins of cancers in women. Journal of Oncology. 2010;**2010**:297671. DOI: 10.1155/2010/297671

[142] Goldhirsch A, Wood WC, Coates AS, Gelber RD, Thürlimann B, Senn HJ, et al. Strategies for subtypes–dealing with the diversity of breast cancer: Highlights of the St. Gallen international expert consensus on the primary therapy of early breast cancer 2011. Annals of Oncology: Official Journal of the European Society for Medical Oncology. 2011;**22**:1736-1747. DOI: 10.1093/annonc/mdr304

[143] Sørlie T, Perou CM, Tibshirani R, Aas T, Geisler S, Johnsen H, et al. Gene expression patterns of breast carcinomas distinguish tumor subclasses with clinical implications. Proceedings of the National Academy of Sciences of the United States of America. 2001;**98**:10869-10874. DOI: 10.1073/pnas.191367098

[144] Paik S, Shak S, Tang G, Kim C, Baker J, Cronin M, et al. A multigene assay to predict recurrence of tamoxifen-treated, node-negative breast cancer. The New England Journal of Medicine. 2004;**351**:2817-2826. DOI: 10.1056/NEJMoa041588

[145] Albain KS, Barlow WE, Shak S, Hortobagyi GN, Livingston RB, Yeh IT, et al. Prognostic and predictive value of the 21-gene recurrence score assay in postmenopausal women

with node-positive, oestrogen-receptor-positive breast cancer on chemotherapy: A retrospective analysis of a randomised trial. The Lancet Oncology. 2010;**11**:55-65. DOI: 10.1016/S1470-2045(09)70314-6

[146] Gnant M, Harbeck N, St TC. Gallen 2011: Summary of the consensus discussion. Breast care (Basel, Switzerland). 2011;**6**:136-141. DOI: 10.1159/000328054

[147] Buyse M, Loi S, van't Veer L, Viale G, Delorenzi M, Glas AM, et al. Validation and clinical utility of a 70-gene prognostic signature for women with node-negative breast cancer. Journal of the National Cancer Institute. 2006;**98**:1183-1192. DOI: 10.1093/jnci/djj329

[148] Viale G, de, Snoo FA, Slaets L, Bogaerts J, van 't Veer L, Rutgers EJ, et al. Immunohistochemical versus molecular (BluePrint and MammaPrint) subtyping of breast carcinoma. Outcome results from the EORTC 10041/BIG 3-04 MINDACT trial. Breast Cancer Research and Treatment. 2017. DOI: 10.1007/s10549-017-4509-9

[149] Aalders KC, Kuijer A, Straver ME, Slaets L, Litiere S, Viale G, et al. Characterisation of multifocal breast cancer using the 70-gene signature in clinical low-risk patients enrolled in the EORTC 10041/BIG 03-04 MINDACT trial. European Journal of Cancer (Oxford, England : 1990). 2017;**79**:98-105. DOI: 10.1016/j.ejca.2017.03.034

[150] Chia SK, Bramwell VH, Tu D, Shepherd LE, Jiang S, Vickery T, et al. A 50-gene intrinsic subtype classifier for prognosis and prediction of benefit from adjuvant tamoxifen. Clinical Cancer Research : An Official Journal of the American Association for Cancer Research. 2012;**18**:4465-4472. DOI: 10.1158/1078-0432.CCR-12-0286

[151] Martín M, González-Rivera M, Morales S, de la Haba-Rodriguez J, González-Cortijo L, Manso L, et al. prospective study of the impact of the Prosigna assay on adjuvant clinical decision-making in unselected patients with estrogen receptor positive, human epidermal growth factor receptor negative, node negative early-stage breast cancer. Current Medical Research and Opinion. 2015;**31**:1129-1137. DOI: 10.1185/03007995.2015. 1037730

Permissions

All chapters in this book were first published in BIAPP, by InTech Open; hereby published with permission under the Creative Commons Attribution License or equivalent. Every chapter published in this book has been scrutinized by our experts. Their significance has been extensively debated. The topics covered herein carry significant findings which will fuel the growth of the discipline. They may even be implemented as practical applications or may be referred to as a beginning point for another development.

The contributors of this book come from diverse backgrounds, making this book a truly international effort. This book will bring forth new frontiers with its revolutionizing research information and detailed analysis of the nascent developments around the world.

We would like to thank all the contributing authors for lending their expertise to make the book truly unique. They have played a crucial role in the development of this book. Without their invaluable contributions this book wouldn't have been possible. They have made vital efforts to compile up to date information on the varied aspects of this subject to make this book a valuable addition to the collection of many professionals and students.

This book was conceptualized with the vision of imparting up-to-date information and advanced data in this field. To ensure the same, a matchless editorial board was set up. Every individual on the board went through rigorous rounds of assessment to prove their worth. After which they invested a large part of their time researching and compiling the most relevant data for our readers.

The editorial board has been involved in producing this book since its inception. They have spent rigorous hours researching and exploring the diverse topics which have resulted in the successful publishing of this book. They have passed on their knowledge of decades through this book. To expedite this challenging task, the publisher supported the team at every step. A small team of assistant editors was also appointed to further simplify the editing procedure and attain best results for the readers.

Apart from the editorial board, the designing team has also invested a significant amount of their time in understanding the subject and creating the most relevant covers. They scrutinized every image to scout for the most suitable representation of the subject and create an appropriate cover for the book.

The publishing team has been an ardent support to the editorial, designing and production team. Their endless efforts to recruit the best for this project, has resulted in the accomplishment of this book. They are a veteran in the field of academics and their pool of knowledge is as vast as their experience in printing. Their expertise and guidance has proved useful at every step. Their uncompromising quality standards have made this book an exceptional effort. Their encouragement from time to time has been an inspiration for everyone.

The publisher and the editorial board hope that this book will prove to be a valuable piece of knowledge for researchers, students, practitioners and scholars across the globe.

List of Contributors

Samuel N. Uwaezuoke
College of Medicine, University of Nigeria/University of Nigeria Teaching Hospital, Enugu, Nigeria

Hakan Altay
Department of Cardiology, Baskent University, Faculty of Medicine, Istanbul, Turkey

Tereza Kačerová,
BIOCEV, 1st Medicinal Faculty Charles University, Vestec, Czech Republic
Grammar School Nad Štolou 1, Prague 7, Czech Republic

Petr Novotný and Ján Boroň
ESSENCE LINE, s.r.o., Prague 5, Czech Republic

Petr Kačer
BIOCEV, 1st Medicinal Faculty Charles University, Vestec, Czech Republic
National Institute of Mental Health, Klecany, Czech Republic

Sofia Esteves, Inês Costa and Nuno Santarem
Instituto de Investigação e Inovação em Saúde, Universidade do Porto, Porto, Portugal
Instituto de Biologia Molecular e Celular, Parasite Disease Group, Universidade do Porto, Porto, Portugal

Anabela Cordeiro-da-Silva
Instituto de Investigação e Inovação em Saúde, Universidade do Porto, Porto, Portugal
Instituto de Biologia Molecular e Celular, Parasite Disease Group, Universidade do Porto, Porto, Portugal
Departamento de Ciências Biológicas, Faculdade de Farmácia da Universidade do Porto, Porto, Portugal

Célia Amorim
Instituto de Investigação e Inovação em Saúde, Universidade do Porto, Porto, Portugal
Instituto de Biologia Molecular e Celular, Parasite Disease Group, Universidade do Porto, Porto, Portugal
Departamento de Quimica, Faculdade de Farmácia da Universidade do Porto, Porto, Portugal

Makoto Aoki, Shuichi Hagiwara and Kiyohiro Oshima
Department of Emergency Medicine, Gunma University Graduate School of Medicine, Maebashi, Japan

Francesca Scionti, Pierosandro Tagliaferri, Pierfrancesco Tassone and Maria Teresa Di Martino
Department of Experimental and Clinical Medicine, Medical Oncology, Magna Graecia University of Catanzaro, Italy

Kemal Turker Ulutas
Department of Clinical Biochemistry, Antakya State Hospital, Hatay, Turkey

Inanc Samil Sarici
Department of General Surgery, Kanuni Sultan Suleyman Training and Research Hospital, Istanbul, Turkey

Ozgul Duzgun
Department of Surgical Oncology, Umraniye Training and Research Hospital, Istanbul, Turkey

Agustin Iskandar and Hani Susianti
Clinical Pathology Department, Faculty of Medicine, Universitas Brawijaya, Malang, Indonesia

Muhammad Anshory
Internal Medicine Department, Faculty of Medicine, Universitas Brawijaya, Malang, Indonesia

Salvatore Di Somma
Department of Medical-Surgery Sciences and Translational Medicine, Sapienza University of Rome, Italy

Sanja Josef Golubic
Department of Physics, Faculty of Science, University of Zagreb, Croatia

Peter Zolotukhin, Viktor Chmykhalo, Anna Belanova, Alexander Dybushkin, Viktor Fedoseev and Dmitriy Smirnov
Biomedical Innovations LLC, Rostov-on-Don, Russia

Harold Moreno-Ortiz and Elkin Lucena-Quevedo
Department of Reproductive Genetics, Fertility and Sterility Colombian Center (CECOLFES), Bogotá, Colombia

Iván Darío Acosta, Luis Alejandro Arias-Sosa, Alix Eugenia Dallos-Báez, Maribel Forero-Castro and Clara Esteban-Pérez
Escuela de Ciencias Biológicas, Grupo de Investigación en Ciencias Biomédicas (GICBUPTC). Universidad Pedagógica y Tecnológica de Colombia, Tunja, Colombia

Serena Bertozzi, Luca Seriau, Roberta Di Vora and Carla Cedolini
Breast Unit, Clinic of Surgery, DAME, University of Udine, University Hospital of Udine, Udine, Italy

Ambrogio P Londero
Clinic of Obstetrics and Gynecology, University Hospital of Udine, Udine, Italy

Laura Mariuzzi
Institute of Pathologic Anatomy, DAME, University of Udine, University Hospital of Udine, Udine, Italy

Index

CPSIA information can be obtained
at www.ICGtesting.com
Printed in the USA
LVHW060851030122
707669LV00002B/89